# Technical Hematology

# Technical Hematology

ARTHUR SIMMONS, L.C.S.L.T. (Canada)

*Clinical Associate Professor*
*Department of Pathology, University of Iowa;*
*Associate Professor of Biology*
*Department of Biology*
*Drake University*
*Des Moines, Iowa*

SECOND EDITION

## J. B. Lippincott Company

*Philadelphia and Toronto*

SECOND EDITION
Copyright © 1976 by J. B. Lippincott Company
Copyright © 1968 by J. B. Lippincott Company

ISBN 0-397-50350-4

Library of Congress Catalog Card No 75-30638

Printed in the United States of America

3 5 4 2

Library of Congress Cataloging in Publication Data
Simmons, Arthur.
  Technical hematology.
  Includes bibliographical references and index.
  1. Blood—Examination. I. Title. [DNLM: 1. Hematology—Laboratory manuals. QY400 S592t]
RB45.S55   1975      616.1'5'075      75-30638
ISBN 0-397-50350-4

# Preface to the Second Edition

Seven years have elapsed since the writing of the first edition of Technical Hematology. During that time, laboratory hematology has changed as much as, or more than, other disciplines in Clinical Pathology. Tests that were unusual and considered esoteric several years ago have in many laboratories become commonplace. These changes have been most apparent in red cell enzyme studies and in the more recent advances in blood coagulation.

Other major changes are reflected in the concept of multiphasic patient screening. The introduction and acceptance of hematology automation has radically altered the routine work load and has brought with it, not only increases in precision and accuracy, but also the spectacle of the laboratory engineer as a potential member of the health team. This automation has enabled the hematology technologist to be freed of many mundane manual chores and has resulted in the expansion of laboratory testing to encompass a more thorough hematology investigation.

It is because of these changing concepts that the Second Edition of this text has been prepared. The addition of a large number of tests and the deletion of obsolete methods and apparatus is, then, necessary to keep this text a functional practical laboratory reference.

The most radical revisions in this text have concerned the blood bank section. Although this text is not meant to be a theoretical book on either hematology or immunohematology, it was thought necessary to revise the previous material to include sufficient theoretical aspects, so as to make the techniques that follow more understandable. In this regard, these methods have also undergone a complete revision and have been updated whenever needed. The net result is that treatment of the blood banking section has been expanded from the original single chapter to the present five chapters in the hope that this clarification will be of practical value to the working medical technologist.

I am indebted to the Medical Graphics Department of the University of Iowa and to the many student, medical technologists and the faculty of the Department of Pathology who have been helpful in this revision. Especial acknowledgements are due to Miss Judy White and Mrs. Joyce Paul for the valuable secretarial skills and patience which they showed in the preparation of the manuscript, and to Mr. George F. Stickley and to Mr. J. Stuart Freeman of the Medical Books Division of J. B. Lippincott Company.

ARTHUR SIMMONS

# *Preface to the First Edition*

This text was written for the working graduate and the student medical technologist. Its aims are twofold: to present as completely as possible the various hematologic techniques that can be used as a diagnostic aid to the physician, and to offer as far as possible some of the alternative methods commonly used. In addition, it is hoped that the medical technologist working in the hematology laboratory will gain more of an insight into the laboratory aspect of some of the hematologic diseases.

There are many ways of determining the same hematologic value, and the method chosen is frequently only a personal preference. This is especially true with the recent surge in the type and range of automatic equipment, which allows the laboratory worker to carry out procedures in vast numbers. The ever-increasing number of laboratories being automated makes it necessary to include all of the standard equipment available on the market, although each student should be grounded in the basic manual principles of a technique before advancing to the automatic aspects.

Brief clinical data has been included, because I believe that the medical technologist, although not practising medicine, should know some of the basic medical reasons for carrying out a test. To produce hematologic data with total disregard to the patient's condition can only lead to boredom, and eventually, to lack of precision and accuracy. One might consider this aspect an accessory to quality control, which is also stressed in the later chapters.

The section on immunohematology contains more theoretical material than other sections, and endeavors to cover the more elementary aspects of this speciality.

My grateful thanks to Dr. K. R. Thornton, my former chief, for his helpful criticisms, encouragement, and reading of the first draft of this text; to Dr. Sloan Wilson, Professor of Medicine and Chief of the Division of Hematology, Kansas University Medical Center; and to Dr. Samuel Hanson, Associate Professor of Pathology, University of Alberta, for helpful suggestions and ideas. I wish to express my sincere appreciation to Dr. James S. Arnold, Associate Professor of Pathology and of Radiology, University of Missouri, for his continual advice and suggestions.

I am indebted to Miss Barbara Ashbaugh and Mr. Roger Odneal of the

Department of Photography and Medical Illustrations, Kansas City General Hospital and Medical Center, for their great help and skill in producing most of the photographs and graphs used, and to Mr. Geoffrey G. Brown, A.I.M.L.T., for the line drawings used.

Acknowledgment is also made to the following companies for giving permission to publish some of their technical procedures, and for providing photographs of their equipment.

American Optical Company
Ames Company
Beckman Instruments, Inc.
Becton, Dickinson and Company
Coulter Electronics, Inc.
Fisher Scientific Company
Hewlett-Packard Company
Hyland Laboratories
Technicon Corporation
Yellow Springs Instrument Company, Inc.

Finally, I would wish to thank Dr. C. J. C. Britton, Dr. H. Foster, and Dr. B. J. Thompson for the training and experience I received under their able guidance. To my wife I owe a great debt of gratitude for the endless hours of typing and retyping, and for suggestions and improvements that she originated.

ARTHUR SIMMONS

# Contents

# Introduction

## BLOOD COLLECTION

The two main methods of obtaining blood samples are finger or heel puncture (capillary blood) and venipuncture.

The first step in the collection of a blood sample is to reassure the patient. With adults it is a relatively easy matter to explain the procedure, but with children extra care should be taken and some endeavor made to win the child's confidence.

### Finger Puncture Method

1. The finger is cleansed with gauze or wool moistened with 70% alcohol or with alcohol-ether mixture, and allowed to dry.

2. A quick puncture is made on the *side* of the finger with a disposable lancet. *Do not* squeeze the finger tightly, because the liberated tissue juices dilute the blood.

3. Wipe away the first drop of blood to avoid tissue juice contamination, and apply *gentle* pressure in a "milking" fashion to obtain a free flow of blood.

4. When the desired amount of blood has been obtained, a clean dry pad is applied to the wound, and the patient is instructed to apply pressure until the bleeding ceases.

### Venipuncture

Blood can be obtained from any of the following sites: (1) antecubital veins of the forearm; (2) ankle veins; (3) wrist or hand veins; (4) femoral veins; and (5) scalp or jugular veins (in infants). This procedure should be carried out by a physician.

### *Syringe Method from Antecubital Veins*

1. The area around the site is cleansed with 70% alcohol or with alcohol-ether mixture, and allowed to dry.

2. A tourniquet is applied around the upper arm, and the patient is instructed to open and close his hand to build up the blood pressure in the vein.

3. A prominent vein is located. If it is not easily seen, the technician's index finger is cleansed as in (1), and the forearm is palpated until a vein is felt.

4. The vein is fixed either by holding it with the finger or by grasping the patient's arm below the elbow and pulling the skin taut.

5. The needle is inserted in the vein obliquely with the bevel upward, and the plunger is slowly pulled back until the necessary volume of blood is obtained.

6. The tourniquet is released, and the patient is instructed to open his hand.

7. A clean pad is applied over the needle puncture and the needle quickly removed in a quick, smooth motion.

8. Pressure is applied to the puncture site with the patient's arm held straight out. *Do not* allow the patient to bend his arm at the elbow, or a large hematoma may form. This is a collection of subcutaneous blood, causing blue and then green skin coloration at the site.

### Vacutainer Method

1. Procedures (1) to (4) are carried out as in the syringe method.

2. The appropriate vacutainer tube is placed in a reusable plastic holder, and a disposable needle is attached by screwing the threaded needle hub to the female end of the holder.

3. The vacutainer tube is inserted into the holder until the top of its stopper is level with the clearly marked guideline.

4. The pressure on the tube is then released, causing the tube to recede slightly.

5. The needle is inserted into the vein as in the syringe method, and the tube base is pushed forward, breaking the vacuum in the tube and enabling the sample to be collected.

6. Procedures (6) to (8) are carried out as in the syringe method.

## ANTICOAGULANTS

Whole blood is necessary for most hematological investigations. The sample must, therefore, be mixed with an anticoagulant to prevent coagulation. The common hematological anticoagulants are listed below.

### Heller's and Paul's Mixture

(syn: double oxalate, Wintrobe's anticoagulant, balanced oxalate)

*Chemical Action.* This anticoagulant removes the free calcium ions from solution through the addition of ammonium and potassium oxalate. Calcium is precipitated as insoluble calcium oxalate.

### Preparation

1. 1.2 g ammonium oxalate and 0.8 g potassium oxalate are dissolved in 100 ml of distilled water.

2. 0.5 ml of this solution is added to each of a series of tubes and evaporated to dryness at 37°C. Higher temperatures decompose the oxalates.

### Notes

1. The dried salts from 0.5 ml of the solution is adequate to stop 5 ml of blood from clotting.

2. The mixture of blood and salts is isotonic. The ammonium salt would give a hypotonic solution, the potassium salt a hypertonic solution.

3. Blood taken into this anticoagulant is unsuitable for morphological examination. The red cells commence to crenate and the white cells exhibit bizarre nuclear patterns.

## Ethylenediaminetetraacetic Acid, Dipotassium or Disodium Salt

(syn: EDTA, sequestrene, versene)

*Chemical Action.* This anticoagulant removes the free calcium ions by chelation.

### Preparation

1. 10 g of the dipotassium salt is dissolved in 100 ml of warm distilled water.

2. 0.1 ml of this solution is added to each of a series of tubes and evaporated to dryness at 37°C.

### Notes

1. The dried salt (0.01 g) from 0.1 ml of the solution is sufficient to stop the coagulation of 5 ml of blood.

2. Blood taken into this anticoagulant can be used for cellular morphology. Platelet counts can also be carried out on 24-hour-old blood.

3. The dipotassium salt is to be preferred to the disodium salt, because it is more soluble.

## Heparin

*Chemical Action.* Heparin acts as an antithrombin and is the only naturally occurring anticoagulant used routinely in the laboratory.

*Preparation*

1. 0.4 g of powdered heparin is dissolved in 100 ml of distilled water.

2. 0.25 ml of this solution is added to each of a series of tubes, and evaporated to dryness at 37°C.

*Notes*

1. 1 mg of heparin—the amount in 0.25 ml of the solution—is sufficient to prevent the coagulation of 5 ml of blood for at least 24 hours.

2. Heparin is valuable when it is important to minimize the chance of hemolysis (e.g., in the osmotic fragility test).

3. Heparin cannot be used when differential white counts and examinations of cellular morphology are to be made, because it imparts a faint blue coloration to the background when the blood smear is stained by any Romanowsky stain.

## Sodium Citrate

*Chemical Action.* This anticoagulant removes the free calcium ions by loosely binding them to form a calcium citrate complex.

*Preparation*

1. 3.8 g trisodium citrate is dissolved in 100 ml of distilled water.

*Notes*

1. For the investigation of coagulation disorders, 9 volumes of blood are added to 1 volume of the anticoagulant.

2. For determining sedimentation rates by the Westergren method, 4 volumes of blood are added to 1 volume of the anticoagulant.

## Sodium Citrate—Citric Acid Buffer

*Chemical Action.* The action is identical to sodium citrate.

*Preparation*

1. 19.2 g of citric acid is dissolved in 100 ml of warm distilled water.

2. 29.4 g of sodium citrate is dissolved in 100 ml of warm distilled water.

3. 23.7 ml of the citric acid solution is added to 26.0 ml of the sodium citrate solution, and the mixture is diluted to approximately 90 ml with distilled water.

4. The pH of the mixture is adjusted to 4.7 and the volume made up to 100 ml with distilled water.

*Notes*

1. For the investigation of blood coagulation disorders, 9.9 volumes of blood are added to 0.1 volume of the buffered anticoagulant.

2. The pH of the anticoagulant is adjusted to 4.7, but when whole blood is added and the plasma is separated, the final pH should be 7.35 ± 0.05.

# 1

# *Hemoglobin*

## METHODS OF ESTIMATION

### Cyanmethemoglobin Method[1]

*Principle.* Hemoglobin is converted to cyanmethemoglobin by Drabkin's reagent. The resulting color is compared photometrically with a known standard.

### Reagents and Apparatus
1. Spectrophotometer
2. Sahli pipet—0.02 ml (+1%)
3. Graduated pipet—5 ml
4. Drabkin's reagent:

   Sodium bicarbonate .................. 1.0  g
   Potassium ferricyanide................ 0.2  g
   Sodium cyanide...................... 0.05 g
   Distilled water......................... to 1 l

### Method
1. 5 ml of Drabkin's reagent is added to a clean tube, and 0.02 ml of well-mixed anticoagulated venous or capillary blood is carefully washed into the reagent.

2. The contents of the tube are mixed and allowed to stand at room temperature for 5 minutes, and the color intensity is compared photometrically at a wavelength of 540 nm or read in a Fisher hemophotometer.

### Notes
1. All forms of hemoglobin are estimated with the exception of sulfhemoglobin.

2. The standards used to calibrate the technique are stable.

3. Some hemoglobin forms (HbS and C) are resistant to lysis and form a turbid solution with Drabkin's reagent. Such turbidity can be elimi-

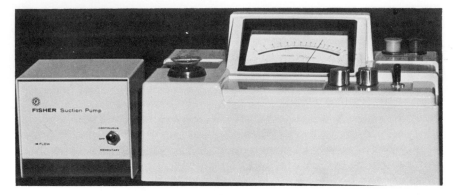

Fig. 1-1. Fisher hemophotometer. (Courtesy of Fisher Scientific Company)

nated by adding 5 ml of water to the mixture and allowing to stand for 5 minutes. The hemoglobin is read normally, doubling the result.

### Standardization

1. Commercially available certified standards with hemoglobin values of approximately 20 g per cent can be purchased. The assayed value is found on the vial label, and is commonly expressed in mg. To convert this label value to hemoglobin in g%, multiply the assay value × the dilution used in the hemoglobin (i.e., label value = 80 mg dilution = 1:251 hemoglobin value = 80 × 251 = 20.08 g).

2. Using a 20 g value as an example, the following series of standards should be set up.

3. The blank tube containing reagent solution is placed in the photometer, so that the optical density reads zero (100% transmission). The photometer is adjusted, if necessary, and the four standard values are read and recorded graphically.

### Notes

1. The stock Drabkin's reagent should be kept away from direct sunlight. It should be stored, preferably, in a dark bottle in a cabinet and made up at least weekly.

TABLE 1-1. Standardization.

| Tube | 1 | 2 | 3 | 4 |
|---|---|---|---|---|
| Standard | 1.5 ml | 2.5 ml | 4.0 ml | 5.0 ml |
| Drabkin's reagent | 3.5 ml | 2.5 ml | 1.0 ml | 0 ml |
| Hemoglobin value | 6 g% | 10 g% | 16 g% | 20 g% |

2. If there is any change in technique (new reagents made, new photometer or photo lamp), the instrument should be recalibrated with new standards.

### Normal Values

Hemoglobin: Male ............. 13.7–18.5 g/dl

Female ............12.0–16.4 g/dl

Infant ............16.2–24.4 g/dl

## Oxyhemoglobin Method[2]

*Principle.* Hemoglobin is converted to oxyhemoglobin by ammoniated water or by sodium carbonate. The resulting pigment is compared photoelectrically against a standard blood or reagent.

### Reagents and Apparatus
1. Spectrophotometer
2. Sahli pipet—0.02 ml (±1%)
3. Graduated pipet—5 ml
4. 0.04% Aqueous ammonia (v/v)

### Method
1. 0.02 ml of well mixed blood is added to 5 ml of 0.04% ammonia in a clean tube.
2. The contents of the tube are mixed and allowed to stand for 2 to 3 minutes at room temperature.
3. The color intensity is compared photometrically at a wavelength of 540 nm.

### Notes
1. The method can be standardized by first determining the hemoglobin by the cyanmethemoglobin method. No commercial oxyhemoglobin standards are available.
2. The original disadvantage of the oxyhemoglobin procedure was that the solution faded because of the high dilution of the solution and the high pH resulting from the use of 0.1% sodium carbonate or strong ammonia solutions. Using 0.04% ammonia, the pigment is stable for a day at room temperature.
3. The rate of fading at alkaline pH is accelerated by traces of copper in the diluent. The substitution of 0.3% tetrasodium ethlyenediaminotetracetic acid for the ammonia helps to further stabilize the solution.

### Standardization. *Thomson's Grey Solution*[3]
1. Stock solution:

Chrome alum ................................. 16.7  g

Copper sulfate hexahydrate .................... 33.3  g

Ammonium cobalt sulfate ...................... 39.5  g
Potassium dichromate ......................... 0.02 g
Distilled water ............................. to 1 liter

2. Allow to stand 6 weeks before using to allow the gray color to develop.

3. Mix 2 volumes of stock solution with 1 volume of distilled water. The resulting color gives an equivalent photometric reading of 14.6 g hemoglobin per cent, at a wavelength of 540 nm.

## Alkaline Hematin Method[4]

*Principle.* Hemoglobin is converted to alkaline hemating by the action of heated sodium hydroxide.

*Reagents and Apparatus*
1. Spectrophotometer
2. Wash-out pipet ($\pm 1\%$)—0.05 ml
3. N/10 sodium hydroxide
4. Boiling waterbath

*Method*
1. 5 ml of N/10 Sodium hydroxide is added to a clean tube, and 0.05 ml of well-mixed blood is carefully pipeted into the reagent.
2. The contents of the tube are mixed and placed in a boiling water-bath for 5 minutes.
3. The resulting color is read photometrically at a wavelength of 540 nm.

*Notes*
1. This method gives a true estimation of total hemoglobin, even if carboxyhemoglobin, methemoglobin, or sulfhemoglobin is present.
2. A true solution is obtained. Plasma proteins and lipoids have little effect on the development of the color, although they can cause turbidity unless the blood and alkali are mixed quickly and thoroughly.
3. Hemoglobin F and Bart's hemoglobin are resistant to alkali denaturation, but normally break down on heating for 5 minutes.

*Standardization*
*Hemin Standard:*
37.5 mg of pure hemin is dissolved in 1 liter of N/10 sodium hydroxide. This is equivalent to a hemoglobin of 7.4 g per cent.
*Gibson-Harrison Standard:*
1. Dissolve the following in 500 ml distilled water:
Chromium potassium sulfate .......... 11.61 g
Anhydrous cobaltous sulfate .......... 13.1  g
Potassium dichromate ................ 0.69 g

2. 1.8 ml N Sulfuric acid is added to the resulting solution and the mixture is boiled for 1 minute, cooled and made up to 1 liter with distilled water.

3. This standard is equivalent to a hemoglobin of 16.0 g per cent.

## Semi-Automated Method

*Principle.* The IL Model 231 Hemoglobinometer measures hemoglobin at 548.5 nm. At this wavelength, human hemoglobin, oxyhemoglobin and carboxyhemoglobin have approximately the same absorption characteristics. The apparatus uses a high precision interference filter with a narrow bandwidth set at 548.5 nm and measures the combined absorbances of hemoglobin, oxyhemoglobin, and carboxyhemoglobin. With this procedure, the three main forms of hemoglobin are measured as they exist, and there is no need to change the various hemoglobin forms to one particular type.

*Reagents and Apparatus*
1. IL Model 231 Hemoglobinometer
2. EDTA or heparinized blood
3. IL Calibrating dye
4. Working diluent (Add 1 volume of IL Diluent Concentrate [No. 33102] to 3 volumes of distilled water.)

*Method*
1. The instrument is set up according to the manufacturer's instructions. (Turn power switch to ON and mode switch to STAND BY.)

3. Turn switch to PUMP.

4. Adjust the hemoglobinometer to zero with the zero control by introducing a diluted buffered hemolysing agent. This is made by adding 1 volume of working diluent to 9 volumes of distilled water.

5. Introduce the calibrating dye and adjust the CALIBRATE control to the correct setting.

6. Introduce the aspirator tube well into the blood sample. Hold the sample in place until the digital readout reaches a steady indication (in approximately 12 seconds).

7. The blood is then removed and the aspirator tube cleaned by wiping with lint-free paper.

8. After the last sample is measured, IL Flushing Agent (No. 33104) is passed through the system for 5 to 10 seconds.

*Notes*
1. The value of the calibrating dye is set by the manufacturer by matching its absorption with that of a known hemoglobin concentration

determined by a routine cyanmethemoglobin method. The dye is stable at room temperature and unaffected by light.

2. Complete standardization is necessary whenever the apparatus has been turned off for any length of time. Recalibration is recommended 15 minutes after initially starting the instrument and approximately every 60 minutes thereafter.

3. Secondary standardization can be carried out using a blood assayed by a conventional cyanmethemoglobin method. Other commercial standards should not be used, since they may not possess the spectrophometric properties needed by stabilizing the hemoglobin with carbon monoxide, and if used can produce appreciable error.

4. Similarly, prepared standards of cyanmethemoglobin possess absorbance spectra unrelated to that of the apparatus and should not be used.

5. Figure 1-2 illustrates the hemoglobin absorption spectra of the hemoglobin pigments measured. In the green region of the spectrum, at 548.5 nm, hemoglobin and oxyhemoglobin have exactly the same absorptivity (they are isosbestic at this point). At the same wavelength, carboxyhemoglobin has an absorptivity approximately 95% of that of both hemoglobin and oxyhemoglobin. The 5% error in measuring carboxyhemoglobin is considered insignificant in the routine measurement of total hemoglobin.

6. Hemoglobin bound with carbon monoxide takes fully an hour to convert completely to the cyanmethemoglobin form. Patients who are heavy smokers, will have as much as 10% of the hemoglobin in the carboxyhemoglobin form. If the total hemoglobin is 15 g/dl as measured

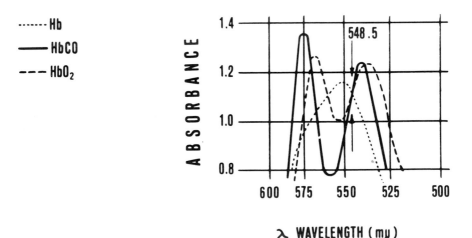

FIG. 1-2. The hemoglobin absorption spectra of the hemoglobin pigments measured.

in a sample having 10% carboxyhemoglobin by the cyanmethemoglobin method, in 3 minutes after dilution the reading will be 15.4 g/dl, 15 minutes after dilution, the hemoglobin will be 15.2 g/dl and after 40 minutes the result will be 15.1 g/dl.

7. Using Unopette accessories (No. 33105) a micro procedure can be carried out. With these pipets, a 1:16 dilution of the blood sample is made. With the switch at the MICRO position, the sensitivity of the apparatus is increased by a factor of ten. The hemoglobinometer is operated as in the normal method, but it is standardized by using the Micro Calibrating Dye (No. 33101), or by using a previously estimated blood and diluting it by the same amount.

## PRIMARY STANDARDIZATION

### Whole Blood Iron Method (Wong)[5]

*Principle.* Iron is detached from the hemoglobin by the action of concentrated sulfuric acid in the presence of potassium persulfate. Proteins are then precipitated by tungstic acid, and the iron is determined colorimetrically in the filtrate by the thiocyanate reaction.

### Reagents and Apparatus
1. Concentrated sulfuric acid
2. Saturated aqueous potassium persulfate: Approximately 7.0 g of reagent grade potassium persulfate is placed in a flask and 100 ml of distilled water is added. Any insoluble material is allowed to settle out.
3. Sodium tungstate (10%)
4. Standard iron solution: 100 mg of analyzed grade iron filings is placed in a 1-liter beaker; 20 ml of concentrated hydrochloric acid and 100 ml of distilled water are added, and the mixture is heated on a steam bath until solution is complete. The mixture is then cooled to room temperature and diluted to exactly 1 liter with distilled water. One milliliter of the standard contains 0.1 mg iron.
5. Potassium thiocyanate 3N: 146 g of reagent grade potassium thiocyanate is placed in a beaker and dissolved in about 300 ml of distilled water; 20 ml of acetone is added as a preservative. The mixture is diluted to a final volume of 500 ml with distilled water.
6. Volumetric flasks—100 ml
7. Volumetric flask—1 liter
8. Volumetric flasks—25 ml
9. Volumetric pipets—20 ml
10. Volumetric pipets—10 ml
11. Volumetric pipets—4 ml
12. Oswald-Folin pipets—1 ml

13. Graduated pipets—10 ml
14. Beakers—2 liter
15. Whatman filter paper (No. 40)
16. Caprylic alcohol
17. Mechanical mixer
18. Spectrophotometer
19. Boiling waterbath

### Calibration Curve

1. 10 ml of the standard iron solution is diluted to 100 ml with distilled water.

2. Four 25-ml volumetric flasks are set up and the following reagents are added in the order given in Table 1-2.

3. The total volume is adjusted to the 25-ml level with distilled water, and the optical density of the dilutions is read at a wavelength of 540 nm within 3 minutes of completion.

4. A calibration curve is plotted on coordinated graph paper, using the values in Table 1-3 to correspond to the standard flasks.

### Method

1. 1 ml of well-mixed whole blood is transferred to a 100-ml volumetric flask.

2. 4 ml of concentrated sulfuric acid is added to the flask, and the contents are mixed for 5 minutes.

3. 4 ml of saturated potassium persulfate, approximately 65 ml of distilled water and 6 ml of 10% sodium tungstate are added to the mixture.

4. The contents of the flask are cooled to room temperature, and 1 drop of caprylic alcohol is added to prevent foaming.

5. The final volume is diluted to 100 ml with distilled water, mixed by inversion, allowed to stand for 5 minutes at room temperature, and then filtered through a Whatman filter paper (No. 40).

TABLE 1-2. Iron Standards.

| FLASK | 1 | 2 | 3 | 4 |
|---|---|---|---|---|
| | ml | ml | ml | ml |
| Diluted iron standard | 0 | 2 | 5 | 8 |
| Concentrated sulfuric acid | 0.4 | 0.4 | 0.4 | 0.4 |
| Distilled water | 10 | 10 | 10 | 10 |
| Saturated potassium persulfate | 1 | 1 | 1 | 1 |
| 3N Potassium thiocyanate | 4 | 4 | 4 | 4 |

TABLE 1-3. Calibration Curve.

| FLASK | 1 | 2 | 3 | 4 |
|-------|---|---|---|---|
| mg% iron | 0 | 20 | 50 | 80 |

6. Into three 25-ml flasks, labeled "test," standard" and "blank," place the substances shown in the amounts given in Table 1-4.

7. The flasks are diluted to the 25-ml mark with distilled water, and the photometer is adjusted so that the blank tube reads zero optical density (100% transmission) at a wavelength of 540 nm.

8. The standard and test are read in the photometer at 540 nm.

9. Calculate the mg iron per cent from the calibration chart.

*Calculation*

$$\frac{\text{milligram iron per cent}}{3.40} = \text{g hemoglobin per cent}$$

*Notes*

Primary hemoglobin standardization by the whole blood method is not used as a routine procedure. Commercial standards are available and are commonly used for the standardization and control of hemoglobin estimations using Drabkin's reagent in the cyanmethemoglobin technique (p. 6).

The whole blood iron method can be utilized if other hemoglobin methods are used. Because of the difficulty and time-consuming aspects of the procedure, it is more often employed as a means of calibrating secondary controls which are then used daily.

Laboratories not wishing to use commercial standards can produce their own by estimating whole blood iron levels, using this value to accurately calibrate their hemoglobin method.

TABLE 1-4. Reagents for Whole Blood Iron Determination of Hemoglobin.

| | TEST | STANDARD | BLANK |
|---|---|---|---|
| | *ml* | *ml* | *ml* |
| Filtrate | 10 | 0 | 0 |
| 1:10 Dilution of iron standard | 0 | 5 | 0 |
| Concentrated sulfuric acid | 0 | 0.4 | 0.4 |
| Distilled water | 0 | 10 | 10 |
| Saturated potassium persulfate | 0 | 1 | 1 |
| 3N potassium thiocyanate | 4 | 4 | 4 |

## ESTIMATION OF PLASMA HEMOGLOBIN

### Method 1

*Principle.* O-Toluidine and hydrogen peroxide in the presence of heme pigment produces a green-blue coloration, the intensity of which is spectrophotometrically compared against a standard hemoglobin.

#### Reagents and Apparatus

1. One Hematest* tablet is crushed and dissolved in 8 ml of warm distilled water, using a magnetic stirrer and vigorous action. The mixture is filtered into a clean bottle and stored at 4°C.

2. The hemoglobin value of a normal blood is determined in duplicate, and an equal volume of distilled water added to the blood to reduce the value to 50% of normal. This dilution is used as the standard by adding 0.1 ml of the dilution to 100 ml of distilled water. For example, if the hemoglobin value is 14 g/dl the plasma hemoglobin standard is 7 mg/dl.

3. All glassware used should be acid washed.

4. Magnetic stirrer

5. Spectrophotometer

6. Micropipet—0.02 ml

7. Graduated pipet—5 ml

8. Heparinized blood; normal control and test

9. Tubes—12 × 75 mm

10. Timer

#### Method

1. Heparinized blood is centrifuged at 2,000 rpm for 15 minutes using a GLC-1 centrifuge (Sorvall).

2. Into each of 4 tubes labeled (a) Blank; (b) Standard; (c) Control; (d) Test, add:

    5.0 ml of aqueous Hematest reagent.

3. Add 0.02 ml of distilled water to the Blank tube; 0.02 ml of the standard to the Standard tube; 0.02 ml of a normal heparinized plasma to the Control tube; and 0.02 ml of the patient's plasm to the Test tube.

4. All tubes are mixed by inversion, left for exactly 10 minutes at room temperature, and the optical density read in a spectrophotometer at 600 nm against the Blank tube.

#### Calculation

$$\text{Plasma hemoglobin} = \frac{\text{Optical Density of Test} \times \text{Standard Value (mg/dl)}}{\text{Optical Density of Standard}}$$

Normal 1 to 7 mg/dl

---

\* Available from Ames Co., Elkhart, Indiana

*Notes*

1. If the optical density of the test is greater than 0.7, it is repeated with a sample diluted with distilled water.

2. The color must be read in exactly 10 minutes after adding the plasma to the Hematest reagent. All readings should be completed within a 2-minute span, since the developing color is unstable.

## Method 2

*Principle.* Acidified benzidine and hydrogen peroxide in the presence of heme pigment produce a green color, which later changes to a blue-violet. This color intensity is compared photoelectrically against a standard hemoglobin.

### Reagents and Apparatus

1. Benzidine 1%. 1 g of benzidine dihydrochloride is added to 90 ml of warm glacial acetic acid and made up to 100 ml with distilled water. An alternate method is to dissolve the salt in 10 ml of hot distilled water and add 90 ml of glacial acetic acid. This variation occasionally produces a better reagent, depending on the quality of the benzidine dihydrochloride used.

2. Fresh 1% hydrogen peroxide (v/v)

3. Standard blood: 0.1 ml of whole blood is delivered into a 100-ml volumetric flask, and distilled water is added to the 100-ml mark. The whole blood hemoglobin of the standard blood is determined by a conventional method.

4. Heparinized plasma: Heparinized whole blood is centrifuged for 15 minutes at 2,000 rpm.

5. 10% Acetic acid (v/v)

6. Volumetric flasks—100 ml

7. Micropipet—1 ml

8. Test tubes—15 ml capacity

9. Volumetric pipets—10 ml

10. Spectrophotometer

11. Centrifuge

### Method

1. Pipet the materials in Table 1-5 into three 15-ml tubes, labeled "test," "standard" and "blank."

2. The contents of the tubes are well mixed and left at room temperature for 30 minutes.

3. 10 ml of 10% acetic acid is added and the tubes mixed by inversion.

4. The color development is read spectrophotometrically at a wavelength of 515 nm using the blank tube as a zero reference.

TABLE 1-5. Reagents for Estimation of Plasma Hemoglobin.

|  | TEST | STANDARD | BLANK |
|---|---|---|---|
|  | *ml* | *ml* | *ml* |
| 1% Benzidine | 1 | 1 | 1 |
| Test plasma | 0.02 | 0 | 0 |
| Standard blood | 0 | 0.02 | 0 |
| Distilled water | 0 | 0 | 0.02 |
| 1% Hydrogen peroxide | 1 | 1 | 1 |

### Calculation

1. $\dfrac{\text{Optical density of the test}}{\text{Optical density of the standard}} \times$ standard value

2. If the standard whole blood hemoglobin is 15 g% then, because the blood is diluted 1:1,000, the resulting standard is equivalent to 15 mg%.

3. Normal plasma hemoglobin values obtained by this method range from 1 to 5 mg%.

### Notes

1. All glassware used should be acid washed.

2. This method is suited for specimens with concentrations of hemoglobin too low to be measured by conventional cyanmethemoglobin methods. Plasma hemoglobin concentrations above 150 mg% can usually be measured by conventional hemoglobin techniques.

3. The collection of the blood sample must be undertaken with great care. Vacutainer tubes should not be used unless the rubber stopper is first removed to destroy the vacuum. The blood should be collected using a syringe or by bleeding directly from the needle into heparin.

## HEMOGLOBIN PIGMENTS

### Oxyhemoglobin

This is the normal state of hemoglobin exposed to atmospheric conditions. Absorption bands at 578 nm and 540 nm are observed in spectroscopic examination.

### Carboxyhemoglobin

1. This is prepared by exposing oxyhemoglobin to carbon monoxide.

2. Carbon monoxide has 200 times the affinity for hemoglobin that oxygen has. The absorption bands of carboxyhemoglobin are similar to those of oxyhemoglobin and are present at 572 nm and 535 nm.

## Reduced Hemoglobin

This is deoxygenated hemoglobin. Absorption bands are present from 540 to 570 nm with a maximum peak at 556 nm.

## Sulfhemoglobin

1. This is produced by adding phenylhydrazine and hydrogen sulfide to oxyhemoglobin. Absorption bands are present at 618 nm, 578 nm and 540 nm.

2. The pigment is found frequently in the blood of patients taking aspirin and codeine.

3 Sulfhemoglobin is usually intracellular and, once formed in the red cells, persists until the cells are destroyed by the reticuloendothelial system

## Methemoglobin

1. This pigment behaves as an indicator, being brown in acidic and red in basic solutions. Absorption bands are present at 630 nm, 578 nm 540 nm and 500 nm.

2. Methemoglobin contains the oxidized form of heme; the iron, being in the ferric state, has no oxygen-carrying capacity.

3. Methemoglobin is most commonly formed from intracellular hemoglobin, but may be present in the plasma if hemolysis occurs.

4. The pigment may be produced by the action of benzene and aniline dyes. Some cases of methemoglobinemia have been attributed to the absorption of toxins or of nitrites from the action of nitrite-producing bacteria in the intestine.

5. Clinically, methemoglobin blood levels of over 5 g/100 ml result in the presence of visible cyanosis.

## Cyanmethemoglobin

This is prepared by adding cyanide ions to methemoglobin. A strong absorption band is present at 540 nm.

## Methemalbumin (Fairley's Pigment)

This pigment can be prepared by incubating hemoglobin with sterile plasma. Absorption bands are present at 624 nm, 540 nm and 500 nm.

## HAND SPECTROSCOPE

*Principle.* When a light beam passes through a prism, it is refracted at the prism surface to produce a spectral image ranging from red to violet.

The hand spectroscope consists of a series of prisms of alternating crown and flint glass, which cause the dispersion of a ray of light without any deviation from the light source.

A series of dark vertical lines is seen throughout the spectrum when the apparatus is held in daylight, and a spectral image when viewed through the eyepiece. These Fraunhofer lines are caused by the absorption of light by oxygen (B 686.7 nm), hydrogen (C 656.3 nm) and (F 486.1 nm), sodium (D 589 nm), iron and calcium (E 527 nm, 518.4 nm) and magnesium (H 450 nm), and are used to show the exact location of unknown absorption bands.

### Method
1. Either daylight or fluorescent light can be used.
2. Fraunhofer D lines are formed at 589 nm with daylight and at 577 nm, 579 nm, 546 nm and 436 nm with fluorescent light.
3. The slit width is adjusted so that a narrow concentrated spectral image can be seen when the spectroscope is held near the light.
4. The intensity of the light source and the concentration of the solution are adjusted by trial and error to give sharp and narrow absorption bands.
5. The bands of the test sample are compared to those of a standard pigment and correlated with the Fraunhofer lines.

## The Spectroscopic Detection of Methemoglobin and Sulfhemoglobin

*Principle.* Heparinized blood is hemolyzed and examined spectroscopically for absorption bands in the red region of the spectrum.

### Reagents and Apparatus
1. Hand or recording spectroscope
2. Heparinized blood
3. Hydrogen sulfide saturated water
4. 10% Aqueous potassium ferricyanide
5. Yellow ammonium sulfide
6. Centrifuge
7. Oswald-Folin pipets—1 ml
8. Graduated pipets—10 ml
9. Micropipets—0.1 ml

### Method
1. 1 ml of heparinized whole blood is added to 9 ml of distilled water, and the dilution is centrifuged for 2 to 3 minutes at 2,000 rpm.
2. The supernatant is examined with a Zeiss hand spectroscope for absorption bands in the red area of the spectrum (620-630 nm), or a

spectral picture is obtained on a recording spectrophometer (e.g., Perkin-Elmer No. 202).

3. If absorption bands are present, 1 drop of yellow ammonium sulfide is added.

4. Absorption bands due to methemoglobin are detected by the disappearance of the band. If sulfhemoglobin is present, the absorption band persists.

### Standards—Sulfhemoglobin

1. 0.1 ml of heparinized blood is added to 9.9 ml of distilled water. 10 ml of this dilution is added to 0.1 ml of a 0.1% aqueous solution of phenylhydrazine hydrochloride.

2. One drop of water saturated with hydrogen sulfide is added to the mixture, and a comparison is made between the test and standard absorption bands. A strong band will be present in the standard at 618 mm.

### Standards—Methemoglobin

1. 1 ml of heparinized blood is added to 4 ml of distilled water. Equal volumes of the hemolyzed dilution and of 10% potassium ferricyanide are then added together.

2. The unknown is compared with the absorption bands produced by this solution. A strong band will be present in the standard at 630 nm.

### Comments

1. An increase in methemoglobin may be due to acetylsalicylic acid, aniline dyes, nitrites, severe sepsis, sulfonamides and other drugs.

2. Methemoglobin is produced when the iron atoms of heme are in the ferric state. It cannot carry oxygen and is useless as a respiratory pigment.

3. The blood of affected patients is brownish in color and cyanosis becomes evident when the level of methemoglobin reaches in excess of 2 g%. The cyanosis is usually present at birth and many persons with methemoglobinemia are first thought to have congenital heart disease.

4. An increase in sulfhemoglobin may be due to phenacetin medication, sulfonamides, sulfur and sulfides and nitrates.


### Quantitative Estimation of Methemoglobin[6]

***Principle.*** Methemoglobin has a maximal absorption at 630 $\mu$m. When cyanide is added, this absorption band disappears and the resulting change in optical density is directly proportional to the concentration of methemoglobin. Total hemoglobin of the sample is measured after complete conversion to cyanmethemoglobin by the addition of ferricyanide–cyanide reagent. The conversion will measure hemoglobin and methemoglobin but not sulfhemoglobin.

### Reagents and Apparatus

1. M/15 Disodium hydrogen phosphate ($Na_2HPO_47H_2O$) 1.78 g of disodium hydrogen phosphate is dissolved in 100 ml of distilled water.

2. M/15 Potassium dihydrogen phosphate ($KH_2PO_4$) 0.91 g of potassium dihydrogen phosphate is dissolved in 100 ml of distilled water.

3. M/15 Double phosphate buffer: 125 ml of the M/15 disodium hydrogen phosphate solution is added to 375 ml of M/15 potassium dihydrogen phosphate. A pH of 6.6 should be obtained. If the pH is too acidic, it should be adjusted by adding additional M/15 disodium hydrogen phosphate solution. If it is too alkaline, additional M/15 potassium dihydrogen phosphate should be added.

4. M/60 Double phosphate buffer: 250 ml of the M/15 Buffer is added to 750 ml of distilled water.

5. 10% Aqueous sodium cyanide

6. 12% Acetic acid

7. 20% Aqueous potassium ferricyanide

8. Volumetric pipets—10 ml

9. "Prothrombin" pipets—0.2 ml

10. Graduated pipets—10 ml

11. Spectrophotometer

12. EDTA blood

### Method

1. 0.2 ml of fresh blood is added to 10 ml of M/60 buffer. The tube is stoppered and inverted several times to mix, and left for 5 minutes.

2. After zeroing the spectrophotometer with distilled water, the optical density of the mixture is read at 630 $\mu$m (OD No. 1).

3. Equal volumes of 10% sodium cyanide and 12% acetic acid are added together, and 1 drop of this mixture is added to the blood-buffer solution. The tube is stoppered, inverted several times, and left for 2 minutes.

4. The optical density of this solution is recorded at 630 $\mu$m (OD No. 2)

5. 8.0 ml of M/15 buffer is placed in a second tube and 1 drop of 20% potassium ferricyanide with 2 ml of the solution from the first tube are added. This mixture is left at room temperature for 2 minutes.

6. One drop of the sodium cyanide-acetic acid mixture is then added, the tube, stoppered and mixed by inversion, and again left for 2 minutes.

7. The final color is read spectrophotometrically at 540 $\mu$m against a blank containing 10 ml of distilled water containing one drop each of sodium cyanide and potassium ferricyanide (OD No. 3).

*Calculation*

$$\frac{\text{OD No. 1} - \text{OD No. 2}}{\text{OD No. 3}} \times 100 = \% \text{ methemoglobin}$$

*Notes*

1. Prepare the neutralized sodium cyanide mixture (sodium cyanide-acetic acid) just prior to use.

2. Take great care not to pipet this mixture or the sodium cyanide by mouth. The solution should be measured by either an automatic pipet or by the use of a rubber bulb. *10% Sodium cyanide is lethal.*

*Normal.* Less than 2%

### Detection of Methemalbumin

*Principle.* Plasma is examined spectroscopically for absorption bands at 624 nm.

*Reagents and Apparatus*
1. Saturated aqueous sodium thiosulfate
2. Saturated aqueous potassium cyanide
3. Centrifuge
4. Hand or recording spectrophotometer
5. Heparinized plasma

*Method*

1. Plasma from a sample of heparinized blood should be used and examined with the hand spectroscope or with a recording spectrophotometer for absorption bands at 624 nm.

2. If a band is present, 1 drop of saturated aqueous sodium thiosulfate is added and the band normally disappears.

3. The absorption band for methemalbumin persists after the addition of 1 drop of saturated aqueous potassium cyanide.

## Schumm's Test

*Principle.* Yellow ammonium sulfide is added to plasma to produce ammonium hemochromogen, which is detected spectroscopically.

*Reagents and Apparatus*
1. Diethyl ether
2. Heparinized plasma
3. Graduated pipets—1 ml
4. Yellow ammonium sulfide
5. Hand or recording spectroscope

*Method*

1. Ether is carefully layered over 2 ml of fresh heparinized plasma, and 0.2 ml of saturated yellow ammonium sulfide is added.

2. The solution is mixed and observed with the hand spectroscope or recording spectrophotometer.

3. If methemalbumin is present in the original plasma, absorption bands of ammonium hemochromogen are present at 558 nm.

*Notes*

1. Methemalbumin is found in the plasma in cases of hemolytic anemia in which hemolysis is mostly intravascular.

2. If liver disease is associated with the hemolytic anemia, the level of methemalbumin rises rapidly.


## HEMOGLOBIN ELECTROPHORESIS (CELLULOSE ACETATE)

*Principle.* Red cells are lysed and applied to cellulose acetate strips, which are then immersed in a barbital buffer. A constant voltage is applied to the system, allowing the various hemoglobin moieties to migrate at different speeds.

The rate of migration along the cellulose acetate is measured by marking the positions of the migration with a staining technique and comparing them with known abnormals.

*Reagents and Apparatus*

1. Hemolysate preparation: 1 ml of oxalated blood is pipeted into a 15-ml graduated centrifuge tube. The tube is filled with normal saline, the solution mixed by inversion, and centrifuged at 2,500 rpm for 10 minutes. The buffy coat is bypassed with a pipet, and an adequate volume of red cells (0.2-0.3 ml) is withdrawn. The red cells are washed 3 times with normal saline, and 6 to 10 volumes of distilled water are added to the volume of packed red cells along with one-half of a volume of toluene to aid lysis. The contents of the tube are mixed by inversion and the cells allowed to hemolyze for 5 to 10 minutes. The hemolysate is centrifuged for 5 to 10 minutes to sediment out the stromal material, and the clear supernatant is transferred to a clean tube, stoppered and stored in the refrigerator.

2. Barbital buffer: Ionic strength 0.05, pH 8.6 ± 0.1. Dissolve 20.6 g of sodium barbital and 3.5 g of barbital in 700 ml of distilled water. Dilute to 2 liters in a volumetric flask with distilled water.

3. Bromphenol blue: 1 g of bromphenol blue is dissolved in 1 liter of 10% alcoholic mercuric chloride.

4. 5% Acetic acid (v/v)

5. Spinco microzone electrophoresis*
6. Oswald-Folin pipet—1 ml
7. Centrifuge
8. Saline
9. Toluene

### Method[6]

1. The electrophoresis cell is filled with fresh barbital buffer. The fluid level siphon is tilted to a horizontal position and the buffer poured into one end of the siphon tube.

2. Enough buffer is allowed to flow through to eliminate any bubbles in the tube, the siphon is slowly released, and the cell is filled to a point between the two lines marked "fluid level."

3. Any buffer which has splashed onto the center partition of the cell around the siphon is wiped away. A film of buffer on the center partition will conduct current between the two reservoirs when the power is applied to the cell, thus decreasing the current through the membrane.

4. The cellulose acetate membrane is floated on the surface of the buffer. Care should be taken not to splash any buffer onto its top surface. Allow the buffer to be drawn up through the membrane by capillary action.

5. One end of the membrane is picked up with forceps, placed on the bridge of the electrophoretic cell and attached securely to the membrane mounts.

---

* Available from Beckman Instruments, Inc., Palo Alto, Calif.

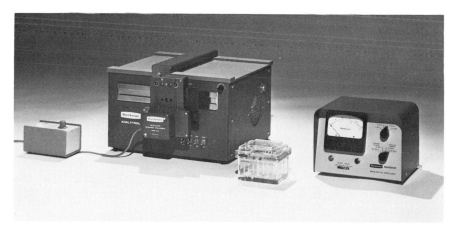

FIG. 1-3. Beckman, micro Spinco electrophoresis apparatus. (Courtesy of Beckman Instruments, Inc.)

6. Ensure that the membrane is fairly taut as described by the manufacturer, and that no air bubbles have formed under it.

7. The bridge is replaced in the cell. Make sure that the membrane ends are immersed in the buffer without touching the cell surface.

8. The buffer and membranes are allowed to equilibrate in the closed system for 10 minutes, and the hemolysate sample is applied with an applicator.*

9. A series of known control hemoglobins (Hb, C, F, S, and A) are also applied to the membrane in the same way, the power supply is connected and the cell run for one hour at 200 volts constant voltage.

10. After the run is completed, the strips are carefully placed in a staining pan containing the bromphenol blue for 15 minutes.

11. The strips are rinsed in two changes of 5% acetic acid for 15 minutes each and rerinsed in 5% acetic acid containing 0.3% sodium acetate.

12. They are again rinsed in water, blotted carefully and dried at room temperature.

### Evaluation of Results

1. The relative mobilities of the unknown samples are compared with the control hemoglobins. Alternatively, the sample strips can be scanned and recorded graphically with a densiometer.

### Notes

1. The buffer solution should be made up *fresh* for every determination. Its pH is critical and for precise work should be routinely checked prior to use.

2. Hemoglobin controls A and F should always be used. Other controls (HbS and HbC) can be commercially obtained, through such controls frequently deteriorate with time. Acid samples result in distortion and streaking of the fractions. Hemolysates prepared by the laboratory should be used only when fresh and should not be stored for more than 3 months in the frozen state.

## HEMOGLOBIN ELECTROPHORESIS (STARCH BLOCK)

*Principle.* Red cells are lysed and the hemoglobin separated by using a starch gel support. The gel is in contact with a barbital buffer through which a constant voltage is passed. The isolated fractions are separated and quantitated at a wavelength of 540 nm.

---

* Available from Beckman Instruments, Inc., Palo Alto, Calif.

### Reagents and Apparatus

1. Potato starch (Fisher Scientific)
2. Phosphate buffer: Ionic strength 0.2, pH 7.4.; 26.70 g of disodium hydrogen phosphate are dissolved in 1 liter of distilled water (1.m); 13.65 g potassium dihydrogen phosphate are dissolved in 1 liter of distilled water (1.M); 496 ml of 1.M potassium dihydrogen phosphate are added to 112 ml of 1.M disodium hydrogen phosphate and diluted to 8 liters. The pH is checked and adjusted to 7.4 as necessary.
3. Barbital buffer: Ionic strength 0.05 pH 8.6; 82.4 g of sodium barbital and 14 g of barbital are dissolved in 1 liter of distilled water, the solution is warmed and diluted to 8 liters with distilled water. The pH is checked and adjusted to 8.6.
4. Gelman Power Pack
5. Casserole dishes (4 glass baking dishes approximately 9½ × 4 × 2 in).
6. Wire coils (Nichrome wire, diameter 0.01 inches)—2 (3 ft in length, having coils approximately 3 in. in diameter)
7. Cellulose sponge cloths—2 (8 × 5 in)
8. Spatula
9. 2% Sodium cyanide
10. 5% Potassium ferricyanide
11. Tuberculin syringe
12. Glass sheet—18 × 10 in
13. Fitted glass funnel—2 liter
14. Whatman filter paper (No. 3)

### Preparation of the Hemolysate

1. 5 ml of heparinized or EDTA anticoagulated blood is centrifuged for 5 minutes at 2,000 rpm (Sorval GLC-1), and the plasma discarded. The red cells are washed 3 times with 0.85% saline and the packed red cell volume estimated.
2. 1.4 ml of distilled water and 0.4 ml of toluene are added for each ml of packed red cells obtained. The tube is stoppered, shaken vigorously for 5 minutes, and centrifuged at 3,000 rpm for 15 minutes.
3. The toluene layer is removed by absorbing with cotton swabs. The hemolysate is also removed using a Pasteur pipet and inserting it below the plug of red cell stroma. If care is taken to remove the hemolysate, it can be stored frozen indefinitely. If the hemolysate is cloudy, it is recentrifuged and stored frozen.

### Preparation of the Starch and Plate

1. A sheet of heavy glass (approximately 18 x 10 in) is thoroughly washed with soap and water, rinsed and dried. Strips of masking tape are placed along the long side of the plate so that they extend to about 2 in

around the corners. The tape should be placed so that it is ¼ to ½ inch above the plate. Blotter pad are placed against the open ends of the plate and temporarily held in place by a heavy object. The plate is now ready for the application of the starch.

2. Approximately 500 g of purified potato starch is placed in a 1-liter beaker, and barbital buffer added until a uniform paste is formed. This paste is filtered through a 2-liter fritted glass funnel attached to a vacuum line or to a water pump.

3. The washed starch is mixed with 400 ml of barbital buffer and allowed to settle for several minutes. The foam and excess buffer are removed with a pipet and discarded.

4. The starch paste is poured onto the prepared plate. The consistency should be similar to that of freshly prepared plaster of Paris. All air bubbles are removed and the block allowed to dry at room temperature.

### *Method*

1. The prepared hemolysate is first converted to the cyanmethemoglobin state; 0.3 ml of the hemolysate is placed in a tube and 0.05 ml of 5% potassium ferricyanide solution added. The mixture is allowed to stand for 5 minutes.

2. 0.05 ml of a mixture composed of 11 volumes of 2% sodium cyanide and 3 volumes of 10% acetic acid is added to the hemolysate-ferricyanide mixture. This is left for 5 minutes.

3. Slits are cut in the starch block using a spatula blade. Each slit is ⅝ in in length and situated about an inch apart. All slits are placed 4 in from one of the short sides of the block. If after the slits are cut, the starch refuses, allow the block to dry for a longer period of time. The block is ready for use when a spatula can be inserted into the starch and the slit remains discrete.

4. 0.02 ml of the cyanmethemoglobin hemolysate is drawn into a 1 ml tuberculin syringe and injected through a 22-gauge needle. The hemolysate should spread evenly through the slit. If the starch block is too wet, the slits will fuse; if too dry, the hemolysate will not spread evenly. If the hemolysate does not spread evenly, spread a few drops of buffer around the slit.

5. After the last hemolysate has been injected, the tape is removed from the plate, and the slits are closed by gently moving the spatula in the slits and applying phosphate buffer simultaneously. The starch will flow together when sufficiently wet.

6. Three thicknesses of Whatman (No. 3) filter paper are cut into strips (4 x 8 in) and soaked in barbital buffer. One inch of the long side of the filter paper is placed over the ends of the starch block and the other end is folded down ready to be placed in the barbital buffer dishes of the apparatus.

7. The 4 glass dishes are placed in the refrigerator. The 2 center dishes are half filled with phosphate buffer, and the outside 2 dishes are half filled with barbital buffer.

8. The Nichrome wire coiled electrodes are placed in the phosphate dishes and the paired buffered dishes (1 barbital and 1 phosphate) are joined by immersing the cellulose sponge cloths in each dish.

9. The starch block level is set on the dishes so that the 3 thickness of filter paper are immersed into the barbital buffer.

10. The wire coils are connected to the power pack so that the negative pole is connected to the coil on the side of the plate nearest the hemolysate applications. The positive electrode is connected to the remaining coil. (The power pack leads should be threaded toward the rubber gasket of the refrigerator door).

12. Electrophorese for 18 hours at 500 milliamps and at 410 volts.

13. After the run is completed, remove the plate and examine on the *underside* of the block. It is possible to invert the starch block without disturbing either the block or the hemoglobin migrations.

14. If quantitative estimates are to be made of the hemoglobins, cut out the bands and elute by washing 4 times with equal volumes of distilled water.

15. Pool all 4 washings and read spectrophotometrically at 540 $\mu$m.

*Notes*

1. If quantitative determinations are not required, record by photographing the underside of the plate. If this is attempted, be sure to photograph within 30 minutes of discontinuing electrophoresing, since the discrete hemoglobin bands tend to diffuse into the surrounding starch.

2. The best resolution may be obtained by diluting a portion of the hemolysate so that the hemoglobin approximates 3 to 4 g%.

3. For the identification of small amounts of minor components, the hemolysate concentration should be between 10 to 12 g%.


## AGAR-GEL HEMOGLOBIN ELECTROPHORESIS[8]

*Principle.* Agar-gel in a phosphate buffer of pH 6.25 can be used to separate hemoglobin C from O, E and $A_2$; hemoglobin D and G from S and hemoglobin O from C, E and $A_2$.

*Reagents and Apparatus*

1. Power supply tray and electrodes as previously described under starch block electrophoresis

2. Buffer: 0.07M, pH 6.25

6.08 g of disodium hydrogen phosphate ($Na_2HPO_4$) (anhydrous) and 22.99

g of sodium dihydrogen phosphate ($NaH_2PO_4H_2O$) are dissolved in distilled water and made up the volume to 3 liters

3. Glass plates (3¼ x 4 in)
4. Bacto-agar (Difco)
5. Concentrated ammonium hydroxide
6. Staining solution:

0.1 g of bromphenol blue is dissolved in 10 ml of glacial acetic acid and added to dissolved water to a total volume 1 liter

7. Whatman (No. 3) filter paper, 1.7 mm strips
8. Hemolysate as prepared for the starch block electrophoresis

### Method

1. 0.5 g of agar is gently added to 50 ml of the buffer solution and heated until the agar is dissolved.

2. The 1% agar is allowed to cool to approximately 50°C, poured onto clean glass plates so that the layer is 0.5 to 1.0 mm thick, and allowed to gel.

3. The Whatman filter paper strips are saturated in the hemolysate and blotted lightly to remove excess solution.

4. The strips are placed flat on the gel parallel to the larger side, about 1 in. in from the edge.

5. The electrophoresis trays are filled with phosphate buffer. A support is placed between them that is slightly narrower than the glass slide and just high enough to be above the sides of the buffer vessels.

6. The gel slide is then layed on this support and connected to the buffer with a single thickness of filter paper wick, but to overlap the gel by 2.0 cm and dipped into the buffer by 1.5 cm.

7. The anode is connected to the side closest to the origin, and electrophoresed for between 45 and 90 minutes at 270 volts. The electrophoresis time depends on the agar thickness, the current used, the concentration of the specimen, and the number of gels run at the same time.

8. The power pack is disconnected and the gels placed flat in a staining dish, and stained with bromphenol blue for 15 minutes.

9. The stain is removed by suction and the gel gently washed in distilled water for 20 minutes.

10. The gel is removed from the dish, trimmed, and carefully blotted with filter papers to remove excess water.

11. The plate and gel are inverted over ammonium hydroxide fumes until the hemoglobin bands begin to turn blue. Excessive exposure should be avoided, since it causes the background to turn blue.

12. The gel is allowed to dry overnight and filed for permanent record.

## HEMOGLOBINOPATHIES

1. The difference between the various hemoglobinopathies lies in the globin part of the hemoglobin molecule and not in the heme. The main differences appear to be centered around the amino acid composition and the number of amino acid residues per molecule.

2. Hemoglobin F has an increased isoleucine content, in addition to possibly altered proportions of other amino acids.

3. The difference between HbS and HbA is in the substitution of a valine residue for a glutamic acid residue in one position of the amino acids forming the polypeptide chain.

4. Normal adult hemoglobin is known as HbA, fetal hemoglobin as HbF, sickle cell hemoglobin as HbS. Other hemoglobins are either designated alphabetically or by geographical location (Hb C, D, E, G, H, I, N, M, Norfolk, Bart's, Lepore).

## ESTIMATION OF HEMOGLOBIN F BY ALKALI DENATURATION

### Method 1

*Principle.* Alkaline hematin is estimated by measuring the increasing optical density of a hemoglobin solution at a wavelength of 540 nm, after the addition of an alkali.

### Reagents and Apparatus

1. N sodium hydroxide
2. Timer
3. Spectrophotometer
4. Hemoglobin solution: The test red cells are washed 3 times in normal saline, and an equal volume of distilled water is added to the red cell mass. The mixture is repeatedly frozen and thawed. The resulting solution is treated with one-fifth volume of $C\gamma$ aluminum hydroxide gel or with washed asbestos pulp and centrifuged for one hour at 5°C at 10,000 rpm. The hemoglobin filtrate can then be stored at refrigerator temperature.
5. Graduated pipets—5 ml
6. Graduated pipets—1 ml

### Method

1. 4.8 ml of the hemoglobin solution are placed in a cuvet of a suitable spectrophotometer, and 0.2 ml of N sodium hydroxide is added to the solution, which is stirred rapidly.

2. On the addition of the alkali, start the timer and record the optical

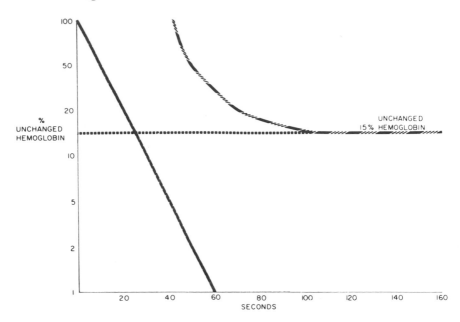

FIG. 1-4. Plasma hemoglobin. Diagonal line represents normal adult hemoglobin. Two-component curve represents adult hemoglobin in initial slope and fetal or unchanged hemoglobin in horizontal section.

density of the solution spectrophotometrically at 10-second intervals until the conversion of oxyhemoglobin to alkaline hematin is complete.

*Normal.* In adults, denaturation is complete in 100 seconds.

*Notes*

1. In the newborn, denaturation is often not completed for 2½ to 3 hours, due to the high hemoglobin F level.

2. If the optical densities are plotted against time on semilog graph paper, a linear relationship is obtained with adult blood containing no fetal hemoglobin.

3. Two-component curves are found with blood containing fetal hemoglobin, an initial steep slope due to the presence of adult hemoglobin, followed by a slow component due to the fetal hemoglobin. By extrapolation back, the fetal hemoglobin can be calculated (Fig. 1-4).

**Method 2[9]**

*Principle.* This modification is similar to that described in the preceding technique. Hemoglobin is converted to alkaline hematin by the action of sodium hydroxide. After one minute, this conversion is stopped by the addition of acidified ammonium sulfate, the acid halting the reaction and the salt precipitating the whole blood proteins. The amount of resistant hemoglobin is measured photometrically.

### Reagents and Apparatus

1. 0.083 N Sodium hydroxide (pH 12.7)

8.3 ml of 1 N Sodium hydroxide is made up to 100 ml.

2. Arresting-precipitating reagent

A saturated solution of ammonium sulfate is prepared by placing excess of the salt in a 2-liter beaker (approximately one-quarter full), adding 1,500 ml of distilled water, mixing and allowing to stand at room temperature for 1 to 2 hours; 400 ml of the clear supernatant, 400 ml of distilled water and 2 ml of 10 N hydrochloric acid are then combined.

3. 0.04% Ammonium hydroxide

4 ml of 0.880 N Ammonium hydroxide is made up to 1 liter with distilled water.

4. Patient's blood (EDTA)

Calculate the hemoglobin of the patient's blood by the cyanmethemoglobin method. Adjust an aliquot by removing either packed cells or plasma so that the final hemoglobin concentration is approximately 10 g.

5. Spectrophotometer
6. Stopwatch
7. Whatman filter paper (No. 1)
8. Graduated pipets—5 ml
9. Micropipets—0.1 ml
10. Micropipets—0.2 ml
11. Tubes—(10 × 75 mm)

### Method

1. Add 0.1 ml of patient's unadjusted whole blood to 5 ml of 0.04% ammonium hydroxide. Mix and allow to stand at room temperature for 2 to 3 minutes.

2. Record the optical density in a spectrophotometer at a wavelength of $540\mu$. This is the standard.

3. 3.2 ml of 0.083 N sodium hydroxide is pipeted into a 10 × 75 mm tube.

4. 0.2 ml of the patient's adjusted blood is added to the alkali and mixed well.

5. Start the stopwatch on the addition of the blood.

6. After exactly 60 seconds, 6.8 ml of the arresting-precipitating solution is added and mixed well by inversion.

7. The mixture is filtered through a Whatman (No. 1) filter paper, and the optical density of the filtrate is read in a spectrophotometer at 540 nm. This is the test.

**Calculation**

$$\frac{\text{Optical density of the test}}{\text{Optical density of the standard}} \times 100 = \% \text{ resistant hemoglobin}$$

*Normal.* Less than 4% resistant hemoglobin.

**Notes**

1. This technique can be used to detect fairly large amounts of resistant hemoglobin, particularly in cord blood. It is not sufficiently sensitive to detect small amounts of hemoglobin F found in many cases of thalassemia minor.

2. Hemoglobin Bart's is also classified as a resistant form of hemoglobin, which is structurally related to hemoglobin F.

3. Neonates have 60% or more hemoglobin F. This level declines rapidly in the first 3 months of life and then more gradually to puberty when it reaches adult levels.

## Demonstration of Hemoglobin H[10]

*Principle.* Hemoglobin H undergoes denaturation in the presence of brilliant cresyl blue.

**Reagents**

1. 20 ml of 3% sodium citrate is added to 80 ml of 0.85% sodium chloride.

2. 1 g of brilliant cresyl blue is dissolved in 100 ml of the citrate-saline dilution.

**Method**

1. Equal volumes of whole blood (direct from the syringe) and 1% brilliant cresyl blue in sodium citrate-saline are mixed together in a small tube and left for 3 hours at room temperature.

2. Blood smears are made as in the reticulocyte count and the red cells are examined without counterstain.

*Results.* Hemoglobin H appears in the form of multiple pale blue spherical inclusion bodies, varying in size from 0.5 to 1 $\mu$. Most of the cells are affected.

## Heat Stability Test for Unstable Hemoglobins[11]

*Principle.* If unstable hemoglobin is heated at 50°C for 2 hours it will precipitate. By comparing the optical density of the supernatant before and after heating, the percentage of unstable hemoglobin can be calculated.

### Reagents and Apparatus
1. EDTA anticoagulated blood
2. TRIS buffer, pH 7.4, 0.1 M:
12.1 g of TRIS (2-amino-2-(hydroxymethyl)
-1-3 propanediol is added to 25 ml of 0.1N hydrochloric acid, and the volume adjusted to 1 liter with distilled water.
3. Cyanmethemoglobin diluent:
1.0 g of sodium bicarbonate, 50 mg of potassium cyanide, and 200 mg of potassium ferricyanide are dissolved in 1 liter of distilled water
4. Spectrophotometer
5. Centrifuge (GLC-1 Sorvall)
6. Toluene
7. 50°C Waterbath
8. 0.85% Sodium chloride
9. Graduated pipets—5.0 ml
10. Micropipet—0.1 ml

### Method
1. 3 ml of freshly collected EDTA blood is washed 3 times with 6 ml volumes of saline.
2. The washed packed red cells are lysed by adding 5 volumes of distilled water, and 1 volume of toluene is added.
3. The solution is well mixed and centrifuged at 3,000 rpm for 15 minutes.
4. Remove the clear supernatant in the center of the tube, using a Pasteur pipet.
5. Add 3 ml of the hemolysate to 3 ml of TRIS buffer, and pipet 2 ml volumes of this mixture into each of 2 tubes.
6. Place tube No. 1 in the refrigerator at 4°C and the tube No. 2 in a 50°C waterbath. Leave for 2 hours.
7. Centrifuge both tubes at 3,000 rpm for 10 minutes, and from each tube remove 0.1 ml of the supernatant and dilute it with 5 ml of cyanmethemoglobin reagent. Leave 10 minutes and centrifuge at full speed for 30 to 45 minutes.
8. The clear supernatants are carefully removed and their optical densities read in a spectrophotometer at 540 $\mu$m, using a blank consisting of 0.1 ml of this buffer and 5 ml of the cyanmethemoglobin diluent.

### Calculation

$$\text{Opt. Den. Tube No. 1} - \left( \frac{\text{Opt. Den. Tube No. 2}}{\text{Opt. Den. Tube No.1}} \right) \times 100$$

= % precipitated hemoglobin

*Normal.* Less than 5% of normal hemoglobin precipitates at 50°C.

*Notes*[12]

1. Phosphate buffers retard precipitation of hemoglobins at 50°C and should not be used for the test.

2. Most unstable hemoglobins have the following characteristics:

a. They have sustained an amino acid substitution in an area which is critical for the normal binding of heme to globin.

b. The resulting unstable molecule is associated with chronic hemolytic anemia which may be exacerbated by infection or the administration of drugs.

c. The unstable hemoglobin precipitates and results in intracellular Heinz bodies.

d. The heme group is lost and degraded to produce urinary excretion of dipyrrolic compounds.

e. The iron is oxidized to the ferric state to produce methemoglobin.

f. The hemoglobin denatures at 50°C.

g. When the mutation involves the $\beta$-chain, free $\alpha$-chain are frequently released and may be detected by starch-gel electrophoresis

3. Alpha-chain abnormalities include hemoglobins, Torino, Bibba, Etobicoke, Columbia and Sinai. Beta-chain abnormalities include hemoglobins Zürich, Köln, Ube, Seattle, St. Mary's, Genova, Hammersmith, Sydney, Freiburg, Gun Hill, Philly, Santa Ana, Wien, Leiden, Riverdale-Bronx, Kings County, Sabine, Tacoma, Boras, Bristol, Shepherds Bush, and Savannah.

### Hemoglobin in Disease

1. Normally, hemoglobin is intracellular, but in some pathological conditions, such as hemolysis from burns and hemolytic anemias, it is found extracellularly.

2. When hemoglobin is found in the urine, the condition is known as hemoglobinuria; when it occurs in the plasma, the condition is termed hemoglobinemia.

3. Normally, adult hemoglobin (HbA) is present in red cells, but other abnormal hemoglobin forms are occasionally found. The protein portion of hemoglobin, the globin, may vary within the same species, producing abnormal hemoglobins with different isoelectric points and amino acid compositions. The heme moiety remains constant. Proteins are amphoteric (in acid solution they are positively charged, in alkaline solution they are negatively charged). At certain intermediate pH value, a protein is electrically neutral, carrying equal numbers of positive and negative charges. This pH is termed the isoelectric point.

4. Abnormal hemoglobins can be differentiated by the rate of alkali denaturation and by their electrophoretic mobility. Fetal and Bart's hemoglobin are more resistant to denaturation by alkalis than is adult hemoglobin. At room temperature and pH 13, adult hemoglobin is converted to alkaline hematin within 100 seconds, whereas fetal hemoglobin takes more than 100 seconds to convert.

5. Diurnal variation in hemoglobin of at least 10% between the hours of 5 p.m. and 7 a.m., a postprandial fall in hemoglobin of 5 to 10%, and seasonal variations in hemoglobin, up to 10% in winter months, have been reported.

6. An indication of relative mobility is given in Table 1-7. An important differentiating point between A and F is that they possess distinctive antigenic groups, making possible the preparation of a specific differentiating antiserum. This antigenic method is not applicable to A and S, because these have so many antigenic factors in common.

7. In practice, most of the abnormal hemoglobins can be detected by cellulose acetate, starch block, or agar-gel electrophoresis

TABLE 1-6. The Effect of Age and Sex on the Hemoglobin Levels in Infants and Children.[13]

| AGE | SEX | HEMOGLOBIN RANGE (g/dl) |
|---|---|---|
| Birth | Male | 17.2—22.6 |
| | Female | 16.2—24.4 |
| 1 month | Male | 8.0—15.8 |
| | Female | 9.1—17.1 |
| 2 months | Male | 8.9—14.1 |
| | Female | 9.2—13.2 |
| 3 months | Male | 9.9—14.5 |
| | Female | 9.4—13.3 |
| 6 months | Male | 11.0—14.3 |
| | Female | 10.9—14.4 |
| 9 months | Male | 10.0—14.0 |
| | Female | 10.1—13.8 |
| 12 months | Male | 10.0—14.5 |
| | Female | 9.9—14.2 |
| 18 months | Male | 11.2—14.6 |
| | Female | 9.9—14.6 |
| 24 months | Male | 10.6—13.8 |
| | Female | 11.3—15.2 |

TABLE 1-7. Cellulose Acetate Electrophoretic Mobility of Abnormal Hemoglobins.

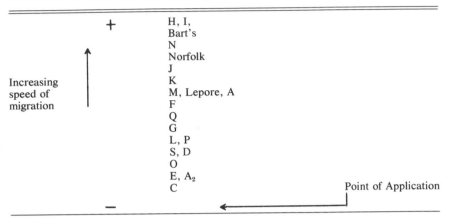

8. The effect of posture and other physiological variants influence the total hemoglobin level in an individual. Recumbent posture is reported to lower the hemoglobin and hematocrit approximately 6%, and severe dehydration producing falsely elevated results are also commonly found.

9. Hemoglobins vary with age. The hemoglobin level in a newborn being between 17.2 and 22.6 g/dl,[12] and falling to 8.9 to 14.1 g/dl in males and 9.4 to 13.3 g/dl in females at 2 and 3 months of age respectively. Other age breakdowns are shown in Table 1-6.

10. Differences in hemoglobin levels in the sexes are believed due to the inhibitory effect of estrogens on erythropoiesis, there being little difference between levels found prior to puberty or after menopause.

11. Residents at high altitudes usually are found to have a secondary polycythemia characterized by elevated hemoglobins. Such elevations are secondary to hypoxia.

12. Hemoglobin $A_2$ (Hb$A_2$) can be separated from hemoglobin A (HbA) by starch block and starch-gel electrophoresis. The normal range of Hb$A_2$ using starch block varies between 1.8 to 3.2%. The concentration of Hb$A_2$ is usually increased in $\beta$-thalassemia, and is often reduced in $\alpha$-thalassemia. An absence of Hb$A_2$ is believed to be diagnostic of $\delta$-thalassemia.

13. Hemoglobin F is immunologically different and possesses different oxygen dissociation properties from HbA. Increased levels of HbF have been reported; the homozygous state showing 100% HbF, the heterozygous state showing between 15 to 35%. In the homozygous form of thalassemia, the HbF is frequently increased in excess of 20%, and it is also increased in sickle cell anemia. Levels of HbF in this disorder are usually below 8%, but are normal in sickle cell trait.

14. An association between HbF and red cell hexokinase Type II is believed to exist. Hexokinase Type II is found only in infants and in adults with hereditary persistence of HbF.

15. HbF may persist or reappear in other hematological disorders. These include myeloma, untreated pernicious anemia, aplastic anemia, myeloproliferative diseases, congenital spherocytic anemia and paroxysmal nocturnal hemoglobinuria.

16. Hemoglobin S (HbS) is characteristic of red cells which sickle when exposed to reduced oxygen tension. It has been shown by electron microscopy, that the formation of reduced HbS parallels the presence of rodlike "tactoid" forms. These are arranged in a linear fashion, thus causing the cell membrane to follow the altered structural shape of the hemoglobin molecule (sickle shape). Most sickled cells form reversible tactoid forms, but a few are sickled irreversibly. The molecular abnormality differentiating this form from HbA is the substitution and replacement of a valine residue for glutamic acid in the sixth position of the β-chain.

17. Hemoglobin C (HbC) is characterized by the substitution of and replacement of lysine in place of glutamic acid in the 6th position of the β-chain. Unlike HbS, HbC does not form tactoid forms, but occasionally intracellular hemoglobin C crystals are observed.

18. Hemoglobin D (HbD) is differentiated from HbS on agar-gel electrophoresis. On both cellulose acetate and starch block electrophoresis both of these hemoglobinopathies migrate at the same speed. The abnormality is found at the 121st position of the β-chain where glutaminyl is substituted for a glutamic acid residue. Unlike HbS and HbC, HbD is not found in any ethnic population. Other differentiating features between HbD and HbS are the absence of sickling and the high ferrohemoglobin solubility of HbD.

19. Hemoglobin E (HbE) is also a β-chain variant. Structurally, the abnormality is at the 26th position of the chain, where lysine is substituted for glutamic acid.

TABLE 1-8. Starch Block Electrophoresis Mobility of Abnormal Hemoglobins pH 8.6.

| + | |
|---|---|
| | H. I. |
| Increasing ▲ | J. N. |
| speed of | A. M. |
| migration | F |
| | G. P. |
| | S. D. L. |
| | E. O. A.$_2$ |
| | C    Point of Application |
| − | ← |

TABLE 1-9. Agar-Gel Electrophoretic Mobility of Abnormal
Hemoglobins pH 6.25.

|  |  |  |
|---|---|---|
| + |  | Point of Application |
|  | ← ——————————————┘ |  |
| Increasing<br>speed of<br>migration ↓ | C<br>Q<br>L<br>H<br>S<br>O<br>A, D, E, A$_2$, G<br>F |  |

## REFERENCES

1. Cannan, R. K.: Proposal for a certified standard for use in hemoglobinometry: Second and final report. Am. J. Clin. Path., *30*: 211, 1958.
2. Sunderman, F. W., *et al.*: Clinical Hemoglobinometry. Baltimore, William & Wilkins, 1953.
3. Thomson, L. C.: An inorganic grey solution. Trans. Faraday Soc., *42*: 663, 1946.
4. Clegg, J. W., and King, E. J.: Estimation of hemoglobin by the alkaline hematin method. Br. Med. J., *11*: 329, 1942.
5. Wong, S. Y.: Colorimetric determination of iron and hemoglobin in blood. J. Biol. Chem., *77*: 409, 1928.
6. Evelyn, K. A., and Malloy, H. T.: Microdetermination of oxyhemoglobin, methemoglobin and sulfhemoglobin in a single sample of blood. J. Biol. Chem., *126*: 655, 1938.
7. Manual of the Beckman Instrument Company, Palo Alto, Calif.
8. Vella, F.: Acid-agar gel electrophoresis of human hemoglobins. Am. J. Clin. Pathol., *49*: 440, 1968.
9. Singer, K., Chernoff, A. I., and Singer, L.: Studies on abnormal hemoglobins. 1. Their demonstration in sickle cell anemia and other hematologic disorders by means of alkali denaturation. Blood, *6*: 413, 1951.
10. Dacie, J. V., and Lewis, S. M.: Practical Hematology. ed. 3, p. 153. New York, Grune & Stratton, Inc., 1963.
11. Schneiderman, L. J., Junga, I. G., and Fawley, D. F.: Effect of phosphate and non-phosphate buffers on thermolability of unstable hemoglobins. Nature, (London), *225*: 1041, 1970.
12. Comings, D. E.: Hemoglobinopathies associated with unstable hemoglobin. In Williams, W. J. *et al.* (eds.): Hematology. p. 440. New York, McGraw-Hill, 1972.

# 2

# *Erythrocytes (Red Blood Cells)*

## RED CELL COUNT

### *Manual Methods*

*Principle.* The number of red cells in a sample of diluted blood is counted in a hemocytometer of known dimensions. From the number of cells seen, the total red cell count of an undiluted sample is calculated.

### *Reagents and Apparatus*
1. Diluting Fluids.
   a. *Dacie's fluid:*
      Trisodium citrate (30%) ............. 99 ml
      Concentrated formalin .............. 1 ml
   b. *Hayem's fluid:*
      Mercuric chloride................. 0.25 g
      Sodium chloride .................. 0.5 g
      Sodium sulfate .................. 2.5 g
      Distilled water .............. to 100.0 ml
   c. *Normal saline:*
      Sodium chloride .................. 0.85 g
      Distilled water .............. to 100.0 ml
   d. *Strong's fluid:*
      Sodium citrate..................... 1.0 g
      Sodium chloride .................. 0.6 g
      Formalin.......................... 1.0 ml
      Distilled water .............. to 100.0 ml
   e. *Gowers' fluid:*
      Sodium sulfate .................. 6.75 g
      Acetic acid (3%)................. 3.5 ml
      Distilled water .............. to 115.0 ml

f. *Toison's fluid:*

Sodium chloride ................. 1.0    g
Sodium sulfate .................. 8.0    g
Methyl violet 5B................. 0.025 g
Glycerol ........................ 30.0   ml
Distilled water.................. 180.0  ml

2. Thoma red cell pipet

3. Hemocytometer. Improved Neubauer ruling: This consists of a thick rectangular glass slide with an H-shaped trough forming two counting areas. It has raised supports to hold the coverglass the proper distance above these areas and a concave indentation on the back. The slight concavity on the underside, directly under the rulings, is present so that scratches, which would impair efficiency, will not appear when seen under the microscope.

When an optically flat coverslip is placed on the raised supports, it forms a chamber having a depth of exactly 0.1 mm.

**Method 1**

1. Anticoagulated or capillary blood is pipeted to the 0.5 mark on the Thoma pipet, and the external surface of the pipet is wiped clean of blood.

2. The diluting fluid is then taken to the 101 mark, care being taken to avoid the introduction of air bubbles into the bulb.

3. The pipet is shaken to mix and the first few drops of dilution are expelled.

4. The hemocytometer is prepared by placing the coverslip on the

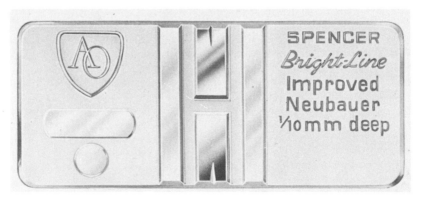

FIG. 2-1. Macroscopic view of hemocytometer, showing H-shaped troughs. (Courtesy of American Optical Co.)

transverse bars. If it is accurately placed, the chamber is transparent, and gentle pressure on the coverslip will produce concentric "Newton's rings." These are seen when there is an optically flat attachment between the hemocytometer and the coverslip, thus ensuring that the depth of the chamber is uniform.

5. With the index finger controlling the end of the pipet, allow one drop of diluted blood to fill one side of the chamber by capillary attraction. Be sure that the drop is of sufficient size to completely fill the area. It should not overflow into the surrounding moat.

6. The cells are allowed to settle in the ruled area for 2 to 3 minutes (depending on the diluting fluid used).

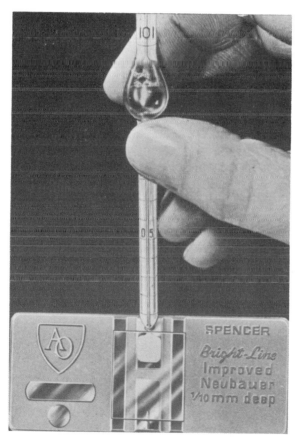

Fig. 2-2. Correct method of filling the counting chamber by capillary apparatus. (Courtesy of American Optical Co.)

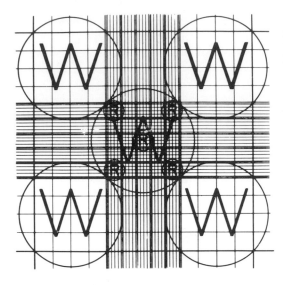

FIG. 2-3. Ruled area of the improved Neubauer hemocytometer, showing the *four* large corner squares usually used in the white cell count (W) and *one* large center square that can be additionally used. The *five* smaller squares (R) are used in the red cell count. (Courtesy of American Optical Co.)

7. With the 10× objective of the microscope, the cells seen in 5 groups of the 16 smallest squares (R) are counted.

## Method 2

### Additional Apparatus
1. Sahli pipet—0.02 ml ± 1%
2. Rubber-stoppered tubes—75 × 10 mm

### Method
1. 0.02 ml of blood is washed into 4 ml of red cell diluting fluid.
2. One drop of this dilution is used to charge the hemocytometer as described above, using a Thoma pipet.
3. The procedure is followed as described in Method 1.

### Normal Values
Adult Male . . . . . . . . . . . . . . . . . . . . 4,500,000-6,500,000/cu mm
Adult Female . . . . . . . . . . . . . . . . . 4,000,000-6,000,000/cu mm
Infants . . . . . . . . . . . . . . . . . . . . . . . 6,500,000-7,250,000/cu mm

### Notes
1. If the coverslip is not placed correctly on the hemocytometer, or if the chamber is incorrectly charged, the coverslip should be removed, the chamber cleaned and dried, and the procedure repeated.
2. In counting the cells, a start should be made at the top left square, and only those cells which lie within the square on the left and top should

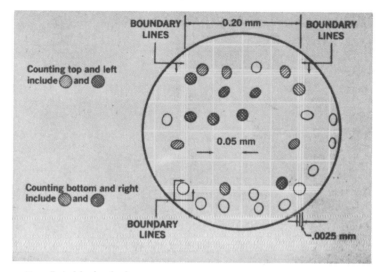

Fig. 2-4. Method of counting cells. (Courtesy of American Optical Co.)

be counted. The cells touching the right or bottom lines should be excluded from the total count.

## The Use of Self-Filling, Self-Measuring Dilution Micropipets*

*Principle.* The pipet consists of a straight thin-walled uniform-bore glass capillary tube, fitted into a plastic holder, and an attached plastic reservoir containing a premeasured volume of diluent. The pipet is closed with a tight-fitting solid plastic plug.

### Method

1. The reservoir is opened by forcing the plug into the main chamber with the thumb.

2. Blood is drawn into the tube immediately on contact with the tip of the capillary. The blood flow into the tube stops when it has reached the end of the capillary.

3. The dilution is made by introducing the capillary into the reservoir. The walls of the reservoir are squeezed slightly before inserting the capillary holder, so that a negative pressure is created when the walls are released. Blood is then drawn from the tube into the diluent.

4. The capillary tube is rinsed with the diluent by gently squeezing the reservoir, forcing the fluid into the capillary and overflow chamber. When the pressure is released, the diluent is again drawn back into the reservoir.

---

* Unopette, available from Becton, Dickinson and Co., Rutherford, N.J.

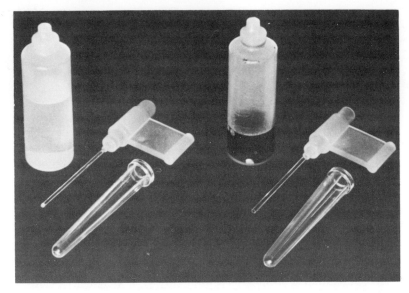

F<small>IG</small>. 2-5. Unopette showing main reservoir and capillary pipet with detached plastic shield. (Courtesy of Becton, Dickinson and Co.)

5. After shaking the diluted blood, the dilution pipet is assembled by removing the capillary tube from the reservoir, reversing it and reattaching it to the reservoir.

6. The reservoir is squeezed gently to charge the hemocytometer, thus forcing diluted blood out of the capillary in uniform drops.

*Note*

Similar pipets can be obtained with diluents suitable for red cell, white cell and platelet counts. The dilution factor when using these pipets is:

1:100 for white cell counts

1:200 for red cell counts and platelet counts

### Hemocytometers

*Improved Neubauer Ruling*

1. The total ruled area is 9 sq mm (3 mm × 3 mm) and the depth is 0.1 mm.

2. Four corner squares, 1 mm × 1 mm, are subdivided into 16 smaller squares and are used for total white cell counts.

3. The center square (1 sq mm) is subdivided into 25 smaller squares; each of these again subdivided into 16 squares, each side being 0.05 mm in length, the total area of the smallest square being 1/400 sq mm. This is

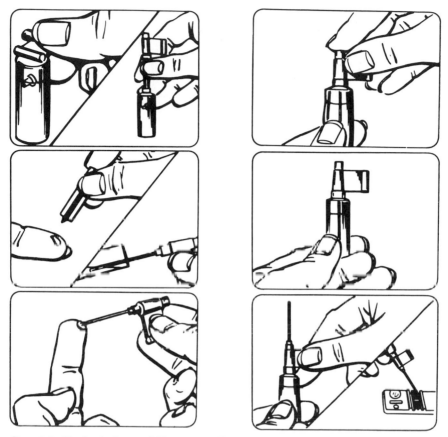

Fig. 2-6. Method of use of Unopette. (Courtesy of Becton, Dickinson and Co.)

the same area as in the original ruling, and is achieved by removing the wide treble ruling of the original chamber and substituting treble ruling lines 0.01 mm apart.

### Original Neubauer Ruling

1. The total ruled area is the same as in the improved ruling.

2. The rulings are also the same as in the improved chamber, with the exception of the center square. This is divided into 16 squares, which are further subdivided into 16 smaller squares. The larger squares measure 0.25 mm × 0.25 mm and are indicated by a treble line.

3. The sides of the smallest squares measure 0.05 mm and their area is 1/400 sq mm.

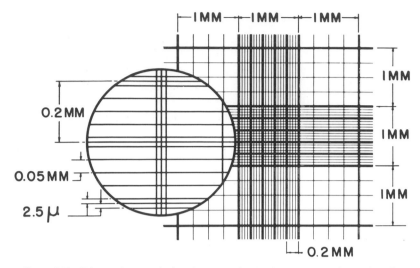

FIG. 2-7. Dimensions of the improved Neubauer counting chamber. (Courtesy of American Optical Co.)

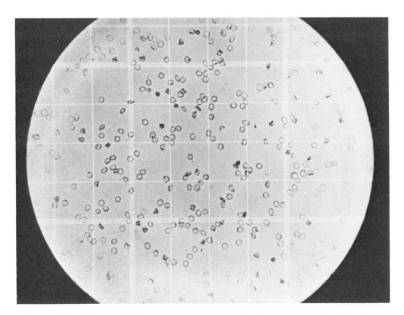

FIG. 2-8. Part of the center square of the improved Neubauer ruling showing red cells as they appear microscopically. (Courtesy of American Optical Co.)

### Calculation

1. As blood is drawn to the 0.5 mark and diluted to the 101 mark, it would appear that the final dilution is 1:202. This is not true, because the fluid in the stem of the pipet does not mix with the blood and is discharged prior to charging the hemocytometer. Since the volume of the stem is 1, this leaves the total bulb volume as 100.

2. 0.5 Volume of blood, when made up to 100 volumes of diluent, produces a final dilution of 1:200.

3. The area of the smallest square is 0.05 mm × 0.05 mm = 0.025 sq mm (1/400).

4. Inasmuch as 5 groups, each consisting of 16 small squares, are counted, the total area counted is 5 × 16 × 0.0025 sq mm = 80 × 0.0025 sq mm = 0.2 sq mm.

5. The depth of the hemocytometer is 0.1 mm.

6. Thus the total volume used in the count is 0.2 sq mm × 0.1 mm = 0.02 cu mm.

7. If 500 red cells are counted in a total volume of 0.02 cu mm, the number of red cells in 1 cu mm = 500/0.02 cu mm = 25,000.

8. But, because the original blood was diluted 1:200, the corrected number of red cells expressed per cu mm is 25,000 per cu mm × 200 = 5,000,000 per cu mm.

9. An abbreviated system of calculating the total red count is N × 10,000, where N is the number of cells counted.

### Faults in Technique

1. Bad sampling of the blood, due to inadequate flow from a capillary puncture.

2. Inaccurate pipeting and the use of poorly calibrated pipets and hemocytometers.

3. Inadequate mixing.

4. Incorrect filling of the chamber and careless counting of the cells.

### Inherent Errors of the Manual Cell Count

1. The gross error of manual counts can be reduced by determining the count in duplicate. This helps to reduce the error, if the two results are averaged, because the larger the number of cells counted, the closer the result will be to the true count.

2. The personal bias in the procedure influences the result. Technologists subconsciously tend to select areas the content of which seems to fit in with a preconceived idea of the result.

3. It has been shown that there is an uneven distribution of cells in the chamber, depending on the momentum given to the cells as the chamber is filled. This uneven distribution is present even in a perfectly mixed sample. It is known that the cells settling in certain areas conform to

mathematical formulae. If $\sigma$ is the standard error of the distribution of the cells, and M is the mean number of cells counted, then: $\sigma = \pm \sqrt{M}$.

4. Therefore, if 200 cells were counted, in 95% of the counts made the expected range of the cells counted would be 172-228 (i.e., $M \pm 2 \sqrt{M} = 200 \pm 2 \propto 200 = 200 \pm 2 \times 14 = 200 \pm 28 = 172\text{-}228$).

In 66% of the counts, the number of cells would be in the range 186—214 (i.e., $M \pm \sqrt{200}$).

*Notes*

1. All apparatus should be thoroughly cleaned after each use. By using a suction pump, pipets are well washed with a sequence of water, ether or alcohol, and dried by blowing air through them. Hemocytometers and coverslips are rinsed in tap water and kept in a small jar of 70% alcohol until used.

2. Hayem's fluid tends to clump the red cells in Hodgkin's disease, multiple myeloma, nephritis and cirrhosis, and Toison's fluid has the disadvantages that it acts as a culture media for some saprophytic fungi and that, due to its high specific gravity, red cells take a long time to settle. Dacie's fluid is the most suitable general red cell diluent.

3. The coverslips must be optically flat and thicker than those used in the routine work of the laboratory. The normal thickness is 0.4 mm. It is important to place the coverslip centrally over the ruled area of the hemocytometer.

**Thoma Hemocytometer**

This chamber is ruled exactly like the improved Neubauer, except that it has no ruled areas in the four corners. This restricts its use to red cell counts.

**Fuchs-Rosenthal Hemocytometer**

This chamber is considerably larger than the Neubauer or Thoma chambers. The ruled area is 4 mm $\times$ 4 mm, and the depth is 0.2 mm. It is divided into 16 smaller squares, each having dimensions of 1 mm $\times$ 1 mm. Each of these squares is subdivided into 16 smaller squares. This chamber is used for counting low cell counts, such as are found in spinal fluid, total eosinophil counts, and leukopenic bloods.

## AUTOMATED METHODS

**Coulter Counter, Model S\***

*Principle.* The counter is designed on the same principle as other earlier model Coulter counters. Using a mercury siphon, a specific volume of an

---

\* Available from Coulter Electronics, Inc., Hialeah, Florida.

electrolyte suspension of particles can be drawn through an aperture of specific dimensions. An aperture current exists between an electrode inside of the tube and another electrode outside the aperture, thus, the particles change the resistance between the two electrodes and produce a voltage drop. The magnitude of the voltage drop is proportional to the volume of the particle. The voltage pulses are fed into a threshold circuit, which discriminates between them by generating voltage count pulses for only the particles that exceed the threshold level, thus counting the number of particles in passage. The voltage pulses are amplified and displayed on an oscilloscope screen as distinct vertical spikes. Relative size is indicated by the relative height of the spikes. Pulses are also fed to a threshold circuit, allowing selection of a level which if reached by a pulse causes the pulse to be counted.

The Counter consists of five separate interconnected units: diluter, analyzer, power supply, pneumatic power supply and printer. The blood is aspirated into the diluter, mixed, lysed, diluted and sensed. The information obtained is processed by the Analyzer where the counting, measurement, and computing functions take place. From the Analyzer unit, signals in the form of voltages representing values are applied to the electronic circuits located in the power supply. These signals are then converted from voltage information to digital data for use by the printer where a numerical printout takes place.

The power supply provides the electrical power for all circuits as required, while the pneumatic power supply provides vacuum pressure for the diluter.

### Description of Model S Coulter Counter

EDTA anticoagulated blood is placed under the aspirator and the touch control bar is depressed. Approximately 1.0 ml of blood is aspirated into the system.

In the blood sampling valve, a measured amount of blood and 10.0 ml of diluent are forced into the WBC Mixing Chambers. The blood and diluent are slowly mixed in the chamber, providing a first dilution of 1:224. A portion of this first dilution is siphoned out of the WBC Mixing Chambers into the Blood Sampling Valve, where a measured amount of the first dilution is forced out by 10.0 ml of diluent into the RBC Mixing Chambers. Here, the first dilution slowly mixes with diluent to provide a second dilution of 1:50,000.

From the WBC Mixing Chambers, the first dilution is forced into the Lysing Chamber, where it is mixed with 1.0 ml of lysing agent, producing a 1:250 dilution. This dilution remains in the chamber for a sufficient amount of time for the red cells to hemolyze and release hemoglobin. The suspension is then passed into the WBC Aperture Counting Bath con-

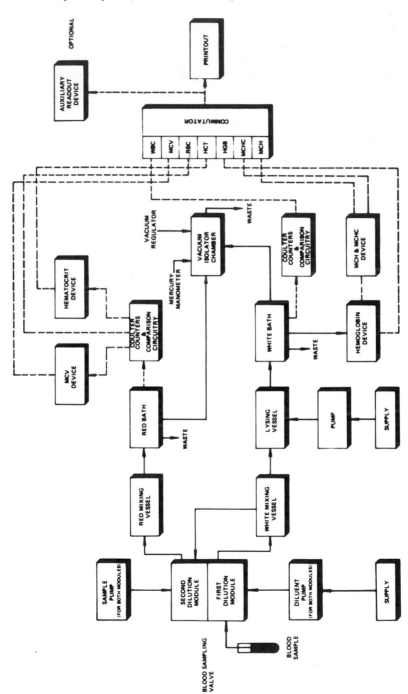

FIG. 2-9. Diagram of the Coulter Counter, Model S. (Courtesy of Coulter Electronics, Inc., Hialeah, Florida)

taining three aperture tubes. By means of a constant fluid vacuum, the sample is drawn into all three aperture tubes simultaneously for 4 seconds. Each aperture tube is provided with an internal electrode, and there is a common electrode in the bath acting as a ground. Three signals are obtained simultaneously by the passage of the WBC's into each aperture tube. In this manner, each count is done in triplicate and the average of the three counts recorded. Each aperture has its own set of electronics. Electronic circuitry contained in the analyzer unit provides an output from these circuits which directly displays an average white cell count.

Because free hemoglobin is present in the WBC count suspension, the hemoglobin measurement may be accomplished in the same bath. A beam of light is passed through the suspension and into a photosensitive device which measures the amount of light passing through the fluid. Electronic circuitry to the output of the photocell provides the hemoglobin reading.

Simultaneously, the red cell suspension passes into a similar bath having three aperture tubes. As in the WBC arrangement, the scanning occurs for a 4-second period representing a flow of a given volume of liquid into all three aperture tubes. The counting is carried out in the same manner as the white count; in triplicate and the results averaged. The mean cell volume measurements are electronically derived from the red count and are recorded.

The remaining red cell indices are electronically derived from the hemoglobin, red cell count and mean red cell volume. The hematocrit is calculated from the formula: Hct = Red Cell Count × M.C.V./100.

The model S is also capable of testing capillary blood. A small volume (44.7 $\mu\ell$) of capillary blood is diluted with 10.0 ml of filtered buffered saline or Isoton diluent. The whole blood 1:224 dilution switch is turned into position and the blood aspirated through the capillary blood aspirator. The results are obtained as previously outlined.

The Pneumatic Power Supply provides for the filling and emptying of the various vessels as well as for discharging waste. Once started, the operations are continuous and automatic, and the respective samples do not contaminate each other.

### Reagents and Apparatus
1. Model S Coulter Counter
2. EDTA anticoagulated blood
3. Cell diluting fluid (Isoton)*
4. Cleaning reagent (Istoterge)*
5. Lysing agent (Lyse S)*

---

* Available from Scientific Products, Evanston, Illinois

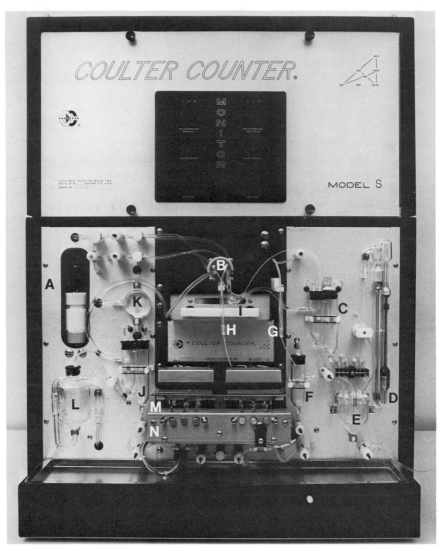

FIG. 2-10. On the Coulter Counter, Model S, operating panel the following points are indicated: A, Diluent dispenser assembly; B, Blood sampling valve; C, white cell mixing chambers; D, manometer; E, vacuum chamber; F, lysing chamber; G, capillary aspirator; H, whole blood aspirator; I, touch bar; J, red cell mixing; K, bubble trap; L, wastechamber; M, aperture tubes; N, hemoglobin photo-optics. (See text for discussion.)

## Method

1. The instrument is set up as in the manufacturer's instructions.

2. A tube of EDTA anticoagulated blood is placed under the aspirator tip, and the touch control gently pressed.

3. Approximately 1.0 ml of whole blood is aspirated and in 20 seconds the results are recorded by the printer.

## Maintenance Procedures

### Daily

1. The blood sampling valve should be cleaned with diluent or distilled water at the end of any large batch of tests. Cycling the unit several times using Isoterge will remove blood from the blood sampling valve.

2. The fluid section of the system should be cleaned daily by depressing the aspirator primary button on the diluter unit control panel several times in succession. This causes Isoterge to be distributed through the fluid section.

3. The Bath Rinse button should also be depressed several times to clean the aperture baths. They may also be cleaned by first turning off the power and raising the aperture. Isoterge is then passed directly into the baths.

4. At the completion of the day's work follow the procedure below to ensure that all fluid lines, plungers and aperture tubes are free of foreign debris.

   a. A 100 ml beaker of diluted Isoterge is placed under the aspirator and the aspirator button depressed 15 to 20 times. At this point the aspirator cylinder should be clear of all blood and filled with clean green Isoterge.

   b. The touch control bar is then depressed drawing Isoterge through the blood sampling valve in the same manner as blood would normally be run. This step is repeated two additional times.

   c. The aperture baths are drained, rinsed, and finally redrained.

   d. The rinse button is then depressed twice so that each aperture bath is filled with 20 ml of rinse fluid. The count button is then depressed and held down for 45 seconds. The baths are finally drained.

   e. The aperture tube assembly is lifted and both counting baths filled with Isoterge. Push the count button and hold for 45 seconds.

   f. The aperture is left in this solution for 30 to 45 minutes. Before starting up the Model S, procedures (c) and (d) are again carried out.

   g. The blood sampling valve is removed and all flat surfaces cleaned with a lint-free tissue and Isoterge, and rinsed in Isoton. Replace the sampling valve when wet.

*Weekly*

1. The glass bowls on the front of the Pneumatic Power Supply Unit should also be checked regularly. The left bowl should not be allowed to collect fluid, and if this does occur it should be unscrewed and drained.

2. The oil in the center bowl (Pneumatic System Lubricant) should be changed when it becomes contaminated or when it drops below the marker.

3. The air filters in the Pneumatic Power Supply Unit should be inspected at regular intervals. If dirty, they should be cleaned and replaced.

*Notes*

1. Blood should never be left in the blood sampling valve when the unit is turned off for more than a few minutes.

2. The operating location should be as free as possible from airborne dust, loud noises and electrical interference (brush type motors, calculating machines, flickering fluorescent lights, etc).

## Hemac 630L*

*Principle*. The Hemac 630L utilizes a 90 $\mu$l sample of whole blood to determine seven hematologic parameters; red cell count, white cell count, hematocrit, hemoglobin, mean cell volume, mean cell hemoglobin, and mean cell hemoglobin concentration.

The prepared blood sample enters a flow chamber in the center of a laminar flow sheath of water. The sheath water, its diameter progressively diminished by the narrowing of the chamber interior, in turn constricts the central core of specimen, thus elongating it, narrowing it and accelerating its flow.

At maximal constriction, the specimen core is reduced to 18 $\mu$. The cells are maintained within the central core by the steady force of the surrounding laminar flow, and pass through the 20 $\mu$ thickness of a focused laser beam at the rate of 2,500 cells/second.

As each cell passes through the beam, the detector and associated electronics generate a "pulse" which is representative of the cells narrow-angle laser diffraction. The pulses are displayed as individual oscilloscope traces, accumulated for printout of the count, and electronically processed for determination of hematocrit. After the red cell count has been completed, a second aliquot of specimen enters the flow chamber for the white cell count.

Hemoglobin is estimated by conventional cyanmethemoglobin methodology, and hematocrit by the sum of pulse aplitudes produced by the narrow angle diffraction measurements.

---

*Available from Ortho Instruments, Raritan N.J.

### Hemalog-8[2]*

*General Principle.* The Hemalog-8 analyzer automatically determines at a rate of 60 samples an hour, the hemoglobin, hematocrit, red cell count, white cell count, platelet count and calculates the mean cell volume, mean cell hemoglobin, and mean cell hemoglobin concentration. The tests are recorded and automatically printed out.

Vacutainer tubes of EDTA anticoagulated blood are placed on the sample tray and locked into place. The operator, by depressing the power push button, starts the flow of pressurized reagents through the system. After approximately 2 minutes, the Ready lamp lights and the operate

* Available from Technicon Instrument Corp. Tarrytown, N.Y.

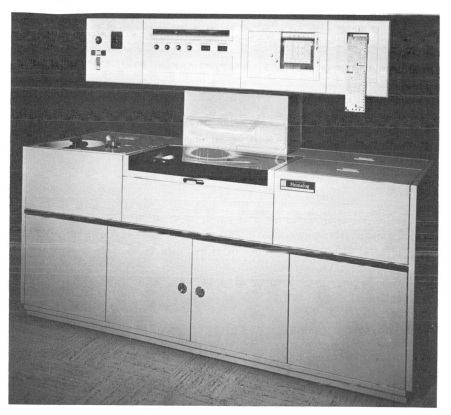

FIG. 2-11. The Hemalog-8, showing (*left to right on upper console*) operator controls, triple oscilloscope, standardization controls, functional brush recorder, and printout module; (*lower console*) sample turntable and optics bench, manifold and pump, and centrifuge. The double doors at the base of the unit house all reagents under pressure. (Courtesy of Technicon Instrument Corp.)

button should be depressed. After the blood is aspirated it is split to provide samples for the platelet count, white count, red count, hemoglobin and hematocrit tests. In the hemoglobin stream, the sample is first combined with a buffered saline reagent which lyses the red cells. The stream is then combined with Drabkin's reagent to convert the hemoglobin to cyanmethemoglobin which is measured by a standard colorimetric technique.

The diluted streams for the platelet, red cell, and white cell counts enter three separate optical benches where the cell counting is carried out.

The sample for the hematocrit test is passed through the manifold without dilution and enters a constantly spinning centrifuge where the cells are packed. During this process, an optical system constantly monitors the height of the packed cell mass.

As the tests are carried out, the results are presented sequentially on the digital display panel. A five-channel single-pen chart recorder serves as a function monitor for the hematocrit, hemoglobin, red cell count, white cell count and hematocrit tests. The graphs produced allow the operator to observe and evaluate the tests in progress as the sample enters, achieves steady-state, and leaves the applicable detection device. That portion of the steady-state plateau from which test results will be taken is shown in the form of a notch on the curve. The red cell indices are calculated by electronic circuitry utilizing the results of the tests carried out by the apparatus.

*Hematocrit Unit.* The hematocrit centrifuge is constantly spinning at 23,000 rpm. Blood samples are loaded, centrifuged, and eliminated by use of a small J-shaped tube mounted in the centrifuge head. Whole blood is pumped to a storage chamber and, using a series of pinch valves, 0.1 ml is admitted to the J tube. The optics detect the line of separation between the packed red cells and the plasma. A light beam is detected through a condensing lens onto a movable tracking mirror. From this mirror the beam is directed through a focusing lens and onto a fixed mirror. The beam is then reflected through a tracking window in the centrifuge head where it scans the length of the J tube window. Whole blood appears opaque to the photomultiplier tube so that when the blood initially flows onto the J tube there is no passage of light pulses through the J tube. The light beam then moves to the top of the window. While scanning that portion of the J tube that contains plasma, the light beam is momentarily passed to the photomultiplier tube (PMT) as the centrifuge head spins. When these pulses are being received by the PMT, the light beam is caused by the control circuit to scan toward the bottom of the window in the J tube. The clear plasma area which appears at the top of the window allows light pulses to reach the PMT. As long as the PMT receives light pulses, the control circuits will cause the optical system to scan toward the bottom of the J tube window.

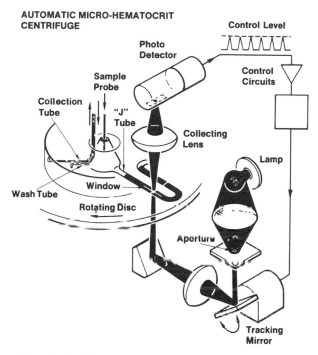

AUTOMATIC MICRO-HEMATOCRIT
CENTRIFUGE

Control Level

Photo
Detector

Control
Circuits

Sample
Probe

Collection
Tube

"J"
Tube

Collecting
Lens

Lamp

Window

Wash Tube

Rotating Disc

Aperture

Tracking
Mirror

FIG. 2-12. The principle of the centrifuge unit of
Hemalog-8. (Courtesy of Technicon Instrument Corp.)

After about 20 seconds, approximately 90% of the red cell packing has been achieved and the light beam becomes almost stationary when the red cells reach full packing.

The reagent delivery system is controlled by an air compressor producing a pressure of 9 lbs/in². This pressure forces the fluids out of the container and through a series of filters to the manifold.

*Hemoglobin Unit.* The hemoglobin reaction employs a standard cyanmethemoglobin technique. The ferricyanide component of the Drabkin's reagent converts the hemoglobin iron from the ferrous to the ferric state to form methemoglobin, which in turn combines with potassium cyanide to produce the stable cyanmethemoglobin. The color development in the system is catalyzed by a sensitizing lamp to insure conversion of resistant hemoglobin and is pumped to the colorimeter where absorbance is recorded at 550 nm$\mu$.

*Cell Counting Unit.* Red and white cells and platelets are counted using three separate optics benches.

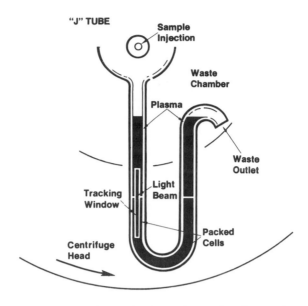

FIG. 2-13. The J tube from above, showing tracking window. (Courtesy of Technicon Instrument Corp.)

The white cell count stream is first reacted with glacial acetic acid and the platelet stream reacts with urea to lyse the red cells. The red cell stream is diluted 1:14,000 with saline prior to counting. At this dilution the white cell contamination becomes negligible.

Particles are counted using a standard dark field principle. Light passes through a condensing lens uniformly illuminating the primary aperture. A projection lens detects light passing through this aperture and forms a reduced image of the aperture in the center of the flow cell. This results in a small brightly illuminated view volume, sharply defined by the reduced aperture image and the sides of the flow passage in the flow cell. The light then emerges from the flow cell, and is blocked by a dark field disc which prevents any direct light from striking the photomultiplier tube. This is known as reverse dark field illumination.

If a clear fluid passes through the flow cell, the light rays are blocked by the dark field disc as described above. However, if particles, such as cells, are dispersed in the fluid stream, they are illuminated as they pass through the view volume. When illuminated, they become secondary sources of illumination, scattering light in the forward direction, toward the objective lens. This collects and focuses the light through a small aperture in front of the PMT. Thus, as each particle passes through

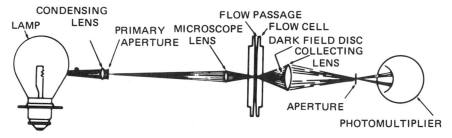

CONDENSING
LAMP   LENS   FLOW PASSAGE
PRIMARY  MICROSCOPE  FLOW CELL
/APERTURE  LENS   DARK FIELD DISC
COLLECTING
LENS

APERTURE
PHOTOMULTIPLIER

FIG. 2-14. The basic principle of the optical system of particle counting.

the view volume, an electrical pulse is generated, which can be viewed on the oscilloscope screen on the front panel of the apparatus.

***Reagents and Apparatus.***
1. EDTA anticoagulated blood
2. Hemalog-8
3. Buffered saline
4. Diluting fluids* (a) red cell, (b) white cell, (c) platelet
5. Drabkin's reagent*

***Method***
1. The instrument is set up as in the manufacturer's instructions.
2. The Power button is depressed. After 4 to 5 minutes the ready indicator is illuminated and the apparatus is loaded with EDTA Vacutainer sample tubes. A metal pin is placed in a stop position following the last sample (end-of-run pin).
3. The Operate button is then depressed and the sampler, after a time interval of less than 1 minute, will begin aspirating samples.
4. After the results are recorded and printed out, the system automatically detects the end-of-run pin and stops with the sample probe in a waterwash receptacle. The end-of-run indicator is illuminated and the system returns to the ready mode.
5. If no more samples are to be run, the Auto Shut Down button is depressed and the apparatus washes itself out automatically for 10 minutes and turns itself off.

***Maintenance Procedures***
*Daily*
1. The sample probe should be inspected for signs of clotted blood and clean as needed.

* Available from Technicon Instrument Corp., Tarrytown, N.Y.

2. The manifold and pump tubes should be inspected to check on wear and the silicone tubing is correctly seated under the air bar notches.

3. All pump tubes and waste lines should be checked for correct bubble patterns, and for a sufficient supply of printout forms and brush recorder paper.

*Weekly*

1. All pump tubes should be replaced as soon as they first appear flattened or after no longer than 300 hours of cumulative running time.

2. If there is any protein buildup in any fitting (especially in the white cell channel) remove with 0.1N hydrochloric acid solution and 1% pepsin by washing out with both of these reagents. If the protein buildup is still evident, soak the fittings in the acid following by the enzyme for two periods of 15 minutes each.

3. Check for loose fittings on (a) the optics bench, (b) the reagent lines, (c) manifold pump tubes.

4. All flow cells should be cleaned by flushing with 0.1N hydrochloric acid, 1% pepsin, and 1:12 commercial liquid detergent.

*Monthly or Greater*

1. All air filters should be cleaned monthly and the lamp replaced on the optics bench every 3 months.

2. Every 6 months, the reagent lines should be replaced and the silicone tubing replced on the manifold.

3. Pumps should be lubricated on a yearly basis.

**Calibration of Automated Apparatus**

In general controls of all automated equipment can be obtained from the manufacturer of the apparatus. While these controls are believed to be run only on the apparatus in question, they can, depending on the situation, occasionally be rechecked using other methods. The drawback of using controls obtained from the apparatus manufacturer is one of cost. It is important to standardize both the Coulter Model S and the Hemalog at least on a daily basis. If large numbers of blood samples are being tested, it may be prudent to recalibrate or recheck the valves twice or three times a day.

An excellent practice is to designate short time periods on a daily basis in which to perform all maintainence checks and to check calibrations.

**Important Differences Between the Coulter, Model S and the Hemalog**

1. The Model S operates almost entirely on the alteration in electrical conductance when a solid particle is introduced into an electrolyte. The Hemalog is a modification of the SMA 7 apparatus which uses flexi-

ble pump tubing to deliver the act as pipets, both blood samples and reagents. The basic principle of particle counting is a dark field system whereby particles refract light around a dark field, the light pulses being collected and recorded.

2. The Model S does not directly measure the hematocrit but mathematically computes it from the mean cell volume. This parameter is directly measured from the height of the pulses recorded on the oscilloscope screen, and directly depends upon the volume of electrolyte displaced when the particle is drawn into the aperture tube. The Hemalog directly measures the hematocrit using a high-speed centrifuge, spinning at 23,000 rpm. It mathematically computes the mean cell volume from this result, as well as the mean cell hemoglobin concentration.

3. The Model S is a semi-automated instrument which allows for an operator to manually present blood samples for analysis as needed. The Hemalog is equipped with a sample tray allowing for up to 40 different tests and controls to be loaded, tested, and automatically recorded. Theoretically, once loaded, it can be left to print out results. Experience has shown, however, that in a very busy laboratory one and occasionally two technologists are needed to keep track of loading and recording results.

4. The Model S is equipped to test micro blood samples obtained from capillary blood. The Hemalog is not so equipped.

5. The reagents in both systems are similar in action.

### Coulter Counter, Model Z*

*Principle.* Particles or cells, suspended in an electrolyte can be sized and counted by passing them through an aperture with a specific path of current flow for a given length of time.

As particles of cells pass through the aperture and displace an equal volume of electrolyte, the resistance in the path of current changes, resulting in corresponding current and voltage changes. The magnitude of this change is directly proportional to the volumetric size of the particle. The number of changes within a specific length of time is proportional to the number of particles of cells in the suspension.

Opening the control stopcock introduces vacuum to the system. This draws sample through the aperture and unbalances the mercury in the manometer, causing it to flow past the start contact, resetting the electronic counter for a zero readout. When the stopcock is closed, the mercury begins to travel back to its balanced position still acting as a siphon and drawing sample through the aperture. As the mercury column passes the start position, it initiates the electronic counting, and when

---

* Available from Coulter Electronics, Inc., Hialeah, Fla.

it passes the stop position, the count ceases. The distance the mercury must flow between the start and stop contacts is calibrated to represent a reproducible sample volume.

The Model Z passes current from the aperture current supply card through the electrodes in the sample stand and back to the preamplifier card in the unit.

Each current pulse, representative of each particle counted, is detected, amplified, and fed to the threshold card. It is here that actual sizing occurs, depending upon upper and lower limits set with the threshold controls. These count pulses are then sent to the readout card for an illuminated display on the unit front panel.

An Aural Monitor card provides a cadence for every thousand counts, allowing the operator to monitor the count.

### Reagents and Apparatus

1. Model Z Coulter Counter, 100 $\mu$ aperture tube
2. EDTA anticoagulated blood
3. Red cell diluting fluid; normal saline filtered to remove background particles or Isoton*
4. Sahli pipet—0.2 ml
5. Volumetric pipet—10 ml
6. Automatic pipet and diluter

### Method[3]

1. The instrument is set up as in the manufacturer's instructions.
2. A 1:50,000 dilution of whole blood is made by pipeting 0.02 ml of blood to 10 ml of filtered saline or Isoton. An additional 20 ml of diluent is added to 0.2 ml of the dilution.
3. Place the beaker containing the sample on the sample stand, immersing the aperture tube and external electrode in the diluted sample. Move the beaker so that the orifice of the aperture tube lies against the side of the beaker. This ensures a good projection of the orifice onto the micro projection screen.
4. Open the vacuum control stopcock setting up a negative pressure. The mercury column will fall and come to rest approximately 1 cm below the horizontal section of the manometer.
5. Close the control stopcock. As the mercury rises, an equal volume of diluted sample is drawn through the aperture tube. When the mercury column passes the first electrode, the count commences, and stops when the column passes the second electrode.
6. If the count is above 10,000 it should be corrected for coincidence

---

* Available from Scientific Products, Evanston, Illinois.

loss by referring to charts supplied by the manufacturer. A red cell count reading 40,000 would be corrected to 44,000. The corrected figure is multiplied by 100 to produce the total red cell count per mm³, that is

$$44,000 \times 100 = 4,400,000/mm^3$$

*Notes*

1. Coincidence correction. In some counts, a loss of count may occur because two or more cells enter the aperture simultaneously and are registered as a single pulse and count. High dilution will reduce this loss. However, when coincidence cannot be reduced by sample concentration, a correlation factor must be employed. Coincidence is negligible when the count is less than 10,000 cells per 0.5 ml of sample. This range includes normal white counts. All red cell counts and higher white cell counts should be corrected.

2. When the machine count is less than 1,000 cells per 0.5 ml, it is advisable to repeat the counts using a larger quantity of blood (e g , 1:200 dilution ratio for white cell counts; 1:20,000 for red cell counts).

3. Extremely high counts may be rendered inaccurate because of the number of cells passing through the aperture exceeding the maximal speed at which the counting mechanism operates. Repeat all counts when the machine count exceeds 70,000 per mm³ at a higher dilution. For polycythemic bloods the red cell count may be adjusted by taking 5 or 10 ml of the 1:50,000 dilution and adding an equal volume of electrolyte. The count so obtained is corrected in the usual way and the result is multiplied by 200 to give a total red cell count per mm³.

4. The outside of the aperture tube should be cleaned by standing it in electrolyte for a short time before placing the 1:50,000 dilution on the sample stand. If this is not done, the result obtained will be too high because of the cells left on the tube following immersion in the first dilution.

5. Blood can be used from a finger stick or venous blood can be taken into a suitable anticoagulant. EDTA is the anticoagulant of choice, but heparin can also be used.

6. Saline is a common medium for dilution. There is less than 1% count loss from settling of the cells within the first 5 minutes. However, it is desirable to perform the counts as soon as possible, because the red cells will slowly swell and hemolyze on standing. A better diluent is buffered Eagle's solution (Isoton).

7. The apparatus should be located so that spillage or splashing on the cabinet is avoided, because potential sources of current leaks can cause signal interference.

8. The aperture tube and external electrode holder, aperture current shortening lead, and manometer controls should also be dry and clean.

Electrical leakage paths, formed by encrustation can also be sources of signal interference.

9. The outer electrode must be completely submerged in the electrolyte during all counting periods or the count will be inaccurate. The electrolyte level in the waste flask should be kept below the glass tubing of the hose connection, otherwise saline solution will be sucked into the vacuum pump and will damage it. The waste flask must be emptied at regular intervals to avoid this damage.

10. There must never be air bubbles in the mercury column. If this occurs, the air bubble activates the on—off terminals producing false results. If air breaks are present, the vacuum stopcock may be opened and the vacuum regulator adjusted until the mercury falls down into the lower bulb. This should reunite the mercury.

11. When the counter is not in use it should be left with Isoterge or Isoton in it.

12. The counting cycle approximates 13 seconds times greater than 15 seconds usually indicate a partially plugged aperture tube, and times shorter than 11 seconds often are found when the orifice of the aperture tube is cracked or enlarged.

13. If the vacuum has to be adjusted, it may be carried out by changing the position of the clamp on the tubing leading to the pump.

To increase the vacuum, the clamp should be moved closer to the pump. To decrease the vacuum, it should be moved in the opposite direction.

### System Controls (Coulter, Model Z)

*Upper Threshold Control.* This determines the upper size limit of the count. The control disengages the upper threshold limit when turned fully counterclockwise.

*Lower Threshold Control.*   This determines the lower size limit of the count. When set too low, extraneous matter is counted.

*Amplification Switch.* This switch adjusts the sensitivity of the Pre-Amp.

*Aperture Current Switch.* This regulates the current flow through the aperture.

*Separate/Locked Switch.* This is located on the left side of the unit. When in the separate position, the unit will count all particles between those lower and upper threshold levels as determined by the respective dial settings.

When in the locked position, the thresholds no longer operate independently. The upper setting will be numerically one-tenth of its value, and the upper threshold level will always be that amount above the lower threshold dial setting.

*Matching Switch.* This is located inside the unit on the left. The switch setting matches the input resistance of the unit to the aperture-electrolyte resistance of the sample stand.

## VARIATIONS IN THE TOTAL RED CELL COUNT

*Age.* The red cell count in infants is normally higher than that found in adults. The count drops rapidly after birth and reaches its trough about the fourth month, after which it gradually rises until puberty. The count then maintains a plateau until old age, when it slowly drops.

*Exercise.* Extreme physical activity or excitement produces higher red cell counts than obtained under normal conditions. This activity can lead to accelerated destruction of cells, which may then serve as a stimulus to erythropoiesis.

*Sex.* Women have lower counts than men, probably because the erythropoietic activity is depressed through estrogen influence. This persists from the age of puberty until old age. In mammals in which menstrual blood loss does not take place, the red cell counts in both sexes are the same.

*Dehydration.* Severe dehydration produces false high counts, as seen in continual vomiting and in severe burns.

*Altitude.* In people living at high altitudes, increased cell counts are found; this condition is termed secondary polycythemia. The higher the altitude, the lower the oxygen tension, resulting in increased erythropoiesis due to hypoxia. Natives of high altitudes often show an increased red cell iron turnover rate, but red cell life span is not increased. When these people come down to sea level, their blood acquires the same morphological characteristics as that of the people habitually residing there.

*Climatic Conditions.* Seasonal variations in the numbers of red cells have been observed. Red cell mass appears to be lowered during summer or warmer months, although Wintrobe feels that data relating to such temperature variations are unconvincing.

*Diurnal Fluctuations.* Under normal conditions of activity, variation of red cell mass and hemoglobin have been recorded. These variations have been found to be inconsistent in relation to meals except in conditions in which excessive volumes of fluid have been absorbed.

## RETICULOCYTE COUNTS

Reticulocytes are young red cells, containing, within the cell membrane, a proportion of ribonucleoprotein which was present in larger amounts in the cytoplasm of red cell precursors. This basophilic material has the property of reacting to certain dyes and forming a blue granular precipitate. The most mature cells are those with the least granulation.

## Methods of Counting

### *Reagents and Apparatus (Indirect Methods):*

1. Diluting fluid: 0.4 g of brilliant cresyl blue or new methylene blue are added to 80 ml of normal saline and 20 ml of 3% sodium citrate. Filter before use.
2. Pasteur pipet
3. 1% Aqueous eosin
4. Eyepiece stocks
5. Tube—10 × 75 mm

## Method 1

1. Approximately 1 ml of filtered stain is delivered into a 10 × 75-mm tube.
2. One to two drops of blood is added to the stain and the mixture is incubated at 37°C for 30 minutes.
3. The tube is centrifuged for 1 minute at 1,000 rpm, the supernatant decanted and an aliquot of the packed cells is withdrawn with a Pasteur pipet.
4. Smears are made from the deposited red cells, in the same way as in differential white cell counts, allowed to dry in air and counterstained with 1% eosin for 30 seconds.
5. Eyepiece stocks are placed in the microscope oculars, reducing the field of view, and at least 1,000 red cells are counted. The number of reticulocytes seen in the 1,000 red cells are totaled and the results expressed as the number of reticulocytes per 100 red cells.

### *Notes*

1. Counterstaining the smear is optional. Many technologists prefer to view the smear without counterstain.
2. Care should be taken in filtering the stain before use, since stain precipitate can be confused with the cell reticulum.
3. A variation of the above method is to spread a grease-free slide lightly with the stain, allow to dry in the air and superimpose a drop of blood onto the dried film. A coverglass with a greased perimeter is placed over the blood, and the preparation is left at room temperature for 15 minutes. Care must be taken to see that the blood smears are thin and spread evenly.

## Method 2

1. Approximately 0.01 g of brilliant cresyl blue or new methylene blue is added directly to anticoagulated whole blood.

2. Mix the blood and stain, and leave at room temperature for 10 minutes.

3. Blood smears are prepared in the same way as in the previous method, and step 5 is carried out as previously described.

### Normal Values
```
Adults ....................................... 0.2—2%
Infants ....................................... 2.0—6%
```

### Notes
1. An area of the smear should be counted where the cells are undistorted and where the staining is good.

2. The cells should be counted using a high power oil immersion lens 97×.

3. If the brilliant cresyl blue is increased in strength, the reticulum fragments appear larger and more easily defined.

4. If the stain is warmed, the reticulum appears with fine granulation and can be easily missed.

5. Ensure that the stain has an alkaline pH; an acid pH results in a fine granular reticulum.

6. The presence of glucose or sodium salts inhibits the staining reaction.


## Morphological Abnormalities of Red Cells

### Alteration in Cell Size

*Anisocytosis.* This term denotes large variations in the size of a single red cell population. The term is often misused and applied to cells that are larger or smaller than normal and to slight clinically insignificant variations. Small fluctuations in size from one cell to another are often seen and should not be commented upon. Degrees of anisocytosis can be expressed according to the number of cells varying from the norm: Thus, 1+ anisocytosis is reported if between 15 to 20% of the cells vary in size; 2+ is reported if 25 to 50% of the cells vary; and 3+ is reported if over 50% of the red cells show variation in size.

*Macrocytosis.* A macrocyte is a red cell having a fixed diameter in excess of 7.7 $\mu$. The cell usually has a full complement of hemoglobin and is frequently the end product of abnormal erythropoiesis or the result of premature release of red cells in the circulation because of excessive oxygen requirements.

*Microcytosis.* These red cells are smaller than normal, having a diameter of less than 6.5 $\mu$. The hemoglobin content of the cell may be normal or reduced, although commonly the cell shows reduction in hemoglobin, especially in iron deficiency anemias.

### Alterations in Cell Shape

*Poikilocytosis.* A poikilocyte is classically a pear-shaped or teardrop red cell, and often represents an old cell ready for erythrofragmentation and phagocytosis. The cell is frequently found together with anisocytosis in severe anemias of most etiologies.

*Elliptocytosis.* Elliptocytes are red cells which vary in shape from elongated forms to true ovals. The cells are inherited as a simple Mendelian dominant trait and are usually unconnected with any clinical state. In rare cases, mild hemolytic anemias have been reported because of the presence of these cells, and occasionally they are found in the peripheral blood of patients with thalassemia and in sickle cell anemia. Abnormal hemoglobins are not usually present in such cells.

*Spherocytosis.* This red cell is globular and possesses an increased thickness and decreased diameter. It appears in blood smears as a small deeply staining cell lacking the normal red cell central pallor. The spherical shape results from a developmental defect, which occurs after the erythroblastic stage and in which a normal cell volume is enclosed within a diminished surface area. Normal red cells become thicker as they take up water, but because the spherocyte is already thick, it requires less water to hemolyze and is hence more fragile.

Two types of spherocytes exist. The congenital type found in hereditary spherocytosis and the acquired form resulting from the contraction and reduction of the surface area of the cell caused by antibody damage. These morphological changes are often seen in ABO erythroblastosis fetalis and less frequently in patients with congenital nonspherocytic hemolytic anemia, leukemia, and in conditions of stasis within the spleen. The abnormality is believed to be caused by a loss of cholesterol and phospholipids from the cell membrane, resulting in the biconvex shape, and predisposing the cell to splenic sequestration. These membrane changes are thought to result in the passive transport of more sodium into the cell than normal.

*Sickle Cells (Drepanocytes).* A sickle cell is a red cell that undergoes bizarre changes in shape when exposed to a reduced oxygen atmosphere. The tendency is to form sickle, holly-leaf, or irregular spiny shaped forms in vitro and in vivo. The sickling phenomenon is due to the formation of tactoid forms of hemoglobin crystals within the cell. This characteristic is usually reversible, but on rare occasions it has been reported to be an irreversible phenomenon.

*Schistocytes.* These cells are disintegrating erythrocytes in the process of fragmentation. They are often seen in severe burns, in disseminated intravascular coagulation, and in other hemolytic processes. They appear to be more common in lipemic blood than in nonlipemic. The cell usually takes the form of triangular or small elliptical shapes which are removed from the circulation by splenic action.

*Burr Cells*. These are mature red cells similar in appearance to crenated cells. They differ in that they possess one or more spiny projections along their periphery and do not exhibit the typical wrinkling of the crenated state. Burr cells are thought to be a form of poikilocyte and have been associated with impaired renal function, hemolytic anemia, and thrombocytopenia. They appear in infants having drug-induced hemolytic anemias and often are paralleled by the presence of Heinz bodies.

*Acanthrocytes*. These are red cells having several irregularly spaced large coarse projections varying in width. They are associated with underlying metabolic defects, amongst those reported being an increased tolerance to carbohydrates, deficiencies of vitamin E, and defective absorption of lipids. These abnormalities are also associated with retinal degeneration, uremia, steatorrhea and retarded growth. Analysis of the red cell membrane shows abnormal lipid content, an increase in sphingomyelin and a decrease in phosphatidyl choline. The osmotic fragility of the cell is normal or slightly decreased, and both the mechanical fragility and the autohemolysis tests are both increased.

*Target Cells*. These cells are flatter than normal, and have a slightly increased diameter, normal volume and subsequently a decreased cell thickness, except at the cell center where there is a bulging of the cell membrane. On cross section, the cell resembles a Mexican hat. The abnormality is believed to reflect cholesterol abnormalities between the cell and the plasma due to the inhibition of bile salts of cholesterol esterification. The cell is frequently found in nonspecific liver disease, and is commonly present in hemolytic anemias, HbC disease, sickle cell disease, sickle cell—HbC disease, thalassemia, sickle cell-thalassemia, iron deficiency anemia, and following splenectomy.

### Alternations in Cellular Staining

*Hypochromia*. Hypochromic red cells are erythrocytes which when viewed microscopically from above, appear to show more pallor in the center than at the periphery than do normal cells. In this state, the cell is usually iron deficient and when present in moderate numbers indicates a reduced mean cell hemoglobin concentration (MCHC).

*Polychromasia*. Red cells which stain a purple-red with Romanowsky stains are termed polychromatic. The staining reaction is due to the presence of RNA and is related to the degree of reticulocytosis and basophilic stippling. This relationship appears to result from technical differences in the preparation of the smear, and consequently the differences can be considered artifactual in origin. Rapid cell fixation can produce increases in polychromasia and basophilic stippling disappears on treatment with ribonuclease.

### Alterations in Structure (Inclusion Bodies)

*Basophilic Stippling (Punctate Basophilia).* This condition applies to red cells having fine blue or violet-blue granules in the cytoplasm of poly-chromatic cells when stained by Romanowsky dyes. The intracellular granulation is not stained by the Prussian blue reaction for iron (Perl's stain) or by the Feulgen stain for DNA. The stippling represents regeneration or immaturity of the cell and is associated with chronic anemia, leukemia, lead poisoning and thalassemia.

*Siderocytes.* These are red cells having multiple iron-containing granules. They vary in size, occasionally reaching $2\mu$ in diameter. In Romanowsky stained smears they appear as faint blue inclusion representing ferric iron aggregates. They are stained by the Prussian blue reaction, and are occasionally seen as fine granules or rods.

Siderocytes are found in moderate numbers in normal blood and in the bone marrow but are characteristically increased in hemolytic anemias, infections, and following splenectomy. They are decreased in iron deficiency anemia. The pathophysiology of these cells can most likely be explained by abnormal erythropoiesis. Normally, iron not yet utilized in heme synthesis is found in the nucleated red cell cytoplasm. Usually this iron is fully used up in heme production and does not appear in the mature red cell. When red cell production is greatly enhanced, terminal mitotic divisions of the red cell line are sometimes missed and incomplete hemoglobin synthesis results in the carry-over of these iron stores as siderocytic granules. When these inclusions are present in nucleated red cells, the cells are termed sideroblasts.

*Pappenheimer Bodies.* These inclusions are seen as fine granules or rods when stained by Romanowsky dyes. They can be differentiated from siderocytes by a negative iron stain (Perl's reaction).

*Heinz Bodies.* These bodies are round protein-containing granules, $1$-$2\mu$ in diameter, found at the periphery of the red cell. They can be detected by supravital techniques, using brilliant cresyl blue or methyl violet, but not by routine Romanowsky stains. They are easily seen as refractile bodies in wet unstained preparations and are believed to be agglomeration of denatured globin, verdohemoglobin, and stromal material. The presence of Heinz bodies in abnormal numbers incidates red cell injury and can serve as an index of existing anemia. Many drug-induced anemias are associated with the presence of these bodies, and they are frequently found in hemolytic anemias, leukemias, and following splenectomy. The inclusion is thought to represent severe toxication of the red cell and is thought to represent severe intoxication of the red cell and is more easily seen when there is an intrinsic cell defect.

*Howell-Jolly Bodies.* These inclusions are purple violet masses, 1 $\mu$ in diameter, occurring singly or doubly and situated in an eccentric position within the cell. They are stained by Romanowsky dyes and by Feulgen's reaction for DNA. The origin of these inclusions is believed to be abnormal mitosis in the metarubricyte stage of cell maturation. When a single chromosome becomes detached and fails to become included in the formation of the nucleus. It then remains free in the cytoplasm as a nuclear remnant.

### Red Cell Artifacts

*Hyperchromia.* In this state, it is postulated that the red cell is supersaturated with hemoglobin. This is a physiological impossibility. According to common usage, hyperchromic cells contain an abnormal increase in hemoglobin and can be identified in many macrocytic conditions. The term "hyperchromia" should be avoided.

*Cabot's Rings.* These inclusions are blue figure-eight or circular bodies once believed to be related to Howell-Jolly Bodies. They are presently thought to be artifacts resulting from damage to the lipoprotein of the cell stroma. The rings are not visible by phase contrast microscopy, but they stain by Romanowsky dyes.

*Crenated Red Cells.* If peripheral blood smears dry slowly, the erythrocyte envelope becomes exposed to a hypertonic environment, causing typical seration of the cell. Occasionally, the wrinkling is accompanied by spiny projections. The abnormality has no clinical significance and is purely artifactual.

## ESTIMATION OF HEMATOCRIT (PACKED CELL VOLUME)

*Principle.* Whole blood is centrifuged and the total volume of the red cell mass is expressed as a percentage of the whole blood volume.

### Micro Method

*Reagents and Apparatus*
1. Capillary tubes—75 mm × 1.5 mm. These tubes are used for anticoagulated venous blood. If capillary blood is used, the tubes are coated with ammonium heparinate. They can be commercially obtained.
2. Microcentrifuge
3. Hematocrit reader
4. Plastic vinyl putty or "critoseal"*

---

* Available from Scientific Products, Evanston, Ill. Cat. No. B 4425.

### Method

1. The capillary tube is filled to within 10 to 15 mm of the end with capillary or well-mixed venous anticoagulated (EDTA) blood.

2. The tube is capped with either a small plastic cap (critoseal) or by placing the dry end of the tube into a tray of plastic vinyl putty. Ensure that the putty seal forms a straight edge across the interior of the tube.

3. The exterior of the tube is wiped free of blood and centrifuged for 5 minutes at full speed (12,000 rpm).

4. The volume of packed red cells is read as a percentage of the total volume of whole blood from the hematocrit reader, following the manufacturer's instructions.

### Normal Values

Male . . . . . . . . . . . . . . . . . . . . . . . . . . . . . . . . . . . . . . . . . . . . 40–54%

Female . . . . . . . . . . . . . . . . . . . . . . . . . . . . . . . . . . . . . 34–49%

Infants . . . . . . . . . . . . . . . . . . . . . . . . . . . . . . . . . . . . . 44–64%

## Macro Method

### Reagents and Apparatus

1. Wintrobe tube. This is a narrow, hard, thick-walled tube, graduated from 0 to 100 mm and having an internal diameter of 2.5 mm and a length of 100 mm.

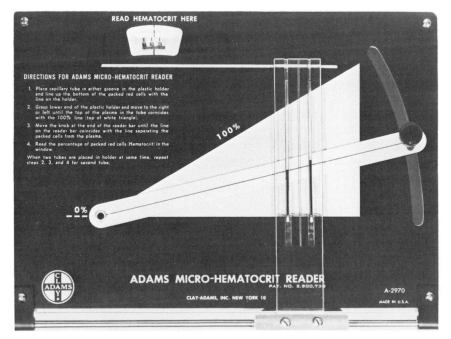

FIG. 2-15. Adams micro-hematocrit reader. (Courtesy of Clay-Adams Co.)

2. Bench model centrifuge, having a speed of at least 3,000 rpm and an internal radius of 15 cm
3. Pasteur pipet—15-cm stem
4. Venous blood

### Method

1. A Wintrobe tube is carefully filled from the bottom with a Pasteur pipet so as to exclude any air bubbles.
2. The tube is centrifuged at exactly 3,000 rpm for 30 minutes, and the packed cell volume is read from the scale on the right side of the tube. (The figures begin at 100 at the top and end at 0 at the bottom).
3. Take care to read the level at the junction of the red cell layer. *Do not* include the "buffy coat" of white cells or the platelet layer in the result.

### Notes

1. With a suitable centrifuge, the hematocrit of a blood sample can be reproduced to within ±1%.
2. The hematocrit reading, obtained by the micro technique, is from 1 to 3% lower than with the macro method, because the volume of "trapped" plasma in the macro method varies up to 4% on any given blood. Centrifuging at a higher speed increases the rate of gravity exerted on the blood, thus reducing the "trapped" plasma value.
3. In addition to the centrifugal force applied, the speed of packing depends upon the density and the size of the cells, the viscosity of the suspending fluid, and the relative densities of cells and fluid.
4. Thirty minutes of centrifugation in the macro technique is just sufficient to produce a constant red cell mass. If the blood is centrifuged for a full hour, the packed cell volume is reduced by between 1% and 3%.
5. Errors occur when the concentration of disodium or dipotassium EDTA exceed 2 mg/ml whole blood. When the vacutainer system is used, the EDTA is designed to provide 1 mg/ml of whole blood. When the volume of whole blood added to the tube is less than 7 ml, the concentration of EDTA exceeds 1 mg/ml. Observed hematocrits become progressively lower as the concentration of EDTA increases. The error reaches 5% when 2 ml of blood is added to the tube, 10% with 1 ml and 17% with 0.5 ml. Hemoglobin values are unaffected. The hematocrit of a sample of blood that has been aerated is about 1% less than that of venous blood.

## Electronic Techniques

*Principle.* The electronic hematocrit operates on the principle that red blood cells act as electrical insulators, whereas serum behaves as a temperature-dependent conductor. The resistance of a calibrated volume of blood is then a function of the relative volume concentration of the insulating blood cells.

### Reagents and Apparatus
1. Heparinized blood
2. Electronic micro-hematocrit*

### Method[4]
1. The power switch is turned to ON and the front dial adjusted until the meter pointer indicates the red line at the 49 position on the scale.

2. 0.02 ml of blood is drawn into the cell to fill the area between the electrodes. The cell is inserted into the clip on the top of the instrument by pushing back the slider, aligning the metal contacts and releasing the slider.

3. The PUSH TO READ button is depressed on the top of the instrument and the hematocrit reading recorded.

4. To ensure that the calibration is unchanged, make sure that the meter pointer is on the red line when the button is released.

### Notes
1. The cell is cleaned immediately after use by drawing saline and acetone through it, using a rubber tube attached to one end of the cell. Do not allow blood to clot in the cell.

2. For maximal accuracy, the cell should be clean, dry and at room temperature.

3. The most accurate and stable readings are obtained 15 to 30 seconds after inserting the cell into its clip.

4. Only fresh whole blood or heparinized blood can be used. Use of other anticoagulants changes the conductivity of the mixture and introduces significant errors.

5. Heparinized blood should be well mixed, but care should be taken to prevent foaming, which could result in air bubbles in the cell.

6. The electronic estimation of hematocrit can be affected by high white cell counts of over 25,000 or by high platelet counts of over 1,000,000. Another variable that can lead to a miscalculation is a determination carried out in dysproteinemia.

*Principle.* The computer measures the average height of the oscilloscope pattern on the Model Z Coulter Counter, which is proportional to the average mean cell volume. From this and the total red count, hematocrit is mathematically determined.

### Reagents and Apparatus
1. Model Z Coulter Counter
2. MCV computer

---

* Available from Yellow Springs Instrument Co., Yellow Springs, Ohio.

FIG. 2-16. Electronic hematocrit, Model 30. (Courtesy of Yellow Springs Instrument Co.)

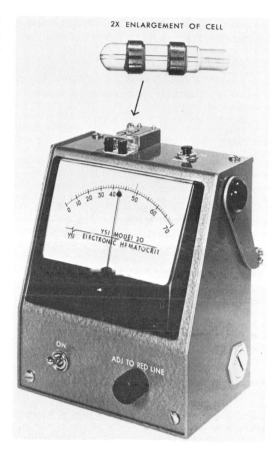

2X ENLARGEMENT OF CELL

3. Hematocrit computer

4. Additional reagents as described on page 61 for the automatic red cell count.

### Method

1. The computer is set up, following the manufacturer's instructions.

2. The start switch is turned to AUTO and, in this position, both the MCV and hematocrit computers will automatically and simultaneously read out the results, as the red cell count is being determined.

### ABSOLUTE INDICES (VALUES)

An estimation of the hematocrit is useful as a screening test for anemia. Also, in conjunction with the hemoglobin and red cell count, it makes possible the determination of mean cell volume (MCV), mean cell hemo-globin (MCH) and mean cell hemoglobin concentration (MCHC).

*Note*

The hematocrit can be estimated by three different principles. True red cell hematocrit (packed cell volume) is calculated by expressing the volume of red cells per unit volume of whole blood. Within certain restraints, the hematocrit when measured by this method is reproducible, although it depends greatly on the gravitational force exerted on the blood. The greater the speed, the larger the centrifugal radius, and the longer the time centrifuged, all combine to produce more efficient packing and result in a lowered hematocrit.

Cell conductivity methods (electronic hematocrit YSI) are not as spe-cific as centrifugal methods. The conductivity of whole blood is affected by variables other than the red cell mass. Such variable factors include the presence of other cells (leukocytes, platelets), the ratio of anti-coagulant/blood used, the presence of intravenous medications (Dextran, Ringer's lactate, saline, etc.) that may be used in treating the patient during the time period the blood sample was obtained, and the presence of abnormal proteins (multiple myeloma, macroglobulinemia).

The estimation of hematocrit by volume displacement (Coulter Counter) likewise cannot be consistently compared to the other two methods. The isotonic buffered saline used to suspend and dilute the red cells does not result in comparable mean red cell volumes and produces normal MCV values of up to 103 cu $\mu$. Because the hematocrit is not measured directly, being a product of the mean cell volume and the red cell count, this method of estimating hematocrit produces slightly higher volumes.

$$\text{Hematocrit } \% = \frac{\text{Mean Cell Volume (cu } \mu) \times \text{Red Count (in millions)}}{10}$$

**Mean Cell Volume (MCV)**

*Definition.* This is the volume of the average red cell, expressed in cubic microns. If the mean cell thickness is normal, it bears a linear rela-tionship to the diameter of the cell.

*Factors Required to Calculate MCV*
1. Hematocrit
2. Red cell count

*Calculation*
1. If the hematocrit is 45%, there is 0.45 cu mm of red cells in 1 cu mm of blood.

If the red cell count is 5,000,000/cu mm, these cells occupy a total volume of 0.45 cu mm.

The volume of 1 red cell (MCV) is then 0.45/5,000,000 cu mm

$$= \frac{0.45 \times 10^9 \text{ cu } \mu}{5 \times 10^6} \qquad \frac{0.45 \times 10^3 \text{ cu } \mu}{5} = 90 \text{ cu } \mu$$

2. A short method of calculating the MCV (in cu $\mu$) is:

$$\frac{\text{hematocrit (as a percentage)}}{\text{red cell count (in millions)}} \times 10 = \text{MCV}$$

## Mean Cell Hemoglobin (MCH)

*Definition.* This is the weight of hemoglobin in the average red cell, expressed as micro micro grams ($\mu\mu$ g) of hemoglobin. If the cell is large, the MCH is raised, unless the cell is iron deficient. If the cell is small and iron deficient, the MCH is reduced.

### *Factors Required to Calculate MCH*
1. Hemoglobin
2. Red cell count

### *Calculation*
1. If the hemoglobin is 15 g per 100 ml of blood, there is 15/100 g of hemoglobin per ml of blood. This is equivalent to 15/100 × 1,000 g of hemoglobin per cu mm of blood. If the red cell count is 5,000,000 per cu mm, the average weight of hemoglobin in 1 red cell is 15/100 × 1,000 × 5,000,000 g per cell = $15/5 \times 10^{11}$ g hemoglobin per cell = g hemoglobin per cell × $10^{12}$ $\mu\mu$ g of hemoglobin = $3 \times 10$ $\mu\mu$ g of hemoglobin per cell = 30 $\mu\mu$ g per cell.

2. A short method of calculating the MCH is:

$$\frac{\text{hemoglobin (g \%)}}{\text{red cell count (in millions)}} \times 10 \ \mu\mu \ g = \text{MCH}$$

## Mean Cell Hemoglobin Concentration (MCHC)

*Definition.* This is the concentration of hemoglobin per unit volume of red cell, expressed as a percentage. Values below 30% are indicative of iron deficiency, whereas values above 36% are physiologically impossible. At this percentage, the red cell is saturated with hemoglobin; thus, concentrations above this figure postulate supersaturation.

### *Factors Required to Calculate MCHC*
1. Hemoglobin
2. Hematocrit

*Calculation.* If the hemoglobin is 15 g per 100 ml of blood and the red cells occupy 45% of the total blood volume, the hemoglobin concentration is $15/45 \times 100\% = 33.3\%$.

### Normal Values For Absolute Indices

MCV ......................................... 83-97 cu $\mu$
MCH ........................................ 27-33 $\mu\mu$ g
MCHC ....................................... 32-37%

### Notes

1. The advantages of absolute indices are that the results are calibrated on observed figures, without reference to arbitrary fixed normals. Absolute indices analyze the condition of the peripheral or venous blood in exact terms of red cell volume, diameter, thickness and hemoglobin concentration.

2. In disease, the absolute indices are changed. Macrocytic anemias often produce increased MCV and MCH values and reduced MCHC values; in microcytic anemias, the MCV, MCH and MCHC are usually lowered.

3. Since cell volume is a cubic measurement, the volume determination is more sensitive to cell size than to linear measurement of the cell diameter. The MCV, in itself, is a reliable indication of macrocytosis, except in the case of microspherocytosis, when the cell volume and mean cell diameter do not retain their normal relationship, the diameter being reduced and the volume increased.

4. The key to iron therapy is the MCHC. Low concentrations indicate that the cells are unsaturated and in need of iron, whereas normal concentrations, whatever the cell size, show that the cells cannot carry any more iron.

5. The absolute indices obtained are only as accurate as the data from which they were calculated. The MCHC is the most reliable value, because it is computed from accurate determinations. The MCH and MCV are of little value when calculated from manual red cell counts. If the red cell count is determined by electronic methods, the values are more significant.

6. There are numerous methods of assessing the mean cell diameter (MCD) of a stained blood film. Two such direct measurements utilize the method of Price-Jones and the diffraction method using a halometer. Most of these techniques measure the red cell diameter in dried blood smears; these practices are unreliable because there is a 10% shrinkage in the diameter due to the fixation and also to distortion of the cells in the preparation of the smears. In addition, the particular fields chosen must show no artificial distortion, no overlapping of cells, and no obvious crenated cells.

## CLINICAL CONSIDERATIONS

### The Anemias

The term "anemia" is defined as a reduction in the amount of circulating hemoglobin, causing a decrease in the oxygen-carrying capacity of the blood. Morphologically, four main divisions of anemia exist:

*Simple Microcytic.* In this disease, the MCV is less than 83 cu $\mu$, and the MCHC is greater than 30%. Clinical syndromes include the following: subacute and chronic inflammatory diseases; idiopathic microcytic anemia.

*Normocytic.* The MCV is normal, between 83 cu $\mu$ and 97 cu $\mu$, and the MCHC is over 30%, frequently between 32% and 36%. Clinical syndromes include the following: scurvy, hemolytic anemias, aplastic anemia, myelophthisic anemia due to carcinoma of the bone marrow, Hodgkin's disease, leukemia, multiple myeloma, and myelosclerosis.

*Macrocytic.* In this condition, the MCV is greater than 97 cu $\mu$, and the MCHC is greater than 30%. Clinical syndromes include the following: pernicious anemia, nutritional macrocytic anemia, anemia developing from carcinoma of the stomach, macrocytic anemia of pregnancy, idiopathic steatorrhea, and sprue.

*Microcytic Hypochromic.* In these states, the MCV is less than 83 cu $\mu$, and the MCHC is less than 30%. Clinical syndromes include the following: nutritional anemia, alimentary tract bleeding and pregnancy.

Another widely used classification of anemia states is to group them according to their pathology. The three classifications of anemia are: resulting from impaired blood production, increased red cell destruction, and blood loss.

### Deficient Red Cell Production

a. Deficient hemoglobin synthesis. Clinical syndromes include iron deficiency anemia, porphyria, and heavy metal poisons.

b. Delayed nuclear maturation. Clinical syndromes include vitamin $B_{12}$ and folic acid deficiencies.

c. Underproduction of erythropoietin. Clinical syndromes include chronic renal disease and hyperthyroidism.

d. Bone marrow failure. Clinical syndromes include mechanical failure due to tumors, drug sensitivity, and idiopathic aplastic states.

### Increased Red Cell Destruction

a. Congenital hemoglytic anemia. Clinical syndromes include hereditary microspherocytosis. Hereditary elliptocytosis, glucose-6-phosphate dehydrogenase, pyruvate kinase deficiency and erythroblastosis.

b. Acquired hemolytic anemia. Clinical syndromes include paroxysmal cold hemoglobinuria, paroxysmal nocturnal hemoglobinuria, and acquired autoimmune hemolytic anemia.

### Blood Loss Anemia

The two forms of such a mechanism are due to either acute or chronic hemorrhage.

*Pernicious Anemia.* True Addisonian pernicious anemia is a disease of adults, rarely seen under the age of 30. It is probable that it cannot occur in childhood, and is primarily a disease of the white races and found in temperate zones. The deficiency is of the "intrinsic factor," which is necessary for the absorption of vitamin $B_{12}$.

The onset of the disease is insidious, the usual history being one of gastric disturbances, increasing lassitude, headaches, and dizziness. In advanced cases, there is a characteristic yellow tinge to the conjunctiva. A sore tongue is present in about 50% of the cases, and achlorhydria is often found.

A number of other conditions including folate deficiency and sprue present the same blood picture, as given below.

The blood changes are characterized by low red cell, white cell and platelet counts. The blood formation is dysplastic, being altered from the normocyte to the megaloblastic type.

The red cells show considerable anisocytosis and macrocytosis, the Price-Jones curve (Fig. 2-20) being shifted to the right and flattened in shape, showing quantitative degrees of cell size and anisocytosis.

The MCD is increased up to 9.7 $\mu$, with an average of 8.3$\mu$. Polychromatic and stippled cells are found, together with reticulocytes. The characteristic cell is the hemoglobinized megaloblast. Rubricytes may also be present in varying numbers, and nuclear remnants such as Howell-Jolly bodies are also seen. The absolute values are characteristic. The MCV is increased from between 100 cu $\mu$ and 140 cu $\mu$, although in some cases this value may fall within normal limits. The MCHC and MCH are usually normal.

Leukopenia is found, due to the depressive action on the myeloid tissue in the marrow, resulting from megaloblastic proliferation. A frequent finding is a "shift to the right" (an increase in mature leukocytes) as large as 18 $\mu$, with multisegmented neutrophils. These cells are termed macropolycytes. In severe cases, platelets are reduced and the bilirubin and bile pigment levels raised; polyuria is also found.

The sedimentation rate is found to be normal, when corrected for the anemia. The first sign of blood regeneration is an increased reticulocyte count.

The bone marrow aspirations are characteristic of the disease. The tissue is hypercellular and is dominated by the presence of megaloblastic

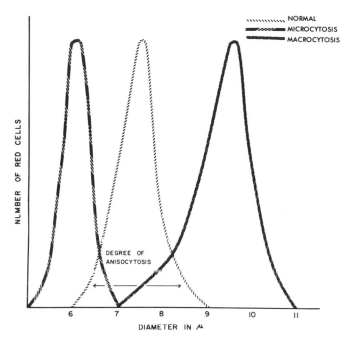

NORMAL
MICROCYTOSIS
MACROCYTOSIS

NUMBER OF RED CELLS

DEGREE OF
ANISOCYTOSIS

6   7   8   9   10   11

DIAMETER IN μ

FIG. 2-17. Price-Jones curve, showing microcytic, normal and macrocytic distribution of cells.

red cells. These cells show definite asynchronism of nuclear-cytoplasmic maturation, the cytoplasm showing a greater degree of maturity than the nucleus of the cell. The cell is larger than normal and typically exhibits earlier hemoglobinization than would normally be expected. The nucleus shows an open-reticular lacy or "clock face" appearance and is often described as "stippled."

A differential diagnosis can be made either by measurement of serum vitamin $B_{12}$ levels or by the use of the Schilling test (see p. 341).

**Anemia Associated with Renal Disease.** Both acute and chronic renal disease are usually accompanied by alterations in erythrokinetics. In some cases bone marrow failure due to reduced erythropoietin production is present and in others, a hemolytic component occurs. The anemia of chronic renal diseases is normocytic and normochromic, but in the more chronically and severely anemic patients, a mild macrocytosis may be present. Usually, only mild anisocytosis is seen, but when the renal function impairment is severe, burr cells, helmet cells, and other bizarre red cell shapes are present. Such alterations in red cell peripheral morphology are not specific to the anemia associated with renal disease but may also be found in malignancy, thrombotic thrombocytopenic purpura, gastrointestinal hemorrhage, and microangiopathic disease.

The severity of the disease is correlated with the degree of evaluation of nitrogen retention, the higher the BUN the lower the hemoglobin. Reticulocytosis may be slightly increased, but it is commonly found to be decreased, especially in severe crises. The red cells show normal osmotic and mechanical fragility. The true marrow picture varies; there may be a marked normoblastic hyperplasia, but often there is depressed red cell activity with poor hemoglobin formation in the nucleated red cells. Sideroblasts are usually present in normal numbers but sideroachrestic anemias have been observed.

The iron-binding protein is usually reduced, but the serum iron levels are inconsistent and vary widely.

*Aplastic Anemia.* This is a rare disease, in which hemopoietic activity is depressed. This loss of activity can be produced by the destruction of the sites of cell formation by toxic agents such as urethane, benzol or chloromycetin, or by ionizing radiation. In most cases, the responsible agent is unknown. The diagnosis is based on a progressive pancytopenia, associated with bleeding and infections. The peripheral red cell morphology is relatively normal, the total red cell count being greatly reduced. Reticulocytes are not increased, and there is a marked reduction in the total white cell count and platelet count.

*Anemia Resulting from Acute Blood Loss.* Large rapid hemorrhages deplete all the formed blood elements of the body. During recovery, the blood volume is rapidly replenished by a shift of tissue fluid into the circulation, resulting in the dilution of red cells and reduced hemoglobin and plasma protein levels. As the body compensates, normoblasts appear in the peripheral blood, together with reticulocytes and polychromatic cells. Normally, a reticulocyte crisis is apparent after approximately 7 to 10 days of hemorrhage.

*Anemia from Chronic Blood Loss.* Constant loss of small volumes of blood slowly depletes the body iron reserves. As long as erythropoietic tissues compensate for this loss, the cell count does not drop markedly, but the plasma proteins and hemoglobin levels become reduced.

**Polycythemia Vera**

This disease is characterized by an increase in the number of red cells, due to an abnormally high erythroblastic activity of the bone marrow, of unknown cause. Clinically, there are headaches, lassitude, visual disturbances, vertigo and a marked congestion around the face. Hemorrhages may occur from the stomach, intestines, kidneys and eyes. Peptic ulcers and congestive cardiac failure are often found in association with the disease.

The red cell count is always raised, sometimes as high as 12 to 15 million cells per cubic millimeter of blood, with a proportional increase in the hemoglobin level. A microcytic blood picture is often produced. The total blood volume and blood viscosity are both greatly increased.

The serum bilirubin level is normal, as are the osmotic fragility and sedimentation rate. The bleeding and clotting times are both normal, and the platelets are usually increased in numbers. Platelet counts of 1 to 3 million cells per cubic millimeter of blood have occasionally been found, and megakaryocytic fragments are often present in the peripheral blood. Leukocytes are ordinarily increased up to 40,000 per cubic millimeter, the predominant cell being the mature neutrophil.

The marrow shows a generalized increase of all precursor elements, especially the normoblastic and granulocytic cells.

Other laboratory findings are an increase in uric acid, increase in plasma iron turnover, and normal oxygen saturation.

Various other diseases have been associated with this disease: myeloid leukemia; leukoerythroblastic anemia; aplastic anemia; myelosclerosis, multiple myeloma

## Secondary Polycythemia

Secondary polycythemia resulting from oxygen deprivation stimulates erythropoietic activity from the kidneys; such an increase results in abnormally high red cell counts, a product of the expansion of bone marrow volume. The increases in hematocrit may not be strictly proportional to the increase in hemoglobin concentration, so that slightly hypochromic and microcytic red cells are seen. Reticulocytosis and hyperbilirubinemia of mild degree are also found. Leukocytosis and leukemoid changes do not occur and the platelet count is normal. Arterial hypoxia is always present. This is best determined by blood-gas analysis and the finding of a hemoglobin saturation of 90% or less. Typical secondary polycythemia can result from any situation that arises from the mixing of arterial and venous blood causing inadequate oxygenation of the tissues. This is found in chronic pulmonary disorders and in individuals residing at high altitudes.

## Relative Polycythemia

In this disorder, the total blood volume is decreased. The change is associated with a decrease in the plasma compartment disproportionate to any change in the total red cell volume, so that there is a relative increase in both the levels of hemoglobin and in the red cell count. The condition frequently is found secondary to other disorders; dehydration, diabetic acidosis, burns, and endocrinopathies are all causes of these findings. Other syndromes associated with relative polycythemia are hypovolemic polycythemia (stress) and Gaisböck's syndrome. Stress polycythemia resulting from the anxieties of daily living can be differentiated from Gaisböck's syndrome. In the former, the red cell mass is normal but the plasma volume is diminished. In the latter, there is an increase in the total red cell mass.

Most patients with relative polycythemia are hyperkinetic males presenting complaints of headaches and giddiness. Most are of stocky build, overweight and hypertensive. The laboratory findings, beside the increase in hemoglobin and red cell count, show normal white cell and platelet counts. Splenomegaly and myeloproliferative complications are not found. Ferrokinetic studies are normal, as are the erythropoietin excretion and leucocyte alkaline phosphatase.

**Erythremic Myelosis (Di Guglielmo's Disease)**

The clinical features of the disease are severe anemia, enlarged spleen and liver, and in irregular fever. The peripheral blood shows a severe normocytic or slightly hypochromic anemia with numerous nucleated red cells, great variations in cellular shape, and occasional myelocytes and metamyelocytes. The reticulocytes are normal and both white cells and platelets are usually decreased.

The bone marrow shows an erythroid hyperplasia with a maturation arrest at the prorubricyte stage and a reticuloendothelial proliferation. The nucleated red cells are of both the normoblastic and macronormoblastic series, many of which show a strongly positive PAS reaction. This staining reaction may be diagnostic.

## REFERENCES

1. Instruction and Service Manual for the Model S Coulter Counter. ed. 5. Coulter Electronics Inc., Hialeah, Fla., 1972.
2. Instruction Manual for the Hemalog-8. Technicon Instruments Co., Tarrytown, N.Y., 1971.
3. Instruction Manual for the Model Z Coulter Counter. Coulter Electronics Inc., Hialeah, Fla., 1973.
4. Instructions for YSI Model 30 Portable Micro Hematocrit. Yellow Springs Instrument Co., Inc., Yellow Springs, O.

# 3

# *Leukocytes (White Blood Cells)*

## WHITE CELL COUNT

*Principle.* The number of white cells in a sample of diluted blood is counted in a hemocytometer of known dimensions. From the number of cells seen, the total white cell count of an undiluted sample is calculated.

### *Manual Methods*

#### *Reagents and Apparatus*
1. Diluting fluids:
 (a) 2% aqueous acetic acid tinged with gentian violet;
 (b) 2% hydrochloric acid.
2. Thoma white cell pipet
3. Hemocytometer (as in the red cell count)

#### *Method*
1. Anticoagulated or capillary blood is pipeted to the 0.5 mark on the Thoma pipet, and the external surface of the pipet is wiped clean of blood.
2. Diluting fluid is taken to the 11 mark, taking care to avoid the introduction of air bubbles into the bulb of the pipet, and the procedure is followed as in the red cell count.
3. By using the 10× objective of the microscope, the cells seen in the four large corner squares of the Neubauer hemocytometer are counted (see Fig. 2-3).

#### *Calculation*
1. Inasmuch as blood is drawn to the 0.5 mark and diluted to the 11 mark, the final dilution is 1:20, not 1:22. The reasons for this apparent discrepancy are the same as in the red cell dilution.
2. The area of each of the four large corner squares is 1 mm × 1 mm = 1 sq mm.
3. The total area of the four squares counted is 4 × 1 sq mm = 4 sq mm.

4. The depth of the hemocytometer is 0.1 mm; thus the total volume used in the count is 4 sq mm × 0.1 mm = 0.4 cu mm.

5. If 100 cells are counted in a total volume of 0.4 cu mm, then 100/0.4 or 250 white cells are present in 1 cu mm.

6. However, because the original blood was diluted 1:20, the corrected number of white cells expressed per cu mm is 250 × 20 = 5,000.

7. An abbreviated system of calculating the total white count is N × 50, where N is the number of cells counted.

### Notes

1. Values outside the normal white count limits are often pathological, although the presence of a normal total count does not always indicate the absence of disease.

2. An increase in the total circulating white cells is termed a leukocytosis. This condition is commonly stimulated by an infection, but myeloproliferative disorders, such as leukemia and related diseases, characteristically produce raised counts.

3. The causes of a leukocytosis are complex. Polypeptide thermolabile and thermostable factors are thought to be present in inflammatory exudates and are called leukocyte-promoting factors. Two leukopenic factors are also present: leukopenin, a thermolabile substance, and necrosin, which is thermostable. The level of the leukocyte count, whether a leukocytosis or a leukopenia, depends on which is the predominant factor.

4. A decrease in the total white count is termed a leukopenia. As in a leukocytosis, the abnormality in the number of cells may be general or specific in nature. Specialized reductions are found in malaria, virus pneumonia, virus hepatitis, and some lipidoses.

### Automatic Methods

### Coulter Counter, Model Z

*Principle.* As described on page 63.

### Reagents and Apparatus

1. Model Z Coulter Counter

2. EDTA or heparinized blood

3. White cell diluent: Saponin, in a dilution of 1:10,000, is added to filtered normal saline, or commercial stromatalyzing agents can be obtained and added to filtered normal saline.

4. Sahli pipet (±1%)—0.02 ml.

*Method*₁

1. A 1:500 dilution of whole blood is made by adding 0.02 ml of blood to 10 ml of white cell diluent.

2. Proceed as in steps 3 to 6 for red cell counts (p. 65).

*Notes*

1. An alternative method of hemolyzing the red cells is to make the 1:500 dilution of blood in filtered normal saline. Immediately prior to estimation, 1 drop of commercially obtained stromatalyzing agent is added to the dilution. Stromatalyzing agents should not be added more than two dilution samples at any one time.

2. Do not breathe saponin dust. If it comes into contact with the skin, quickly wash the area with copious volumes of water.

3. High concentrations of saponin speed the destruction of the red cell stroma but reduce the time before white count loss is noted. Stromatolysis may require 1 to 4 minutes, depending on red cell concentration and temperature. White cell destruction should not occur in less than 30 minutes.

4. Nucleated red cells are not destroyed by saponin and are included in the total white count, but platelets are destroyed, eliminating the possibility of large platelets or platelet clumps being counted.

5. Additional notes on the care and use of the instrument can be found on page 65.

**Coulter Counter, Models (see p. 50)**

**Hemalog 8 (see p. 57)**

*Normal Values*

| | |
|---|---|
| Adults | 3800-10,500/cu mm |
| Infants | 9,000-38,000/cu mm |
| Age: 1 week | 5,000-21,000/cu mm |
| 1 year | 5,000-12,000/cu mm |
| 4 years | 5,000-10,000/cu mm |

## IDENTIFICATION OF HEMOPOIETIC CELLS

The teaching of cellular morphology is one of the more difficult assignments undertaken. One technique is to instruct the student to "dissect the cell with his eyes" and to describe what he sees, beginning with the cell size and working inward to finish with a description of the cellular nucleus.

Often a student, when asked the name of a particular cell, will guess, but, if he is drilled in always describing the cell, he will frequently eliminate certain possibilities and arrive at the correct or most correct solution by a process of elimination.

## White Cell Series

### Myeloblast

*Size.* Two to three times that of a mature red cell (i.e., 14 to 21 $\mu$).

*Outline.* Regular.

*Cytoplasm.* Occupies 10 to 15% of the total cell area. Stains deeply basophilic by Romanowsky stains. No granules are present.

*Nucleus.* Round in shape, having a characteristic reticular network. No chromatin aggregations are normally present, but 2 to 6 nucleoli are usually seen. The nuclear membrane is smooth and even in outline. There is no condensation of chromatin seen near its inner surface as is frequently found in lymphoblasts.

*Main Points of Recognition.* The differentiation is mainly based on the number and distribution of the accompanying cells. Micromyeloblasts are often mistaken for lymphoblasts, the distinguishing feature between these two cells being that the myeloblast commonly has 4 nucleoli, whereas the lymphoblast has 1 to 2.

### Promyelocyte

*Size.* Three to four times that of a mature red cell (i.e., 21 to 28 $\mu$).

*Outline.* Regular.

*Cytoplasm.* Less basophilic than in the myeloblast, often with purple inclusion granules. The total cytoplasm area occupies 20 to 30% of the cell.

*Nucleus.* Round in outline. Nucleoli may still be seen in the early cell.

*Main Points of Recognition.* This cell is larger than its precursor and may show some faint myeloid cytoplasmic granulation. The nucleus may often have faint nucleoli still present.

### Myelocyte

*Size.* Up to twice the size of a mature red cell (i.e., 7 to 14 $\mu$).

*Outline.* Regular.

*Cytoplasm.* Stains pinkish blue with the Romanowsky stains and contains coarse granules. The total area occupies between 25 and 40% of the cell.

*Nucleus.* The outline is regular and occasinally indented. The size of the nucleus is reduced in comparison to that of the promyelocyte and is often asymmetrically placed in the cytoplasm. Some chromatin aggregates are seen.

*Main Points of Recognition.* Typical features are the absence of the nucleoli, the increased cytoplasm—nucleus ratio and the presence of typical coarse granulation.

### Neutrophil Myelocyte

The same general characteristics prevail, except that the granules stain red-blue with the Romanowsky dyes.

### Eosinophil Myelocyte

In this cell, the granules appear as large, spherical orange-brown bodies, more numerous than in the neutrophilic cell, and often mixed with neutrophilic granules.

### Basophil Myelocyte

This cell is generally smaller than the other myelocytes, and the granules less numerous, but larger and more prominent. They stain a deep blue-black with the Romanowsky dyes, making the cell typical in appearance.

### Neutrophilic Metamyelocyte

*Size.* Smaller than the myelocyte (i.e., 7 to 10 $\mu$).

*Outline.* Regular.

*Cytoplasm.* Stains pink-blue with the Romanowsky dyes and occupies 50% to 70% of the cell. Characteristic granulation is present, depending on the lineage of the cell.

*Nucleus.* Typically kidney shaped, but may be only slightly indented. The chromatin structure is more pyknotic than in the myelocyte stage, and no nucleoli are present.

*Main Points of Recognition.* The shape of the nucleus is typical of this stage of maturation of the myeloid cells.

### Neutrophilic Band

*Size.* One to one and one-half times that of a mature red cell (i.e., 7 to 10 $\mu$).

*Outline.* Regular.

*Cytoplasm.* Abundant. Stains pinkish blue with the Romanowsky dyes. A small amount of fine granulation is seen.

*Nucleus.* May be band shaped or deeply indented, with or without constrictions forming rudimentary lobes. For a cell to be classified at this stage of maturation, the nucleus should show a *band* of chromatin connecting the nuclear lobes. If a *filament* is present, the cell is classified as a polymorphonuclear cell.

### Polymorphonuclear Neutrophil

*Size.* One to one and one-half times that of a mature red cell (i.e., 7 to 10 $\mu$).

*Outline.* Regular.

*Cytoplasm.* As in the neutrophilic band.

*Nucleus.* Lumpy, compact chromatin arranged in segments, connected by short bridges of chromatin or by elongated threads. No nucleoli are present.

### Polymorphonuclear Eosinophil

*Size.* One to one and one-half times that of a mature red cell (i.e, 7 to 10 $\mu$).

*Outline.* Regular.

*Cytoplasm.* Abundant. Stains pinkish red with the Romanowsky dyes. A moderate number of coarse red granules are present.

*Nucleus.* Similar to that of the neutrophil.

### Polymorphonuclear Basophil

*Size.* One to one and one-half times that of a mature red cell (i.e., 7 to 10 $\mu$).

*Outline.* Regular.

*Cytoplasm.* Similar to that of the neutrophil, but contains large basophilic-staining granules.

*Nucleus.* Simialr to that of the neutrophil, but normally only 2 or 3 lobes are found.

### Lymphoblast

*Size.* Similar to that of the myeloblast. Microlymphoblasts are not found.

*Outline.* Regular.

*Cytoplasm.* Similar to that of the myeloblast.

*Nucleus.* Similar to that of the myeloblast, with the addition of a slightly coarser reticulum. One or two scanty nucleoli are present, being more prominent than in the myeloblast, and there is often a coarse reticulum present.

*Main Points of Recognition.* This cell is difficult to distinguish from other blast cells. The number of nucleoli and the relative size of the cell, together with the type of accompanying cell, should all be taken into consideration.

### Prolymphocyte

*Size.* Two to three times that of a mature red cell (i.e., 15 to 21 $\mu$).

*Shape.* Round.

*Outline.* Regular.

*Cytoplasm.* Occupies 20 to 25% of the cell and strains basophilic with Romanowsky dyes Scanty azurophilic granules occasionally are present.

*Nucleus.* Appears coarser than that of the lymphoblast and may contain nucleoli or nuclear remnants.

*Main Points of Recognition.* The increased volume of cytoplasm (decreased nuclear—cytoplasmic ratio) and the presence of occasional azurophilic granules provide a fine distinction between this cell and the lymphoblast.

### Large Lymphocyte

*Size.* Up to twice that of a mature red cell (i.e., 7 to 14 $\mu$).

*Outline.* Regular.

*Cytoplasm.* Occupies approximately 30% to 40% of the cell and stains a hyaline blue with the Romanowsky dyes. Small numbers of minute azurophilic granules may be present.

*Nucleus.* Large round structure, sometimes eccentrically placed, staining intensely and showing coarse reticulin masses and chromatin aggregation. Nucleoli are rarely seen.

*Main Points of Recognition.* The clear, pale blue cytoplasm and the lumpy nucleus differentiate this cell from the monocytic series.

### Small Lymphocyte

*Size.* Approximately that of a mature red cell (i.e., 6.8 to 7.3 $\mu$).

*Outline.* Regular.

*Cytoplasm.* Little is seen. Normally, a small rim of cytoplasm is visible at the periphery of the cell, staining pale blue, and often containing azurophilic granules.

*Nucleus.* Occupies almost the complete cell. It stains intensely and contains many chromatin aggregations, thus appearing irregularly dense.

*Main Points of Recognition.* This cell may be confused with the intermediate or early normoblast. The main difference is the extremely scanty cytoplasm.

### Atypical Mononuclear Cells (Reactive Lymphocytes)

*Size.* Two to three times that of a mature red cell (i.e. 14 to 21 $\mu$).

*Shape.* Round.

*Outline.* Regular.

*Cytoplasm.* Occupies between 20 and 50% of the cell and stains a muddy basophilic blue with Romanowsky stains. There is often a wide perinuclear halo surrounding the nucleus and no granules are usually visible. Frequently the cytoplasm stains more intensely at the cellular periphery than elsewhere and exhibits a foamy vacuolated structure.

*Nucleus.* This may be oval, kidney shaped, or slightly lobular. The nuclear chromatin forms a coarse network of strands and aggregates and is described as a "Swiss-cheese" form.

*Main Points of Recognition.* The characteristic foamy cytoplasm having a basophilic periphery is an important morphological feature of this cell.

### Monoblast

*Size.* Two to three times that of a mature red cell (i.e., 14 to 21 $\mu$).

*Outline.* Regular.

*Cytoplasm.* Similar in appearance to that of the myeloblast, occupying between 20 and 30% of the total cell area.

*Nucleus.* Basophilic, showing irregular chromatin patterns, with 2 to 6 nucleoli.

*Main Points of Recognition.* In the early stages, this cell is indistinguishable from other blast cells. The main point of differentiation is in the number and distribution of accompanying cells.

## Monocyte

*Size.* Two to three times that of a mature red cell (i.e., 14 to 21 $\mu$).

*Shape.* Round and sometimes oval.

*Outline.* Regular.

*Cytoplasm.* Occupies 50 to 60% of the cell and has a dull blue "ground glass" appearance when stained by the Romanowsky dyes. Small, irregularly distributed areas of dense azurophilic granules are seen and occasionally larger vacuoles are present.

*Nucleus.* This varies in shape from a round regular outline to the more familiar indented or horseshoe-shaped structure. The chromatin appearance is open and loose. There is a sharp segregation of chromatin and parachromatin, the chromatin being distributed in a linear arrangement of delicate strands, giving the nucleus a stringy appearance. The nuclear membrane is delicate but clear. No nucleoli are seen.

*Main Points of Recognition.* Typical features are the characteristic ground-glass cytoplasm and the indented nucleus.

## Plasma Cell

*Size.* Up to twice that of a mature red cell (i.e., 7 to 14 $\mu$).

*Shape.* Oval.

*Outline.* Regular.

*Cytoplasm.* Intensely basophilic and foamy in appearance. Occasionally, scanty acidophilic granules are seen (Russell bodies). The cytoplasm occupies 30 to 40% of the total cell area.

*Nucleus.* Eccentrically placed, showing typical "cartwheel" chromatin structure. No nucleoli are seen.

*Main Points of Recognition.* The shape of the cell with basophilic cytoplasm and eccentric nucleus is typical.

## Red Cell Series (Normocytic)

### Rubriblast (Pronormoblast)

*Size.* Two to three times that of a mature red cell (i.e., 14 to 21 $\mu$).

*Outline.* Irregular.

*Cytoplasm.* Basophilic and homogeneous in appearance. No granules are present.

*Nucleus.* Oval or round in shape, occupying 85 to 90% of the cell. The nucleus stains irregularly, exhibiting chromatin aggregation. It is surrounded by a thin halo that is sometimes difficult to see. Normally, 1 to 4 nucleoli are present, which are often and hard to see.

*Main Points of Recognition.* The general size and shape of the cell are similar to those of other blast cells, but the cell differs in its nuclear characteristics. The nucleus is smaller and the staining characteristics are more pronounced.

### Prorubricyte (Early Normoblast)

*Size.* Slightly smaller than its precursor, the pronormoblast (i.e, 12 to 18 $\mu$).

*Outline.* Similar to that of the pronormoblast.

*Cytoplasm.* More abundant and less basophilic than that of the pronormoblast, occupying 60 to 70% of the cell. No granules are present.

*Nucleus.* Prominent. Deeply staining chromatin bands are evident, often in a cartwheel arrangement. Nucleoli are sometimes present.

*Main Points of Recognition.* The typical coarse chromatin arrangement of the nucleus with the abundant basophilic cytoplasm typifies this cell.

### Rubricyte (Intermediate Normoblast)

*Size.* Up to twice that of a mature red cell (i.e., 7 to 14 $\mu$).

*Outline.* Irregular.

*Cytoplasm.* Polychromatic. More abundant in relation to the cell size than in the prorubricyte.

*Nucleus.* Reduced in size, with deeply basophilic chromatin aggregation.

*Main Points of Recognition.* Faint purple-blue polychromatic cytoplasm, differentiating it from its precursor cell.

## Metarubricyte (Late Normoblast)

*Size.* Slightly larger than the mature red cell (i.e., 7 to 10 $\mu$).

*Outline.* Regular.

*Cytoplasm.* Hemoglobinized, and abundant and occupying 50 to 80% of the cell.

*Nucleus.* Pyknotic in character. Stains uniformly with the Romanowsky dyes. Occasionally eccentrically placed.

## Reticulocyte

This cell stains as a mature red cell with the Romanowsky dyes. It can be differentiated only by staining by a supravital technique. Using this method, the reticulocyte appears slightly larger than a mature red cell, containing, within its cellular membrane, numerous granules and often a network of reticular material

### *Megaloblastic Series*

## Promegaloblast

*Size.* Three to four times that of a mature red cell (i.e., 21 to 28 $\mu$).

*Outline.* Irregular.

*Cytoplasm.* Varies from a deeply basophilic to a purple-blue when stained with the Romanowsky dyes. No granules are present.

*Nucleus.* Usually occupies 60 to 70% of the cell area, showing a regular chromatin network. 3 to 6 nucleoli are present.

## Early Megaloblast (Basophilic Megaloblast)

*Size.* Two and one-half to three and one-half times that of a mature red cell (i.e., 18 to 26 $\mu$).

*Outline.* Regular.

*Cytoplasm.* Increased in volume as compared to its precursor cell. Basophilic in character with no granules present.

*Nucleus.* This shows a coarse reticular structure. There are no nucleoli, but a fine halo is present around the external surface of the nucleus.

*Main Points of Recognition.* The coarse reticular nucleus is the main point of differentiation between this cell and the prorubricyte. The cytoplasm is more hemoglobinized and there is a lower nuclear cyto-plasmic ratio.

### Intermediate Megaloblast (Polychromatic Megaloblast)

*Size.* Up to twice that of a mature red cell (i.e., 10 to 14 $\mu$).

*Outline.* Irregular.

*Cytoplasm.* Increased in volume in comparison to that of the early megaloblast. Basophilia decreasing and moderate hemoglobinization present.

*Nucleus.* Shows the characteristic cartwheel coarse chromatin structure. No nucleoli are seen.

*Main Points of Recognition.* The coarse open nucleus differentiates this megaloblastic cell from the corresponding normoblatic cell. The hemoglobinization is more complete than in the rubricyute and the nuclear cytoplasmic ratio is reduced.

### Late Megaloblast (Orthochromatic Megaloblast)

*Size.* Similar to that of the intermediate megaloblast.

*Outline.* Regular.

*Cytoplasm.* Hemoglobinized and abundant.

*Nucleus.* Small and densely stained, often homogeneous in appearance. Sometimes a fine reticulum is present.

*Main Points of Recognition.* The size of the cell is the characteristic feature.

### *Platelet Series*
### Megakaryoblast

*Size.* Three to seven times that of a mature red cell (i.e., 21 to 50 $\mu$).

*Outline.* Irregular.

*Cytoplasm.* Appears moderately basophilic. No granules are present.

*Nucleus.* Large, indented and irregular in shape, occupying 70% to 80% of the total cell area. Occasionally 1 or 2 small indistinct nucleoli are present.

*Main Points of Recognition.* The presence of nucleoli distinguishes this cell from the promegakaryocyte.

### Promegakaryocyte

*Size.* Three to twelve times that of a mature red cell (i.e., 20 to 80 $\mu$).

*Outline.* Irregular.

*Cytoplasm.* Appears basophilic, although scattered azurophilic granulation is present, especially in the perinuclear zone.

*Nucleus.* Approximately the same size as that of the megakaryoblast. It may still possess vestigial nucleoli, exhibit an open reticular chromatin structure, and possess a tendency to be multilobulated.

## Megakaryocyte

*Size.* Ten to fifteen times that of the mature red cell (i.e., 70 to 100 $\mu$).

*Outline.* Irregular.

*Cytoplasm.* Abundant, appearing slightly basophilic and containing numerous azurophilic pseudopodia and granules.

*Nucleus.* Lobulated and irregular in shape, staining poorly with the Romanowsky dyes. Often chromatin aggregation is present.

*Main Points of Recognition.* This cell is the largest element in the blood, and has been confused with an osteoclast. The basic morphological difference is in the granular cytoplasm and the lobulated nucleus, the osteoclast having multiple separate nuclei.

## Blood Platelet

*Size.* 2 to 3 $\mu$.

*Outline.* Irregular.

*Cytoplasm.* Blue, with the occasional azurophilic granules.

*Nucleus.* Nil.

*Main Points of Recognition.* This element is the smallest found in the blood.

## DIFFERENTIAL CELL COUNT

### *Preparation of Blood Smears*

## Coverslip Method

1. Two clean grease-free coverslips are held by their edges, one in each hand.

2. A small drop of capillary or venous blood is touched to one coverslip and the other is immediately superimposed diagonally on top.

3. As the blood spreads by capillary attraction between the

coverslips, they are drawn smoothly apart by sliding in the horizontal plane.

**Slide Method**

1. Place a drop of blood approximately 2 mm in diameter at one end of a clean grease-free slide.

2. A smooth spreader slide is placed at 40° angle, touching the drop of blood.

3. As the blood spreads along the edge of the spreader slide, the spreader is evenly and quickly pushed away from the drop.

The value of differential white counts depends on the quality of the smear made and its staining. The quality of smear depends on the following:

a. Only a moderate sized drop of blood should be used.

b. The edge of the spreader should be smooth.

c. Slides should be clean and free from grease and fingermarks.

d. Films should be dried in the air as quickly as possible.

e. The angle of the spreader should be approximately 40°. If the angle is greater than this, a think film is produced. If the angle is smaller, a thick film is produced.

f. The time taken to spread the film. If made quickly, the result will be a thin film, but if the film is spread slowly, a thick smear is produced.

### *Criteria for Good Films*
1. Films of reasonable thickness.
2. Smooth appearance.
3. The absence of a "tail."
4. Clear labeling with patient's name and date.
5. Margin.

If the smears are made too thin, or if a rough-edged spreader is used, many of the leukocytes become aggregated at the edges and in the tail.

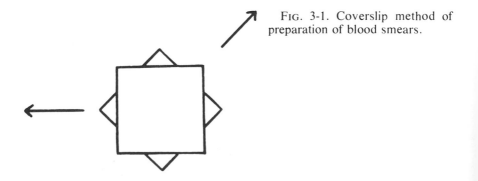

Fig. 3-1. Coverslip method of preparation of blood smears.

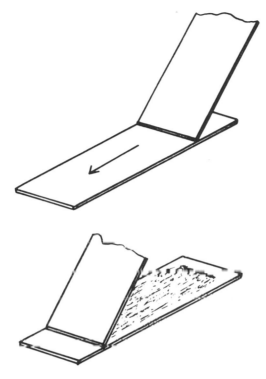

Fig. 3-2. Slide method of preparation of blood smears.

Moreover, polymorphonuclear neutrophils and monocytes predominate at the margins, tail and lymphocytes in the middle of the smear.

One of the problems of the differential white count is to overcome these distributions. Two main methods have been advocated, the longitudinal and the battlement methods.

### Longitudinal Method

The cells are counted in strips running from the head to the tail of the smear. At least three strips should be counted and the percentages calculated from the figures obtained. At least 200 cells should be recorded.

### Battlement Method

The cells in two microscopic fields along the edge of the smear are counted. Those cells in the immediate four fields toward the center, in two fields parallel to the edge, and in four fields toward the edge are counted. The process is repeated until 200 cells are recorded.

### Refinements of the Differential Count

The nucleus of the mature neutrophil is divided irregularly into lobes, which are joined together by 5 chromatin filaments or by broad bands of nuclear material. This lobulation gives an indication as to the cell age, the youngest cells having nuclei shaped like the letter "c" whereas those of the older cells are lobulated, with as many as 6 lobes to each cell.

## Arneth-Cooke Count

Arneth divided the neutrophils into five main groups and then subdivided the group further, depending on their nuclear shape. The technique proved so complicated that it was discontinued in favor of Cooke's modification.

This groups the cells into five areas according to the number of filamentous chromatin threads present. Group I includes all cells in which the nucleus is either unlobed or, if lobed, is joined by a band of definite chromatin. Group II contains those cells having one filament; Groups III, IV and V have 2, 3 and 4 filaments, respectively.

*Method.* One hundred neutrophils are counted and divided into their respective groups.

### Calculation

1. An index can be calculated by adding the totals of Group I and Group II. If this figure exceeds 45, a "shift to the left" is present.

2. Alternatively, if the totals of Group I, Group II and half of Group III are added, the marker figure is 60.

### Normal Values (Arneth-Cooke Count)

Group I ......................................... 10-12%
Group II ........................................ 25-30%
Group III ....................................... 47-53%
Group IV ....................................... 16-19%
Group V ........................................ 2- 3%

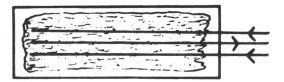

FIG. 3-3. Longitudinal method of counting cells in differential white cell counts.

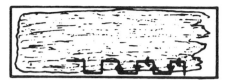

Fig. 3-4. Battlement method of counting cells in differential white cell counts.

## Notes

1. Infections show a shift to the left. The number of monolobed or bilobed cells is increased at the expense of the multilobed. This occurs also in toxemias and after hemorrhage.

2. In some institutions, the differential white count is expressed both as a percentage of 100 cells counted and in relative terms of the number of cells per cu mm of blood. Thus, if there are 50% lymphocytes counted in the differential count, and the total white cell count is 5,000 per cu mm, the relative lymphocyte count is 50% of 5,000 or 2,500 cells per cu mm.

### Calculation of Absolute Differential Count

$$\text{Absolute Differential Cell Count} = \frac{\text{Total White Cell Count}}{100} \times \text{percentage of cells estimated by differential}$$

### Normal Values (Differential White Cell Count)

| ADULTS | % | ABSOLUTE NUMBERS |
|---|---|---|
| Neutrophils ..................... | 40–80 | 1600–88 |
| Bands .......................... | 0–6 | 0–650 |
| Eosinophils ..................... | 1–7 | 40–770 |
| Basophils ....................... | 0–1 | 0–100 |
| Monocytes ...................... | 2–11 | 200–1200 |
| Lymphocytes ................... | 15–50 | 600–5500 |

| AGE          CHILDREN | NEUTROPHILS (%) | LYMPHOCYTES (%) |
|---|---|---|
| Birth ........................... | 60 | 30 |
| 10 days ......................... | 40 | 60 |
| 4–6 months ..................... | 30 | 50 |
| 4 years ......................... | 40 | 40 |
| 6 years ......................... | 60 | 30 |

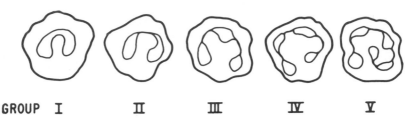

GROUP  I        II        III        IV        V

FIG. 3-5. Arneth-Cooke count.

## AUTOMATED WHITE CELL DIFFERENTIAL COUNTS
## PATTERN RECOGNITION INSTRUMENTS

### LARC*

*Principle.* The basic principle of operation is digital image processing. Using morphological features similar to those taught in hematology training, the apparatus recognizes the normal adult leukocytes found in the peripheral blood. The analyzer distinguishes between band and segmented neutrophils and also identifies abnormal cells and recalls these for the operator's review at the end of the count.

The LARC analyzer is an automated microscope operated by a small digital computer which also performs cell recognition. Its other major function is information output through visual displays. The automated microscope is built around a slide-holding stage, driven by step motors. A blood smear is placed in the holder and oil is applied to the smear. Once oiled, the slide is brought into initial focus manually, but focus is then maintained automatically.

The automatic acquisition of leukocytes is initiated when the technologist commands the apparatus to make a differential count. Starting from a home position, the stage translates in a comblike pattern. When a leukocyte is detected in the field, the stage centers the cell for the TV camera. Once a cell is read into the computer, the stage returns to a center line and renews its comblike pattern search.

The results are displayed through a television console which briefly shows the operator each cell being classified. The final results are presented in a printout form. The LARC analyzer can count any number of cells designated by the technologist. However, 100 cell counts taking approximately 2 minutes (on normal blood smears) are most often used. The LARC analyzer does not accept conventionally prepared wedge-bound smears, since such preparations are not uniformly monocellular, and have areas in which the cells are difficult to differentiate. Blood

---

* Corning Scientific Instruments. Medfield, Mass.

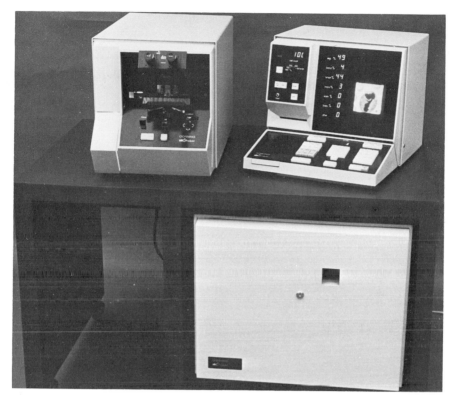

Fig. 3-6. The LARC pattern recognition apparatus. (Courtesy of Corning Scientific Instruments)

smears suitable for use by the LARC can be made by a Corning Slide Spinner, which produces a monocellular blood smear.

A second pattern recognition apparatus, the Hematrak* employs similar principles to the LARC. The major difference in this analyzer is its use of conventional wedge-made blood smears. To allow for consistency in the quality of the smears the manufacturer recommends the use of the Hemaprep* which automatically prepares two standardized conventional wedge-made smears at a time.

### Advantages of Pattern Recognition

1. The sytem offers consistency in screening large normal work loads and speed of operation (25/hour).

2. The LARC classified is an apparatus and is not subject to fatigue or to human error.

---

* Geometric Data Corporation, Wayne, Pa.

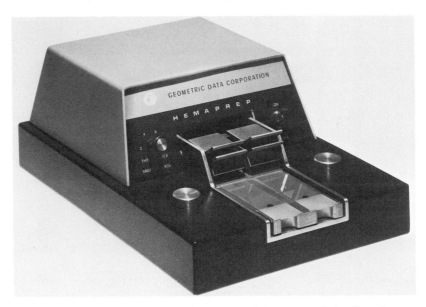

FIG. 3-7. The Hemaprep. (Courtesy of Geometric Data Corp.)

3. Accuracy and precision are as good as a highly skilled morphologist.

### Disadvantages of Pattern Recognition

1. Since the LARC classifier is an integrated system it will not classify slides prepared by the conventional wedge or coverslip technique. The slides must be stained as in the LARC stainer and with LARC stain in order for the cells to be correctly classified.

2. Blood must be spun and fixed within 6 hours.

3. Abnormal cells are placed in the "other" category and must be reviewed by the technologist.

## The LARC Spinner

*Principle.* In this apparatus, a plateau holds a slide in a horizontal plane perpendicular to the shaft of a motor. A low-inertia high torque meter is used to produce a rapid acceleration to the desired spinning speed (5,000 rpm) and a rapid stop (0.25 seconds).

The technologist places a slide on the platen, wets the center of the slides with approximately 0.2 ml of anticoagulated blood and closes the lid. This activates the motor.

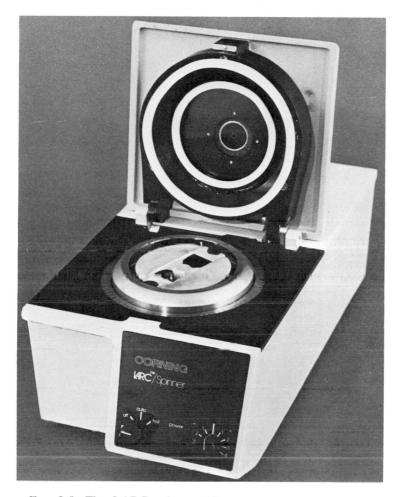

FIG. 3-8. The LARC spinner. (Courtesy of Corning Scientific Instruments)

### Advantages

1. A monolayer is found covering the entire slide surface.
2. The distribution of leukocytes by cell type is more uniform than a wedge preparation.
3. Cell morphology is preserved on the slide.
4. The apparatus is automatic and is not subject to the variations found in manual methods.

### Disadvantages

1. If the slides are dirty, the cells do not adequately adhere to the glass.

2. Hyperlipemic at foaming blood can produce a nonusable starburst pattern.

3. The volume of blood used to flood the slide must exceed 0.15 to 0.2ml. This volume ensures that the monolayer covers the slide.

4. Fresh EDTA anticoagulated blood less than 6 hours old, must be used.

5. Once applied to the slide, the pool of blood must be spun immediately to avoid settling out of the leukocytes and platelets and possible drying around the perimeter which will disrupt the monolayer.

## Flow-through Cytochemical Instrument Hemalog-D*

*Principle.* The Hemalog-D is a multisegmental autoanalyzer which separates, stains, and sizes 30,000 leukocytes in 55 seconds. Designed as a modular unit, it is composed of individual channels, each with its own manifold, flow cell, and photometric counting station.

Leukocytes contain a number of enzymes which are utilized in cytochemical staining and are characteristic of individual cell types. In each channel of the instrument, a cell type is uniquely stained and passed through a photometric counting system, which also determines the cell size. Two optical sensors monitor the flow cell detection slit in each channel. One measures the light absorption resulting from passage of a cell of given size. The other measures light absorption resulting from passage of a cell taking up a given amount of stain.

The specific cytochemistries involved are as follows:

*Basophils.* Alcian blue combines with the heparin of the cell to produce a blue-green color within the cell. Formalin is added to fix the leukocytes and propylene glycol to match the refractive index of the red cell ghosts.

*Monocytes.* In this channel, the cells are mixed with precooled formalin. The stream is then reacted with alpha naphthol butyrate, a substrate for lipase present in monocytes. Diazotized basic fuchsin is added, and combines with the free alpha naphthol released by lipase activity to form a red precipitate within the cells.

*Neutrophils and Eosinophils.* In this stream, the blood sample is mixed with precooled formalin. Following fixation of the leukocytes, the sample passes through a heating coil to inactive interfering enzymes such as catalase. The stream is then cooled again in a jacketed coil, mixed with acetic acid, and reheated with a mixture of hydrogen perioxide and 4-chloro-1-naphthol to stain the peroxidase-positive granules of the neutrophils and eosinophils. Finally, propylene glycol is added to neutralize the refraction of the red cell ghosts. (At the pH of

---

*Technicon Instruments Corporation. Tarrytown, N.Y.

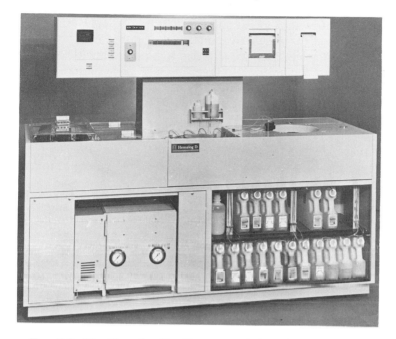

FIG. 3-9. The Hemalog-D. (Courtesy of Technicon Instruments Corp.)

this reaction, pH 3.2, eosinophils are stained more intensely than the neutrophils and can be photo-optically separated.)

*Lymphocytes.* Lymphocytes are not stained, but are measured by an electronic sizing method.

### Differences Between Pattern Recognition and Cytochemistry Flow-through Automated Differentials

1. Pattern recognition apparatus analyzes the peripheral blood smear in a conventional morphological manner, while cytochemical methods use enzymatic cell markers to differentiate the cells.

2. Pattern recognition techniques are limited similarly to manual counts, in that the number of cells counted is frequently 100 or 200 per test. Counting larger numbers of cells imposes a greater delay, and the method loses some of its advantages over manual methods. The cytochemical technique counts 30,000 cells per blood sample, producing greater precision than that achieved by pattern recognition or by manual methods. Differentiated counts on leukopenic blood samples are frequently difficult to carry out by pattern recognition, but may be deter-

mined by the Hemalog-D on counts as low as 500/mm$^3$ (3,000 cells are counted on blood samples between 500-4,000 cells/mm$^3$).

3. EDTA anticoagulated whole blood is used in the Hemalog-D, while specially prepared blood smears are used in cell pattern recognition instruments.

4. The Hemalog-D does not differentiate immature cells by type, but classifies them as LUC (Large Unclassified Cells). Pattern recognition instruments can differentiate immature cells, and possess the ability to recall difficult cells to be reexamined manually.

5. The cytochemical flow-through principle is a fully automated instrument allowing 60 different blood samples to be processed in 1 hour, while the pattern recognition apparatus are not fully automated but merely speed up the manual procedure. (Note: Although the manufacturers of pattern recognition counters state that it takes approximately 60-90 seconds to process a count, this time does not take into account the total "clean-bench-to-clean-bench" time needed, which includes smear preparation and manual reexamination of difficult cells.)

## STAINS

### Romanowsky Stains

These stains depend for their action on compounds formed by the interaction of methylene blue and eosin. The difference between the various stains is mainly in the proportion of the reagents and in the methods of preparation. Most Romanowsky stains are of no value if water is present in the alcohol, because the neutral dyes are then precipitated from solution, or if acetone is an impurity of the alcohol. The mode of action probably depends on partial dissociation of the components after dilution with buffered water. Intensity of staining varies with the extent of dilution with buffered water. Intensity of staining varies with the extent of dilution and with the nature and quality of the derived dyes. The eosin acts as both stain and mordant.

### Wright's Stains

#### *Preparation*
1. 0.2 g of pure Wright's stain is added to 100 ml of anhydrous acetone-free methyl alcohol.

2. The solution is boiled on an electric plate at 60°C until the stain is in solution, allowed to cool and filtered through a dry filter paper into a dry flask. The stain should be kept in a well-stoppered bottle and away from acetone and acids.

### Method of Use

1. The blood smears are fixed by adding 1 volume of the undiluted stain to the slide for 1 minute.

2. Two to three volumes of buffered distilled water is added to the slide (pH 6.4), with care taken to avoid washing off the stain.

3. The diluted stain is mixed either by gently blowing a stream of air on the slide, or by repeatedly sucking the dilution up and down in a Pasteur pipet.

4. Leave the diluted stain for 5 to 10 minutes, determining the exact time by trial and error.

5. The stain is washed off the slide with a stream of distilled water, allowing the water to differentiate the smear for 1 to 2 minutes, or until the edges of the smear become faintly pink. Drain the water from the slide, and allow it to dry in the air. Do not blot the slides; this can cause lint and surface scratches to mar the blood smear.

6. Occasionally it is necessary to wipe the underside of the slide with a damp tissue to remove concentrated stain.

## Giemsa Stain

### Preparation

1. 1 g of powdered stain is added to 66 ml of glycerol, and the solution boiled on an electric plate at 60°C for 2 hours.

2. 66 ml of pure acetone-free methyl alcohol is slowly added and the solution mixed, allowed to stand for 7 to 14 days in direct daylight to ripen, and filtered before use.

### Method of Use

1. The blood smears are fixed by placing in acetone-free methyl alcohol for 1 to 2 minutes, and one volume of Giemsa stain is diluted with 9 volumes of buffered distilled water (pH 6.8).

2. The diluted stain is either added on the slide, or the slide is immersed in a Coplin jar full of the stain. Leave for between 5 and 10 minutes.

3. Wash off the stain with a stream of distilled water, and differentiate as in the Wright's staining procedure.

4. The water is drained from the slide, which is then allowed to dry in air.

## May-Grünwald's Stain

### Preparation

1. 0.25 g of May-Grünwald stain is dissolved in 100 ml of pure acetone-free methyl alcohol by heating the mixture to 60°C on an electric

hot plate. The solution is filtered through dry filter paper into a dry flask and stoppered.

### Jenner's Stain

*Preparation.* This stain is prepared exactly as in the May-Grünwald technique.

### May-Grünwald-Giemsa or Jenner-Giemsa Stain

*Preparation.* 100 ml of stock May-Grünwald or Jenner stain is diluted with 150 ml of buffered distilled water (pH 6.8); 100 ml of the stock Giemsa stain is then diluted with 400 ml of the same buffered distilled water.

#### Method of Use
1. Fix the blood smear by placing in acetone-free methyl alcohol for 5 minutes.
2. The diluted May-Grünwald or Jenner stain is added to the slide, allowed to act for 3 minutes and washed off with a steam of distilled water.
3. The diluted Giemsa stain is then added and allowed to remain for 15 minutes or longer, depending on its maturity.
4. The stain is then washed off with buffered distilled water and the smears are allowed to differentiate for 1 to 2 minutes, or until the edge of the film is a faint pink.
5. Drain the water from the slide and allow it to dry in the air.

### Composition of the Buffer Used to Dilute Romanowsky Stains

1. $M/15$ potassium dihydrogen phosphate. 9.08 g of the anhydrous salt is made up to 1 liter with distilled water.
2. $M/15$ dibasic sodium phosphate. 9.47 g of the anhydrous salt is made up to 1 liter with distilled water.

To prepare a buffered solution of given pH, follow Table 3-1.

TABLE 3-1. Composition of Buffer Solutions.

| pH | POTASSIUM DIHYDROGEN PHOSPHATE (ML) | DIBASIC SODIUM PHOSPHATE (ML) |
|---|---|---|
| 5.2 | 98.2 | 1.8 |
| 6.4 | 73.0 | 27.0 |
| 6.8 | 50.8 | 49.2 |
| 7.2 | 28.0 | 72.0 |

*Notes*

1. Methylene blue on oxidation produces colored compounds termed "azures" which have the ability to combine with eosin. The main difference in the various Romanowsky stains is because of the differences in the preparation of these azures.

2. Nuclear chromatin is acidic and is stained by basic dyes. The neutrophilic cytoplasm of the granulocytes appears pink-violet, being weakly stained by the azure complexes. The eosinophilic granules contain a spermine derivative that has a strong alkaline reaction. These granules stain with the acidic component of the dye.

Conversely, basophilic granules contain heparin, which is an acid ester of a polysaccharide. These granules have an affinity for the basic dye.

**Automatic Slide Stainer***

*Principle.* The slide stainer consists of three elements, a slide conveyer, staining platen and three solution pumps. When a glass slide with a dry blood film is placed at the loading point, it is advanced face down into a position on the staining platen. The leading edge of the slide makes contact with the sensing switch, which activates a cam switch, starting a pump that meters and delivers stain to the capillary space between the blood smear and the platen.

As the stain is delivered through an opening in the platen, it spreads under the surface of the slide. The smear is fixed by the methyl alcohol in the stain. The slide then advances to a position where it triggers a second sensing switch to start the second pump, which delivers buffer and dilutes the film of polychrome methylene blue. The stain and buffer mix as the slide passes over angled baffles. As the slide advances, it triggers a third switch, which starts a third pump delivering a water rinse. The slides are then dried by a stream of warm air at the end of the cycle and are dropped and stacked into a collecting drawer. The apparatus takes approximately 32 minutes to stain 25 slides.

# EOSINOPHILIC COUNTS

*Principle.* Red blood cells are hemolyzed by the diluting fluid and the eosinophils stained with either eosin or phloxine so that they are easily counted in the hemocytometer.

---

* Hema-Tek Slide Stainer, Ames Co., Elkhart, Ind.

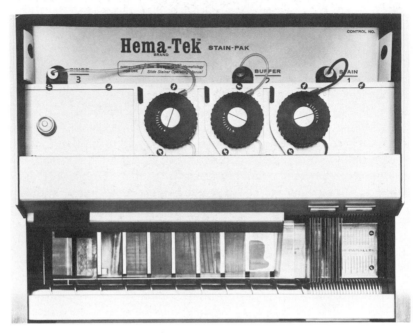

Fig. 3-10. Hema-Tek slide stainer, showing stain, buffer and rinse modules, and slides being stained. (Courtesy Ames Co., Elkhart, Ind.)

### Reagents and Apparatus

1. Diluting Fluids:

   a. *Discombe's modification of Dunger's fluid:*

   | | |
   |---|---|
   | Aqueous eosin | 0.1 g |
   | Acetone | 10.0 ml |
   | Distilled water | 90.0 ml |

   b. *Randolph's fluid:*

   | | |
   |---|---|
   | Phloxine | 0.1 g |
   | 1% Calcium chloride | 100 ml |

   An equal volume of propylene glycol is added to the stock solution before use.

   c. *Manner's fluid:*

   | | |
   |---|---|
   | Urea | 50.0 g |
   | Phloxine | 0.1 g |
   | Trisodium citrate | 0.6 g |
   | Distilled water | 100.0 ml |

   d. *Pilot's fluid:*

   | | |
   |---|---|
   | Phloxine | 0.2 g |
   | 25% Sodium carbonate | 0.4 ml |

Propylene glycerol . . . . . . . . . . . . . . . . . . . . . . . . 50 ml
Distilled water . . . . . . . . . . . . . . . . . . . . . . . . . . . .50 ml
2. White cell Thoma pipet
3. Fuchs-Rosenthal hemocytometer

### Method

1. Anticoagulated or capillary blood is pipeted to the 0.5 mark on the Thoma pipet and the external surface of the pipet is wiped clean of blood.
2. The diluting fluid is taken to the 11 mark, taking care to avoid the introduction of air bubbles into the bulb of the pipet.
3. Set up the Fuchs-Rosenthal hemocytometer in the same way as the Neubauer chamber is set up for red and white cell counts.
4. Using the 10× objective of the microscope, count the cells seen in the complete ruled area (16 sq mm).

### Calculation

1. The blood is diluted 1:20 as in the total white cell count.
2. The total ruled area is 4 × 4 mm = 16 sq mm. The depth of the chamber is 0.2 mm; thus the total volume of the ruled area is 16 × 0.2 = 3.2 cu mm.
3. If 20 eosinophils are counted in a total volume of 3.2 cu mm, there are 20/3.2 or 6.25 eosinophils in 1 cu mm. But, inasmuch as the original blood is diluted 1:20, the corrected number of eosinophils expressed per cubic millimeter is 20/3.2 × 20 = 125.
4. An abbreviated system of calculating the total eosinophil count is N × 6.25, where N is the number of cells counted.

*Normal.* 40 to 440 per cu mm.

### Notes

1. There is a great variation in the number of circulating eosinophils in health. The lowest counts are found in the morning, the highest at night. Elevated counts are found in tuberculosis, asthma, and other allergic conditions and parasitic infections.
2. Eosinophil counts are occasionally used as an index of adrenocortical activity in the Thorn test. A fasting morning absolute eosinophil count is determined, 25 units of ACTH is given intramuscularly and the eosinophil count repeated 4 hours later.

If there is normal adrenal cortex function, the total eosinophil count is 50% or less of the fasting count.

3. Occasionally, Charcot-Leyden crystals are found in secretions from sites having eosinophils in excess, as in bronchial secretions of asthmatics.

The crystals are derived from the disintegration of eosinophils and can be produced from eosinophilic nucleoprotein by the action of laboratory detergents on concentrations of eosinophils.

## BONE MARROW BIOPSY

This technique is used to diagnose many hematological conditions. It is not necessary to describe the technique, because the biopsy is carried out by a physician and not by a technologist. There are three main methods of obtaining a bone marrow:
1. Needle biopsy
2. Rib biopsy
3. Trephine

The sites for needle biopsy are: the sternum, the iliac crest, the cervical spinal vertebrae, and, in children, the tibia. The technologist is frequently asked to assist in the collection of bone marrow specimens and usually makes the smears and prepares histological blocks. Because the technologist is the first to examine the specimen, the question will often be asked whether marrow has been obtained.

Two criteria in the macroscopic examination of bone marrow smears are:
1. The presence of fat spaces when the slide is held to the light.
2. The presence of bone marrow fragments on the "tail" of the smear.

### *Histological Processing and Staining of Bone Marrow Smears*

In cases in which a complete surgical biopsy has been performed, the following method of processing is recommended.

### Modified Hynes' Method

*Principle.* Tissues are fixed so as to kill the cells instantly and render them as lifelike as possible. After decalcification with a weak acid and embedding with wax, the mercury deposits from the fixative are removed with iodine, which in turn is removed with sodium thiosulfate. The tissue is then overstained with heated Wright's stain diluted in an acidic buffer, differentiated and dehydrated in alcohol.

### *Reagents*
1. *Zenker's fluid:*
   Mercuric chloride ............................ 5 g
   Potassium dichromate ....................... 2.5 g
   Distilled water .......................... to 100 ml

5 ml of glacial acetic acid is added to this solution immediately before use.

2. 5% Formic acid
3. 5% Sodium sulfate
4. *Lugol's iodine:*
   Iodine ........................................ 1 g
   Potassium iodide ............................ 2 g
   Distilled water ......................... to 100 ml
5. 5% sodium thiosulfate
6. Wright's stain
7. Buffered distilled water pH 5.0
8. Methyl alcohol

### Method
1. The smears are fixed in Zenker's fluid or any mercuric fixative for 24 hours and decalcified in 5% formic acid for 24 to 72 hours.

2. The acid is removed by placing the tissue in 5% sodium sulfate or 5% lithium sulfate for 1 to 2 hours, and the biopsy is washed well in running tap water, embedded in paraffin wax and sectioned.

3. Soak the section in xylol for 3 to 5 minutes to remove the wax, and wash in 95% alcohol to remove the xylol.

4. The 95% alcohol is removed by rinsing with distilled water for 5 to 10 seconds, and the mercuric salts are removed by placing the section in Lugol's iodine for 5 minutes.

5. The iodine is taken from the section by placing in 5% sodium thiosulfate for 5 minutes and washing in running tap water for 10 minutes.

6. The section is flooded with a mixture of 1 volume of Wright's stain and 2 volumes of buffered distilled water pH 5.0, and the slide is heated until steam rises. It is allowed to stain for 10 to 15 minutes, then differentiated and dehydrated with absolute methyl alcohol for 10 to 30 seconds.

7. Clear by rinsing in xylol for 30 seconds and mount in a neutral medium.

### Barrett's Method[2]

#### Reagents
1. Fixative:
   Mercuric chloride ......................... 5.0 g
   Potassium dichromate ..................... 2.5 g
   Distilled water .......................... 100.0 ml
   Formalin ................................. 10.0 ml
2. Stains
   *Orange solution:*
   1% Erythoxin .................................... 1
   1% Orange G ..................................... 3
   Distilled water ................................. 2

*Blue solution*

1% Toluidine blue .............................. 1
1% Methylene blue ............................. 2
Distilled water .................................. 17

3. Carazzi's hematoxylin:

Hematoxylin ........................... 0.5 g
Potassium iodate........................ 0.1 g
Potassium aluminum sulfate ............... 25.0 g
Glycerol ............................... 100.0 ml
Distilled water ......................... 400.0 ml

4. Buffer solution I:

13.6% Potassium dihydrogen phosphate ..... 4  ml
Distilled water .......................... 250  ml

5. Buffer solution II:ml N Sodium hydroxide ... 1  ml
Potassium dihydrogen phosphate........... 1  ml
Distilled water ......................... 250  ml

For use, 2 volumes of solution I is added to 1 volume of solution II.

6. 5% Formic acid
7. 5% Sodium sulfate
8. Lugol's iodine (see previous technique)
9. 5% Sodium thiosulfate
10. Acid alcohol:

$$ml$$

Absolute ethyl alcohol ........................... 70
Concentrated hydrochloric acid ..................... 1
Distilled water ................................. 29

*Method*

1. The marrow fragments are treated as in Hynes' method up to step 5, then processed by the following steps.

2. Stain the sections in Carazzi's hematoxylin for 5 minutes and rinse in running tap water for 10 to 15 seconds.

3. Differentiate in 1% acid alcohol for 10 seconds and wash in running tap water for 5 minutes to blue.

4. Place the slide in a moist chamber and flood with a solution containing 0.5 ml of orange solution, 0.5 ml of buffer solution and 1 ml of acetone. Leave for 30 minutes.

5. Rinse in running tap water and stain for 24 hours in a solution containing 0.1 ml of orange solution, 0.1 ml of blue solution, 10 ml of buffer solution and 30 ml of distilled water.

6. Wash in distilled water, dehydrate, clean and mount as in steps 6 and 7 of Hynes' method.

## Staining of Bone Marrow Smears

The smears should be fixed in methyl alcohol as soon as possible. One volume of Wright's stain is mixed with 2 volumes of distilled water pH 6.4, added to the slide and left for 15 to 20 minutes. The smears are differentiated for 1 to 2 minutes, using the same buffered distilled water.

If unsatisfactory results are obtained, variations in the volume of stain and water and in the staining time are recommended. The use of acidic water (pH 6.4) produces the best results.

### *Normal Range for Differential Cell Counts on Bone Marrow Smears*

|  | % |
|---|---|
| Reticulum cells | 0.1–2 |
| Hemocytoblasts | 0.1–1 |
| Myeloblasts | 0.1–3.5 |
| Promyelocytes | 0.5 5 |
| Myelocytes | |
| neutrophil | 5.0–20 |
| eosinophil | 0.1–3 |
| basophil | 0.0–0.5 |
| Metamyelocytes | 10.0–30 |
| Polymorphonuclears | |
| neutrophil | 7–25 |
| eosinophil | 0.2–3 |
| basophil | 0–0.5 |
| Lymphocytes | 5–20 |
| Monocytes | 0–0.2 |
| Megakaryocytes | 0.1–0.5 |
| Plasma cells | 0.1–3.5 |
| Rubriblast | 0.5–5 |
| Prorubricyte | 0–5 |
| Rubricyte | 2–20 |
| Metarubricyte | 2–10 |
| Myeloid-erythroid ratio | 2.5–5.0:1 |

## MORPHOLOGICAL ABNORMALITIES IN WHITE CELLS

### Nuclear Abnormalities

*Hypersegmentation.* The nucleus of a mature polymorphonuclear granulocyte normally contains two to five lobes. In hypersegmented states, the cell often contains six to ten lobes. Such cells are rarely seen in health but are found in the blood in the presence of both a folic acid and a vitamin $B_{12}$ deficiency. When such a cell is formed, it occasionally exhibits a diameter between 16 and 25 $\mu$. It is then termed a Macropolycyte.

***Sex Chromatin Bodies.*** The sex chromatin body present in granulocytes is a small mass adjacent to the nuclear membrane, approximately 1.5 $\mu$ in size. These structures are present in 80 to 90% of the somatic cells of normal females. The appendage is attached to the nucleus of polymorphonuclear neutrophils and eosinophils by a thin chromatin filament. They are also found in band and metamyelocyte stages of maturation. Contradictory opinions have been reported concerning the frequency of the drumsticks in the leukocytes of normal males. Some authorities state that they are never found; others feel that they do occur in small numbers. In females, they are found in 0.2 to 8% of the granulocytes.

***Rieder Cells.*** In leukemia proliferation, there are occasionally found irregularities in the nuclear outline of both myeloblasts and lymphocytes. Normally these cells possess a round or oval nuclear outline, and when the nucleus becomes indented, the cell is termed a Rieder cell. This anomaly is thought to represent asynchronism of nuclear maturation compared to that of the cytoplasm.

### Cytoplasmic Abnormalities

***Alder's Anomaly.*** This hereditary condition is manifested by the presence of nonspecific azurophilic granulation of the cytoplasm of all the leukocytes. Nuclear maturation is normal in such states, and the anomaly has been attributed to a cytoplasmic polysaccharide metabolic defect. When all the leukocytes are affected, it is common to find cells with their nucleic obscured by the dense granulation. The condition is clinically insignificant, but occasionally has been associated with gargoylism.

***Pelger-Hüet Anomaly.*** This state is characterized by decreased segmentation of the granulocytes, condensation of the chromatin in all stages of maturation and normal cytoplasmic maturation. The "shift to the left" takes two distinct morphological forms: the spectacle-cell appearance of the granulocytic nucleus and the "Stödtmeister" form, in which the nucleus is round and regular in outline, similar to that of a mature lymphocyte. The anomaly can be divided into congenital and acquired forms, the defect usually being benign and in a heterozygous state, and in transmitted as a dominant non-sex-linked characteristic.

***Döhle-Amato Bodies.*** These inclusions are round, oval or spindle-shaped structure, 1 $\mu$ to 4 $\mu$ in size. Three or four bodies may be present on the periphery of neutrophilic leukocytes. They stain gray-blue with Romanowsky dyes and are considered to ber part of the vestigial cytoplasm left from earlier developmental cellular stages. The inclusions are found in toxic conditions such as scarlet fever, septicemia, peumonia, burns or measles. Differentiation between Döhle bodies and May-Hegglin bodies may be difficult. Döhle bodies are not permanent structures, while those found in May-Hegglin anomaly are inherited as an autosomal dominant trait.

*May-Hegglin Bodies.* These structures are seen in May-Hegglin anomaly. This is characterized by large numbers of inclusions in all leukocytes and also in platelets. The inclusions are similar in morphology to Döhle-Amato bodies (see above) and are light blue spindle-shaped or crescent structures. They can be found in adult neutrophils, eosinophils, basophils, monocytes and in lymphocytes. They are peroxidase- and PAS-negative and are occasionally present in otherwise healthy persons. Giant platelets are frequently associated with this anomaly, and concomitant thrombocytopenia resulting in a hemorrhagic tendency is also found.

*Chediak-Higashi Anomaly.* This is a rare cytoplasmic anomaly. It is inherited as an autosomal dominant trait and is characterized by large numbers of specific granules in granulocytes and lymphocytes. The neutrophils also show faint cytoplasmic inclusions, oval, fusiform, or irregular in shape, green-gray in color and resembling Döhle bodies. Moncoytes in the peripheral blood show large inclusions of phagocytosed material derived from ingested neutrophils and eosinophils. Large azurophilic granules are also present in the lymphocytes and plasma cells. Cytochemical studies show that the granules in the neutrophils, eosinophils, and monocytes are strongly peroxidase-positive, while those present in the lymphocytes are peroxidase-negative.

*Auer Rods.* These inclusions are rodlike structures found in the cytoplasm of myeoloblasts promyelocytes and monoblasts, measuring $1 \mu$ to $2 \mu$ in length and staining a vivid azurophilic color with Romanowsky dyes. The nature of these inclusions is believed to be abnormal development of the cellular lysosomes. The presence of Auer rods is used as presumptive evidence of myelogenous or monocytic leukemia.

*Toxic Granulation.* The normal granules in segmented neutrophils or band cells are fine and stain a pink-violet with Romanowsky dyes. In severe infections, the granules of these cells and of their precursors become coarse and deeply stained. This toxic granulation is thought to be produced when normal cytoplasmic maturation is inhibited, and the resulting transformation of basophilic or acidophilic granules to the mature pink-violet state is arrested. The granulation associated with

Alder's anomaly and with the Chediak syndrome is frequently confused with this state.

**Demonstration of LE Bodies Using Defibrinated Blood**

*Principle.* The patient's white cells are incubated at 37°C with his own serum containing the LE factor. A buffy coat is obtained, and the smears are stained and screened for the presence of the inclusion bodies.

*Reagents and Apparatus*
1. Erlenmeyer flask containing 10 glass beads
2. 37°C Incubator
3. Pasteur pipet
4. Wintrobe tube
5. Centrifuge
6. Slides
7. Romanowsky stain

*Method*
1. 10 ml of venous whole blood is delivered into an Erlenmeyer flask containing the glass beads. The flask is twisted in a swirling motion for 5 minutes to defibrinate the blood and is placed in an incubator at 37°C for 3 to 4 hours.
2. The defibrinated blood is pipeted into a Wintrobe tube and centrifuged at 3,000 rpm for 10 minutes to obtain a buffy coat, which is carefully removed with a Pasteur pipet. Smears are then made and stained by routine methods.

**Demonstration of LE Bodies Using Clotted Blood[6]**

*Reagents and Apparatus*
1. Wire sieve
2. Venous whole blood
3. Centrifuge tube—15 ml
4. Pasteur pipet
5. Centrifuge
6. 37°C Incubator
7. Wintrobe tube

*Method*
1. 10 ml of venous blood is allowed to clot at room temperature and is incubated at 37°C for 2 hours.
2. The clot is mashed through a fine wire sieve. The serum and free cells are expressed from the sieve and centrifiged at 2,000 rpm for 5 minutes.

3. 1 ml of the upper layer of cells is removed and recentrifuged in a Wintrobe tube at 2,000 rpm for 5 minutes to obtain a suitable buffy coat.

4. Thin buffy coat smears are made and the slides stained by routine Romanowsky dye.

## Demonstration of LE Bodies Using Normal Leukocyte Suspensions

### *Reagents and Apparatus*

1. Patient's serum: 10 ml of whole blood is allowed to clot at room temperature and the serum stored frozen at —20°C until used.

2. Normal leukocyte suspension: 5 ml of heparinized group O blood is centrifuged at 3,000 rpm for 5 minutes. Half of the red cell column is removed with a Pasteur pipet and discarded. The remaining cells and the plasma are remixed and allowed to settle at 37°C until 1 to 2 ml of the plasma can be withdrawn. The supernatant plasma, rich in leukocytes and platelets, is centrifuged and washed 3 times for 5 minutes in normal saline at a speed not exceeding 1,000 rpm. After the final washing, the saline is decanted and the leukocytes resuspended in the residual volume of saline.

3. Wintrobe tube
4. 37°C Incubator
5. Centrifuge
6. Pasteur pipet
7. Slides

### *Method*

1. 1 Volume of patient's serum is added to 1 volume of normal leukocyte suspension and left in an incubator at 37°C for 3 to 4 hours.

2. The serum-leukocyte suspension is centrifuged at 1,000 rpm for 5 minutes, a portion of the buffy coat is removed with a Pasteur pipet, and thin smears are made and stained routinely by Romanowsky dyes.

### *Notes*

1. An LE cell is a neutrophil containing a basophilic, opaque homogeneous mass within its cytoplasm. The nucleus of the neutrophil is normally displaced and sometimes appears as a crescent around the ingested material. The LE body usually shows no evidence of chromatin arrangement, but gives a positive Feulgen reaction, indicating nuclear origin.

2. The phenomenon depends upon the presence of three substances:
    a. LE factor
    b. nuclear protein
    c. viable phagocytic leukocytes

3. The LE factor is an IgG antibody to nucleoprotein which combines with cell nuclei to produce swelling and subsequent rupture of the cell membrane. If sufficient antibody is attached to the nuclei, they are phagocytized by neutrophils to produce typical LE cells, this process requiring complement. The nuclear protein source is either a neutrophil or a lymphocyte. While the phagocyte is most often a polymorphonuclear leukocyte, monocytes or eosinophils may sometimes contain inclusion characteristic of the LE cell.

4. LE cells are often confused with tart cells, which are of no clinical significance. They are usually monocytes that have phagocytized another cell. The main morphological difference between LE and tart cells is that the nuclear mass is homogenized in the LE cell, whereas distinct chromatin threads are seen in the Tart cell.

The size of the inclusion is also smaller, appearing about 8 to 10 $\mu$ in diameter rather than the usual 15 to 18 $\mu$. While it does represent nuclear debris, the tart cell does not appear to have been acted upon by the antinuclear antibodies associated with lupus erythematosus.[6,7]

5. Preparations that contain LE bodies may also have extracellular globular material and rosettes present. The extracellular material appears similar to the intracellular ingested LE material, and the rosettes are formed when the neutrophils surround one of the extracellular masses.

6. The association of positive LE preparation with various medications has been reported. Both hydralazine (Apresoline) and procainamide are known to cause such reactions, and the reported cases probably represent an uncovering of a lupus diathesis in an otherwise healthy patient.[8]

**Antinuclear Antibody Test (ANA)**

*Principle.* Antinuclear antibody reacts with various components of the nuclei of tissue cells. Fluorescein-conjugated antihuman gamma globulin reacts with the antinuclear antibody within the nuclei of the tissue antigen. When microscopically viewed, using an ultraviolet light source and a dark field condenser, the nuclei or portions of the nuclei fluoresce.

*Reagents and Apparatus*
1. Fresh mouse liver and kidney
A small section of each tissue is placed on a tissue holder containing a drop of embedding medium. The sections are frozen with $CO_2$ and sections 3 to 4 $\mu$ are cut on a cryostat —20°C. A microscope slide is touched to the cut section so that the tissue adheres, and it is fixed with cold acetone for 10 minutes.
2. Cryostat

3. Fluorescent microscope with dark field condenser and a source of UV light.

4. Serum

5. Phosphate Buffered Saline pH 7.3*

6. Positive control of known titer

7. Negative control

## Method

1. The mouse tissue section is washed twice in cold phosphate buffered saline for 2 minutes.

2. The excess saline is removed from the slide, which is placed on a flat surface. Do not let the slide dry.

3. A 1:10 dilution of the patient's serum is made in the phosphate buffered saline, and the fixed tissue is overlayed with this diluted serum for 30 minutes at 25°C.

4. A positive-control serum (diluted 1:640) and a normal serum (negative-control diluted 1:10) are set up in parallel with the test.

5. After incubation, the sections are washed in cold phosphate buffered saline by gently rinsing them with a fine stream of buffered saline from an overhanging wash bottle. The slides are then placed in three dishes of buffered saline; the first for 10 seconds with continuous movement, the second and third for 5 minutes each.

6. The excess buffered saline is drained from the slides, the tissues are overlayed with fluorescein-conjugated antihuman IgG serum† diluted 1:24 with buffered saline and left for 30 minutes at room temperature.

7. Wash twice in buffered saline, 5 minutes each wash, and coverslip with glycerol mounting media.

8. The sections are read immediately under a fluorescent microscope using a UV light source and dark field condenser.

## Normal

Males: 20-60 years, 3% positive slides
Females: 20-60 years, 7% positive slides
Both sexes: over 80 years, 49% positive slides

## Interpretation

1. A slide is considered positive if the nuclei fluoresce more brightly than the cytoplasm. The nuclei in negative preparations appear as black holes in the cytoplasm.

2. Diffuse staining is characteristic of systemic lupus erythematosus (SLE); peripheral staining of acute stages of SLE, nucleolar staining of

---

* Available from B.B.L. No. 11248, Baltimore, Md.

†Available from Hyland Laboratories, Costa Mesa, Calif.

other collagen diseases (not of SLE), and speckled staining is not usually found in SLE.

### Notes

1. When reporting positive results, one indication should be given of the type of staining characteristic.

2. The frequency of positive tests is:

|                      | %  |
|----------------------|----|
| SLE                  | 99 |
| Lupoid hepatitis     | 99 |
| Scleroderma          | 73 |
| Rheumatoid arthritis | 69 |
| Discoid lupus        | 47 |

## CLINICAL CONSIDERATIONS

### *Classification of Leukemic States*

Proliferative blood disorders include diseases other than the leukemias. A wide range of diseases can exhibit a "leukemic-type" picture. These are termed luekemoid diseases. "The leukemias can be classified on the basis of: (a) the duration of the disease, (b) the predominant cell type present in the peripheral blood and bone marrow (c) the total white cell count in the peripheral blood."

1. Duration of the Disease.

Patients with acute leukemia have a short life expectancy, usually less than 6 months. Chronic leukemia often produces life expectancy of over 1 year and the subacute form of the disease usually incidates a duration between the acute and chronic forms.

2. Predominant Cellular Pattern.

Morphological characteristics of the cells distinguishes between myelocytic, lymphocytic and other forms. In acute blast cell leukemia, a pure population of immature cells is always present, but in general chronic leukemias show large numbers of "cytic" cells (myelocytes in chronic myeloid leukemia; monocytes in chronic monocytic leukemia) and acute leukemias large numbers of blastic cells. (Myeloblasts in acute myeloid leukemia; lymphoblasts in acute lymphocytic leukemia; monoblasts in acute monocytic leukemia.) Morphologically, subacute leukemia resembles the acute form of the disease more than the chronic.

3. Total White Cell Count in the Peripheral Disease.

Two different forms of leukemia can be differentiated: (a) leukemia, (b) aleukemia. In the first form, the total white cell count is always raised. In the aleukemic form, the total count is below the normal limits, but immature and atypical cells are almost always present.

*Acute Myeloid Leukemia.* The disease appears suddenly; fever, body pains, rigors and often a sore throat are tyupical clinical findings. There is a progressive hypochromic anemia with a tendency to hemorrhage from the mucous membranes, this generalized bleeding being due to a reduction in platelets and platelet precursors. The lymphatic glands are usually not enlarged, but the cervical glands are sometimes larger as a result of mouth infections. The liver and spleen are both enlarged.

The blood picture shows characteristic changes. The total white count is rarely as high as in the chronic form, usually between 15,000 and 50,000 cells per cubic millimeter; the majority of cells are myeloblasts. Myeloblasts with indented or bilobed nuclei are occasionally seen, and are known as Rieder cells; when these are present in large numbers, the condition is called a paramyeloblastic leukemia. Auer bodies may also be found in the cytoplasm of myeloblasts and myelocytes.

The red cell elements are reduced, and polychromatic cells, reticulocytes and rubricytes are all present in varying numbers. The general picture is of a severe iron deficiency anemia, with a progressive thrombocytopenia.

Differentiation in the laboratory is accomplished by a careful study of the blood picture and by examining blood and bone marrow films stained by both Romanowsky and peroxidase techniques. Often difficulty arises in differentiating between myeloblasts and lymphoblasts, even with the use of special staining techniques. Occasionally, leukemic infiltrates in the bone marrow and other tissues appear green. This is then known as "chloroma".

*Acute Lymphatic Leukemia.* This is the most common form of the acute leukemias. Clinically, pyrexia, limb pains, headaches and rigors are found. Initially the glands may not be significantly enlarged but may begin to swell in a short time. The cervical glands become swollen first, and gradual pyrexias and night sweats become apparent.

The blood picture often has a total leukocyte count fluctuating between 10,000 and 100,000 cells per cubic millimeter of blood. The predominant and diagnostic cell is the lymphoblast.

The red cells show a progressive decline in numbers, and the hemoglobin falls rapidly and in parallel. Red cell regeneration is evident; polychromatic cells, reticulocytes and rubricytes are present. The mature red cells show marked anisocytosis and poikilocytosis, and there is a generalized thrombocytopenia. The hematological diagnosis is made by careful examination of blood and bone marrow films. Lymphoblasts and myeloblasts are usually differentiated by three main criteria:

1. The predominant type of cell present;
2. The number of nucleoli present; lymphoblasts normally have between 1 and 2 nuceoli, whereas myeloblasts have between 2 and 6.

3. Peroxidase staining.

***Monocytic Leukemia.*** This is a rare disease, two main forms existing:

1. The Schilling type ("the pure form")
2. The Naegeli type ("the mixed form")

The Schilling form is said to arise from the reticulum cells of the reticuloendothelial system. The cells are large with an open chromatin network, bizarre nucleus and irregular cell border.

The Naegeli form is postulated as arising from myeloid tissues, because Naegeli considered monocytes to be derived from myeloblasts. It is now thought that this mixed form is really a variant of acute myeloid leukemia.

The disease is insidious in onset, rapidly becoming acute. A chronic form is extremely rare. Clinically, the symptoms resemble those of the other acute leukemias.

Blood changes show a progressive hypochromic anemia with a marked hemolytic tendency; total leukocytes can increase up to 50,000 cells per cubic millimeter of blood, but may be within normal limits. The differential white count shows a large proportion of well-formed monocytes, which gradually develop into more primitive forms in the terminal stages of the disease. These early cells are difficult to differentiate from myeloblasts.

***Chronic Myeloid Leukemia.*** The onset is often insidious. Clinically, there is lassitude, loss of weight, splenomegaly and anemia. The disease is rare before the age of 20 and most common after the age of 30.

The diagnostic laboratory feature is the increase in the total white count. 250,000 cells per cubic millimeter of blood are often found, and counts up to 750,000 cells per cubic millimeter of blood have occurred. The differential white count shows that the cells are granulocytes, the majority being polymorphonuclear neutrophils, band forms, metamyelocytes and myelocytes.

The diagostic cell is the myelocyte, which shows wide variation in size and shape. A small proportion of myeloblasts is sometimes seen in the peripheral blood, but normally the total number does not exceed 3 or 4 per cent of the white count.

A chronic anemia is present; the red cell count and hemoglobin are both reduced. Polychromasia anisocytosis and poikilocytosis are present to a moderate degree; nucleated red cells, reticulocytes and stippled cells are also present. In severe cases, macrocytes are seen. The platelets are increased in number in the early stages of the disease, but a thrombocytopenia develops as the condition becomes established.

The marrow shows an increase in myelocytes, myeloblasts and undifferentiated cells, and is often characterized by the presence of the abnormal Philadelphia chromosome (Ph'). This unusually small chromosome is believed to be formed from chromosome 21 by deletion or translocation. It has not been found in normal persons and is absent in nonleukemic myeloproliferative disorders. This chromosome marker occurs in a majority of bone marrow cells, including those containing hemoglobin, and suggests that the involved cell is a progenitor of both granulocytic and erythroid cell types.

*Chronic Lymphatic Leukemia.* This form of the disease appears to be the most common. The onset is insidious, the first clinical symptoms being lymphadenopathy, anemia, and splenomegaly.

The blood picture has a total leukocyte count between 30,000 and 200,000 cells per cubic millimeter of blood. Higher values are occasionally found, the predominant cell being a small lymphocyte. Scanty lymphoblasts may also be present.

The red cells and hemoglobin are always reduced; a progressive iron deficiency anemia with polychromasia, poikilocytosis, anisocytosis, and reticulocytosis is also found. A progressive thrombocytopenia results in hemorrhages from the mucous membranes of the eyes, and from the gums in the late stages.

The bone marrow is infiltrated with normal and abnormal lymphocytes.

*Aleukemic Leukemia.* The onset of the disease may be insidious. Splenomegaly and anemia are typical findings. This form of the disease shows a tissue infiltration by the predominant cell, with the total white count of the peripheral blood remaining within or below normal limits. Almost always, persistent and repeated examinations of the blood reveal a few immature cells.

The bone marrow shows normal cellularity, the abnormality being in the cellular distribution.

*Miscellaneous Leukemias.* Cases have been described in which the predominant cells have been eosinophils and basophils. In such conditions, the terms eosinophilic and basophilic leukemia are used. Rare cases of platelet proliferation have been described, the condition being known as megakaryocytic leukemia. Britton[3] states that "there is little or no evidence that a true megakaryocytic leukemia occurs, but the megakaryocytic tissue may well be involved in any myeloproliferative process, thereby exhibiting a relationship to leukemia, polycythemia, and other related disorders."

*Promyelocytic leukemia* is characterized by atypical progranulocytes containing large irregular azurophilic granulation. There is frequently a consumption coagulopathy in which there is a decrease in fibrinogen, abnormal prothrombin and partial thromboplastin times, decreasing platelet counts, and an increase in fibrinolytic acitivity.

*Mast cell leukemia* is an extremely rare form of leukemia. The abnormality is the increase in tissue mast cells, rich in histamine, which is liberated and produces nausea, diarrhea, flushing, and palpitation.

*Multiple Myeloma.* This is a tumor characterized by multiple involvement of the skeletal trunk. The onset is insidious. Bone pain can occur anywhere, but is more commonly found in the lumbar and sacral regions. The bones are tender on palpation, and a fever may occur with loss of weight. The commonest type of tumor cell resembles the plasma cell. The nature of the abnormal cell in the peripheral blood is still uncertain, although many workers have described cases in which they term the condition plasma cell leukemia. Wintrobe[4] takes the opposite view and differentiates plasma cells from myeloma cells. The circulating "plasma cells" appear as modified myeloma cells stemming from the tumors, but Moeschlin[5] considers the cells found in myeloma to be normal reticulum cells of the bone marrow, which resemble plasma cells.

The blood picture shows a hypochromic microcytic anemia, although macrocytes are sometimes found. Anisocytosis, poikilocytosis and nucleated red cells are also usually present. The total white count is generally raised to 15,000 cells per cubic millimeter of blood, but sometimes falls within normal limits. Nongranulocytic cells are increased, and undifferentiated early cells are frequently present in large numbers. Many myeloma "plasma cells" are found in both the peripheral blood and the bone marrow. The cells are 2 to 6 times the size of a red cell and are oval in shape; the cytoplasm is deeply basophic. Various forms of cellular inclusions are seen ranging from large well formed, closely packed vacuoles (Mott or grape cells) to azurophilic protein granules (Russell bodies). The nucleus is eccentrically placed and contains 1 to 2 nucleoli.

Autoagglutination, rouleaux formation, myeloma protein detected by electrophoresis, Bence Jones protein and cryoglobulinemia are other common features of this disease.

## Other Hematological Diseases

*Waldenstrom's Macroglobulinemia.* Macroglobulinemia is a syndrome that may occur in many disease processes (chronic lymphocytic leukemia, myeloma etc.). When it occurs a macroglobulin of approximately 1,000,000 is present in the plasma. The disease occurs more commonly in males over the age of 50 and usually presents with a clinical history of weight loss, weakness, infection, and enlarged lymph nodes. The bone marrow is often replaced with atypical lymphocytes and the peripheral blood frequently shows a normocytic anemia and abnormal cold agglutinins. The total serum proteins are increased together with the sedimentation rate and serum viscosity.

Abnormal beta or gamma globulins are present in the plasma and demonstrated by electrophoresis. The Sia test, based on the insolubility of macroglobulins in water, is often positive.

## Infections

An increase in circulating white cells is most likely to occur in acute infections. This increase is reflected in the numbers of polymorphonuclear neutrophils accompanied by an increase in the more immature forms. A reduced or normal white count in the presence of an increase in immature granulocytes appears to indicate an early stage of an infectious process or a lack of response to the infectious agent.

Severe infections and tissue destruction are often accompanied by toxic granulation, bizarre cytoplasmic vacuolation, and abnormal cytoplasmic basophilia in the granulocytes.

Common causes of neutrophilic leucocytosis include infections with pyrogenic bacteria, chemical intoxications, acute hemorrhage, and neoplasms (leukemia, lymphoma, etc.).

Lymphocytosis can be the result of acute viral (whooping cough, mumps, infectious mononucleosis) and bacterial infections, hyperthyroidism, and lymphocytic leukemia.

Monocytosis is often found associated with infections, especially with gram-negative bacilli, parasitic infections (Kala-azar, malaria), viral infections (rickettsia) and monocytic leukemia.

Eosinophilia is usually present in allergic reactions owing to asthma and hay fever, parasitic infestations, and some neoplasms (Hodgkin's disease, myelocytic leukemia).

*Myelofibrosis.* This syndrome is believed to be the result of the bone marrow and reticuloendothelial response to injury. The laboratory results show an anemia with bizarre red cell morphology and characterized by large numbers of nucleated red cells. Immature granulocytes are also present in the peripheral blood, together with a marked leucocytosis. Increases in eosinophils, basophils, and monocytes are also sometimes found. There is a mild thrombocytosis together with an increase in platelet size. The variable leucocyte alkaline phosphatase stain results are not helpful, but the absence of the Philadelphia chromosome is useful in separating this syndrome from chronic myeloid leukemia.

The bone marrow is hypocellular and shows areas of increased fibrosis.

*Agranulocytosis.* The hematological picture is one of leukopenia, neutropenia, anemia, and thrombocytopenia. The disorder is frequently caused by drugs; those most likely to produce this syndrome include benzol, chloramphenicol, and sulfonanides.

*Infectious Mononucleosis.* This is an acute infection believed to be viral in origin (Epstein-Barr Virus: EPV). The peripheral blood is characterized by the presence of large atypical mononuclear cells varying in both size and shape. These cells possess an oval or kidney-shaped nucleus and a basophilic vacuolated cytoplasm (see p. 94). The total white-cell count varies between 12,000 and 18,000/mm[3]. Other laboratory results include reduced leukocyte alkaline phosphatase activity, a mild thrombocytopenia, and occasional anemia resulting from a hemolytic crisis due to the presence of autoantibodies having anti-i specificity. The presence of high-titered antisheep red cell antibodies, that are unabsorbed by red cells or tissues containing the Forssman antigen, is usually diagnostic.

*Gaucher's Disease.* This is a lipid storage disease producing anemia and thrombocytopenia and is characterized by the presence of Gaucher's cells (foamy histiocytes) in the bone marrow. The morphology of these cells is:

*Size.* Between 3 and 11 times the size of a mature red cell (i.e. 20-80 $\mu$).

*Shape.* Round, oval, or spindle shaped.

*Outline.* Regular

*Cytoplasm.* Occupies 60 to 80% of the cell. Appears fibrillar in form and stains faintly with eosin, but does not stain with Sudan III or oil-red-O stain for fat. In Romanowsky-stained preparation, the cytoplasm has a pale blue-gray color. The fibrillar pattern can be seen most advantageously with Mallory's analine blue dye[8].

*Nucleus.* Moderately condensed, centrally or eccentrically placed.

The disease is primarily found in children and presents a chronic course of splenomegaly skin pigmentation and bone pain. The cytochemical abnormality involves the enzyme glucocerebrosidlase which catalyzes the hydrolysis of glucocerebroside to glucose and ceramide.

Other storage reticuloses include Niemann-Pick disease, Letterer-Siwe disease, and Hand-Schüller-Christian disease.

*Lupus Erythematosus.* The condition is an auto-immune disease affecting connective tissues throughout the body. It is characterized by an erythematous macular rash, nephritis, lymphadenopathy and splenomegaly.

The diagnostic laboratory finding is the presence of LE cells when patients' serum is incubated with any source of white cell. An additional technique used in the confirmation of the disease is the demonstration of an antinuclear factor by fluorescent techniques. The factor has been found in lower titer in other diseases and can be differentiated by heating the patients' serum to 65°C. In lupus, the inactivation does not destroy the factor, whereas in other disorders it is inactivated by heating.

## REFERENCES

1. Instruction and Service Manual for the Model Z Coulter Counter. ed. 5. Coulter Electronics Inc., Hialeah, Florida, 1970.
2. Barrett, A. M.: A method for staining sections of bone marrow. J. Pathol., 56:133, 1944.
3. Britton, C. J. C.: Disorders of the Blood. ed. 9, p. 578. New York, Grune & Stratton, 1963.

4. Wintrobe, M. M.: Clinical Hematology. ed. 6, p. 1192. Philadelphia, Lea & Febiger, 1967.
5. Moeschlin, S.: Untersuchungen Über Geuese und Funktion. Helv. med. Acta, 7:227, 1940.
6. Hargraves, M. M.: Discovery of the LE cell and its morphology. Mayo Clin. Proc., 44:579, 1969.
7. Dubois, E. L.: L.E. cell test and antinuclear antibodies. JAMA, 200:1053, 1967.
8. Dubois, E. L.: Procainamide induction of a systemic lupus erythematosus-like syndrome. Medicine, 48:217, 1969.

# 4

# Tests Used to Detect Hemolytic Anemias

## OSMOTIC FRAGILITY TEST (IMMEDIATE)[1]

*Principle.* The test determines the resistance of the red cells to hemolysis in varying concentrations of hypotonic saline at room temperature.

### Reagents and Apparatus
1. Stock 10% sodium chloride, buffered (pH 7.4):
   Sodium chloride .............................. 180 g
   Disodium hydrogen phosphate ................ 27.31 g
   Sodium dihydrogen phosphate ................ 4.86 g
   Distilled water ........................... to 2 liters
2. Graduated pipets:
   Graduated in 0.01 ml—1 ml
   Graduated in 0.1 ml—10 ml
3. Micropipet—0.1 ml
4. Volumetric pipet—10 ml
5. Volumetric flask—100 ml
6. Spectrophotometer
7. Heparinized venous blood

### Method
1. 1% Saline is made from the stock by diluting 10 ml to 100 ml with distilled water.
2. Serial dilutions of the 1% working solution are made as in Table 4-1.
3. The saline dilutions are mixed well and 0.1 ml of heparinized whole blood is added to each tube.
4. Stopper the tubes and mix by inversion, allow the tubes to stand for 2 hours at room temperature and then remix the same way.
5. Centrifuge the suspensions for 5 minutes at 2,000 rpm. Calculate the percentage of hemolysis in each of the supernatants from the following, using a spectrophotometer at a wavelength of 540 nm.

*134*

6. Zero the galvanometer reading prior to use with the normal saline blank set up in the dilutions.

7. Set up a 100% standard by adding 0.1 ml blood to 10 ml of distilled water.

**Calculations**

$$\frac{\text{Optical density of test dilutions}}{\text{Optical density of the standard}} \times 100 = \text{per cent hemolysis}$$

If the optical density of the 100% standard reads 0.5, and that of one of the dilutions reads 0.3: 0.3/0.5 × 100 = 60% hemolysis

*Normal.* Plot the percentage hemolysis from each tube against the percentage saline, and compare against the known normal range.

**Notes**

1. The proportions of blood and saline and the pH of the dilutions are critical. A proportion of 1 volume of blood to 99 volumes of saline is such that the added plasma has little effect on the tonicity of the mixture. If the ratio of the mixture were decreased to 1:20, the plasma volume would affect the tonicity of the dilution.

2. A pH shift of 0.1 unit is equivalent to altering the tonicity 0.01%, with red cell fragility increasing as the pH falls.

3. A difference of 5°C is equivalent to an alteration of tonicity of 0.01%; as the temperature decreases, the fragility increases.

TABLE 4-1. Serial Dilutions of the Working Saline Solution.

| 1% WORKING SALINE (ML) | DISTILLED WATER (ML) | % FINAL SALINE |
|---|---|---|
| 2.0 | 8.0 | 0.20 |
| 2.5 | 7.5 | 0.25 |
| 3.0 | 7.0 | 0.30 |
| 3.5 | 6.5 | 0.35 |
| 3.75 | 6.25 | 0.375 |
| 4.0 | 6.0 | 0.40 |
| 4.25 | 5.75 | 0.425 |
| 4.5 | 5.5 | 0.45 |
| 4.75 | 5.25 | 0.475 |
| 5.0 | 5.0 | 0.50 |
| 5.5 | 4.5 | 0.55 |
| 6.0 | 4.0 | 0.60 |
| 6.5 | 3.5 | 0.65 |
| 7.0 | 3.0 | 0.70 |
| 7.5 | 2.5 | 0.75 |
| 8.0 | 2.0 | 0.80 |
| 8.5 | 1.5 | 0.85 |

TABLE 4-2. Normal Range of Osmotic Fragilities (Immediate) at Room Temperature.

| % SALINE | % HEMOLYSIS |
|----------|-------------|
| 0.3 | 97–100 |
| 0.35 | 90–97 |
| 0.4 | 50–95 |
| 0.45 | 5–45 |
| 0.5 | 0–6 |
| 0.55 | 0 |

4. A normal control blood should be estimated under the same experimental conditions as the unknown.

5. The sample of blood should be obtained with a minimum of trauma, and the test should be set up as soon as possible after the sample is collected.

6. The use of anticoagulants that osmotically alter the dilutions is undesirable. Heparinized or sterile defibrinated blood can be used.

7. It is important to measure carefully the volume of blood added to each saline dilution, and to ensure that the *blood drops directly into the saline*.

8. The Osmotic Fragility test can be carried out using prediluted saline concentrations. The Unopette (B.D. No. 5830) system employs the disposable pipeting system containing reservoirs of varying buffered saline concentrations. The technique used is identical to that found on page 45.

### Significance of the Test

1. When red cells are placed in a hypertonic solution, they lose fluid until an equilibrium is set up with the surrounding fluid, and they crenate. In hypotonic solutions, the cells take up fluid and swell until either an equilibrium is set up or the cell ruptures.

2. In some hemolytic anemias, the resistance of the red cell to hypotonic solutions is reduced, and in some it is increased. Examples of diseases in which there is a characteristic reduction in such resistance are hereditary spherocytosis and some of the acquired hemolytic anemias. Most of the hemoglobinopathies (sickle cell anemia, thalassemia), iron deficiency anemia, and occasionally myelosclerosis, leukemia, lymphosarcoma, and patients following splenectomy demonstrate an increased red cell resistance.

3. Increased fragility (decreased resistance) of red cells to saline

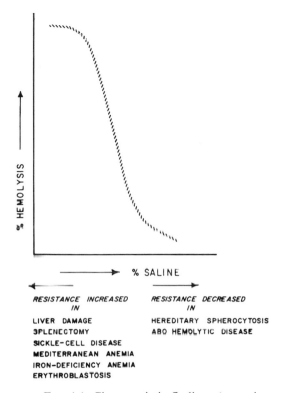

FIG. 4-1. Characteristic findings (osmotic fragility) in various diseases.

solutions is related to cell shape. The more spherical the cell, the greater its fragility to concentrations of saline. Normal hemolysis is preceded by a phase in which the red cell assumes a spherical shape. When the cells have been hemolyzed by saline, the envelope and the stroma may still be seen as "ghosts" while the reticulocyte reticulum is still present and recognized after hemolysis has occurred.

4. Red cells can be dissected in physiological saline without the release of the hemoglobin into solution, but, if the same cells are placed in hypotonic saline, the hemoglobin goes into solution. This is explained by postulating that the hemoglobin lies within and is absorbed by a fibrillary framework of stromatin that extends into the cell. The hemoglobin is held electrostatically, and, when the charge of the stromatin is neutralized by reducing the pH to its isoelectric point, the hemoglobin escapes from the cell.

## INCUBATED OSMOTIC FRAGILITY[2,3]

*Reagents and Apparatus.* As in the immediate osmotic fragility.

*Method*
1. Venous blood is drawn into sterile heparin tubes and incubated at 37°C for 24 hours. The procedure described under immediate osmotic fragility is then carried out.

*Significance of the Test.*[1] The incubated test appears to be more sensitive than the immediate test to mild alterations of cell fragility.

When normal red cells are incubated under sterile conditions for 24 hours, they undergo metabolic changes. It has been shown[4] that during this incubation, the increase in osmotic fragility is directly correlated with loss of red cell cholesterol. This material is usually in equilibrium with free cholesterol in the serum. During incubation a heat-labile serum factor takes part in the esterification of the free cholesterol of the serum, upsetting the cell-serum equilibrium so that cell cholesterol decreases. With this loss, the cell does not change in volume, but the surface area decreases with consequent spheroidicity and increased osmotic fragility.

2. The changes in red cell metabolism during incubation can be prevented if the serum is previously heated at 56°C for 30 minutes and the incubation carried out at pH 7.5.


## MECHANICAL FRAGILITY[5]

*Principle.* The test subjects the red cells to a standard degree of trauma which is applied by shaking whole blood with glass beads.

*Reagents and Apparatus*
1. Matburn rotator
2. Glass beads—4 mm in diameter
3. Tubes—75 × 10 mm
4. Heparinized blood
5. 0.04% Aqueous ammonia
6. Graduated pipets—1 ml
7. Graduated pipets—10 ml
8. Microhematocrit tubes
9. Spectrophotometer


**Method 1**

1. 0.1 ml of blood is added to 9.9 ml of normal saline, centrifuged at 2,000 rpm for 5 minutes. The supernatant is decanted and saved as the blank.

TABLE 4-3. Normal Range of Osmotic Fragilities (Incubated).

| % SALINE | % HEMOLYSIS |
|---|---|
| 0.2 | 95–100 |
| 0.3 | 85–100 |
| 0.35 | 75–100 |
| 0.4 | 65–100 |
| 0.45 | 55–100 |
| 0.5 | 40–85 |
| 0.55 | 15–70 |
| 0.6 | 0–40 |
| 0.65 | 0–10 |
| 0.7 | 0–5 |

2. The hematocrit is adjusted to approximately 45% by the withdrawal of either an aliquot of cells or of plasma.

3. A 2-ml volume of blood and 4 glass beads are placed in each of 2 tubes.

4. The tubes are stoppered and rotated at 33 rpm for 1 hour at room temperature. The contents are pooled, and 0.1 ml of blood is added to 9.9 ml of 0.04% ammonia. The dilution is repeated, using normal saline as a diluent.

5. Allow the dilution to stand at room temperature for 5 minutes and centrifuge at 2,000 rpm for 5 minutes.

6. Decant the saline supernatant and read the degree of hemolysis spectrophotometrically at a wavelength of 540 nm. The saline tube prepared in step 1 is used as the blank and the 0.04% ammonia tube as a 100% standard.

*Normal Value.* 2 to 5% hemoglobin

## Method 2

1. Centrifuge the heparinized blood at 2,000 rpm for 5 minutes and withdraw 0.5 ml of plasma.

2. Carry out procedures 1 to 3 as in the above technique and rotate at 33 rpm for 1 hour. Pool the contents of the tubes and centrifuge at 2,000 rpm for 5 minutes.

3. Determine the plasma hemoglobin of the prerotated and postrotated bloods by the method described on page 16, and express the difference in hemoglobins in mg %.

*Normal.* 0 to 5 mg Plasma hemoglobin

*Notes*

1. High hematocrit values, reduced temperatures, and alkaline blood pH values produce increased mechanical fragilities.

2. Spherocytes, sickle cells, agglutinated cells, and cells from newborn infants are susceptible to mechanical trauma, but poikilocytes are not abnormally fragile by this technique.

## AUTOHEMOLYSIS[6]

*Principle.* The amount of spontaneous lysis in sterile heparinized bloods is estimated after incubation with and without glucose and ATP.

### Reagents and Apparatus
1. Sterile adenosine triphosphate (ATP)
1 g of ATP is dissolved in 4 ml of sterile normal saline
2. Sterile 10% glucose in normal saline
3. Sterile 0.85% sodium chloride
4. Heparinized blood
5. Sterile tubes—13 x 100 mm
6. Drabkin's reagent (see p. 7)
7. Spectrophotometer
8. Centrifuge (GLC-1 Sorval)

### Method
1. 20 ml of blood is heparinized and divided equally into 3 sterile tubes.
2. 0.2 ml of ATP solution and 0.2 ml of glucose solution are added to the first and second tubes.
3. 0.2 ml of sterile saline is added to the third tube. This is used as the blank control tube.
4. All three tubes are gently inverted and incubated for 24 hours at 37°C.
5. At the end of this time, they are again gently inverted and reincubated for an additional 24 hours.
6. All the tubes are then centrifuged at 2,000 rpm for 10 minutes.
7. Routine hemoglobin estimations are then carried out on all three supernatants, using the cyanmethhemoglobin reagent as the zero blank. Alternatively, plasma hemoglobin may be estimated using the technique outlined on page 16.
8. The heparinized blood is resuspended in the third tube and a whole blood hemoglobin determined (p. 7).

*Calculation.* The percent hemolysis of the 3 tubes is obtained by dividing each by the whole blood hemoglobins in g%. The percent hemolysis is reported for each of the 3 tubes.

### Significance of the Test
1. Normal blood undergoes little spontaneous hemolysis when incubated under sterile conditions for 48 hours. The addition of either glucose or adenosine triphosphate reduces the degree of hemolysis.

2. Increased autohemolysis occurs in many types of hemolytic anemia. Three lytic patterns may be seen.

a. Autohemolysis of type I is seen in glucose-6-phosphate dehydrogenase deficiency, hexokinase deficiency, and acquired nonsphenocytic hemolytic anemia.

b. Autohemolysis of type II is observed in pyruvate kinase deficiency and in patients with acquired spherocytic hemolytic anemia.

c. The third type of result is seen in patients with hereditary spherocytosis and in triosephosphate isomerase deficiency.

*Normal Values* (in percent hemolysis)

## SEMIQUANTITATIVE ESTIMATION OF SERUM HAPTOGLOBIN[7,8]

*Principle.* When hemoglobin is added to serum it combines with haptoglobin ($\alpha_2$ globulin). If the amount of hemoglobin added is greater than the ability of the haptoglobin to bind it, free hemoglobin appears in the serum, and this is separated from the hemoglobin-haptoglobin complex by electrophoresis at pH 7.0.

Different concentrations of hemoglobin are added to the serum to be tested. After electrophoresis, the cellulose acetate strips are stained for hemoglobin. The concentration at which free hemoglobin appears is noted. Other electrophoresis strips are stained for protein to determine the positions of $\alpha$ and $\beta$ globulins.

### Reagents and Apparatus

1. Specimens: 2 ml of clotted blood is centrifuged and the serum separated. The sample once separated, can be stored at $-20°C$ for 1 to 2 weeks, but is unsatisfactory if hemolysis is present.

2. Hemolysate prepared from normal red cells

2.0 ml of EDTA anticoagulated normal whole blood is washed 3 times with 0.85% saline. The cells are lysed by adding 1.4 ml distilled water

TABLE 4-4. Normal Values.*

| TUBE | 1 | 2 | 3 |
|---|---|---|---|
| Normal | 0.1–0.8 | 0.1–0.6 | 0.2–0.4 |
| Type I | 0.4–2.0 | 0.5–4.0 | 1.0–6.0 |
| Type II | 0.2–2.0 | 4.0–48.0 | 8.0–44.0 |
| Hereditary Spherocytosis and Triosephosphate isomerase deficiency | 1.0–6.0 | 0.2–14.0 | 6.0–30.0 |

* In percent hemolysis

and 0.4 ml toluene/ml packed red cell mass. The mixture is shaken vigorously for 5 minutes and centrifuged at 3000 rpm for 15 minutes. Using a Pasteur pipet, the dark red hemolysate is removed and the hemoglobin concentration determined by a conventional procedure (p. 7).

Dilutions of hemolysate are then made in saline so that the hemoglobin concentration is 0.5, 1.0, and 2.0 g/dl.

3. Phosphate buffer (0.05M; pH 7.0)

0.68 g of potassium dihydrogen phosphate is dissolved in 100 ml of distilled water; 1.34 g of disodium hydrogen phosphate is dissolved in 100 ml of distilled water; 400 ml of the potassium dihydrogen phosphate solution is added to 600 ml of the disodium hydrogen phosphate.

4. 0-Dianisidine staining mixture

a. 1.46 g of sodium acetate and 0.52 ml of glacial acetic acid are dissolved in 400 ml of distilled water and the volume made up to 500 ml (1.5M; pH 4.7).

b. 1.43 g of 0-dianisidine is dissolved in 100 ml of 95% ethyl alcohol (3.3' dimethoxybenzidine)

c. 3% hydrogen peroxide. 1 ml of 30% hydrogen peroxide is diluted to 10 ml with distilled water. This reagent is prepared fresh.

d. Immediately prior to use, the staining mixture is prepared by adding together

*ml*

| | |
|---|---:|
| 0-dianisidine reagent | 70 |
| Acetic acetate buffer | 10 |
| Distilled water | 18 |
| 3% Hydrogen peroxide | 2 |

5. Centrifuge (GLC-1)
6. Electrophoresis equipment
7. Hot-air oven
8. Ponseau S stain

### *Method*

1. Eight electrophoresis membranes are soaked overnight in the phosphate buffer.

2. 0.02 ml of each hemoglobin concentration are added to 0.2 ml. samples of the control serum and the patient's serum to provide final hemoglobin concentrations of 50,100, and 200 mg/dl.

3. These dilutions are incubated at 37°C for 20 minutes. The 200 mg/dl dilution is further incubated at 37°C overnight with the control serum, to obtain methemalbumin.

4. The electrophoresis equipment is set up following the manufacturer's instructions, and the cell is filled with the phosphate buffer.

5. With a micropipet, deliver 4 ml of each of the following to each of the previously soaked membranes, making sure that the specimens are applied exactly in the center of the strip:

    a. Control serum (no hemoglobin added)

    b. 50 mg/dl (control serum)

    c. 100 mg/dl (control serum)

    d. 200 mg/dl (control serum)

    e. Patient's serum (no hemoglobin added)

    f. 50 mg/dl (patient's serum)

    g. 100 mg/dl (patient's serum)

    h. 200 mg/dl (patient's serum)

6. The applied samples are allowed to equilibrate for 30 minutes and the electrophoresis cell to run at 190 volts for 90 minutes.

7. The membranes (*b, c, d, f, g,* and *h*) are labeled, placed between blotters and dried by placing in a warm hot air oven at 55°C for 20 minutes.

8. The membranes (*a* and *e*) are not dried in this way, but are stained with Ponceau S, as in the routine protein electrophoresis.

9. The remaining dried membranes are stained by immersing in 0-dianisidine dye for 10 minutes and placing in distilled water until ready to be evaluated.

*Normal.* If, in addition to the hemoglobin-haptoglobin band, a second band of free hemoglobin appears, it indicates that more hemoglobin was added than could be bound to the haptoglobin. Normal haptoglobin concentration (expressed as mg hemoglobin-binding capacity) is approximately 100 mg hemoglobin/dl serum.

If free hemoglobin appears in the 50 mg/dl sample, haptoglobin is decreased. If free hemoglobin is absent in the 200 mg/dl sample, haptoglobin is increased.

### Notes

1. Haptoglobins are plasma glycoproteins which show alpha-2 globulin mobility on cellulose acetate electrophoresis. The protein has a strong affinity for free hemoglobin.

2. Haptoglobin begins to disappear when hemolysis exceeds about twice the normal rate. This occurs whether the hemolysis is predominately extravascular or intravascular; but rapid depletion, often with the formation of methemalbumin occurs as a result of small degrees of intravascular hemolysis.

3. Reduced haptoglobin levels are also found in megaloblastic anemias, following hemorrhage into the tissues, and in liver disease.

4. An increased haptoglobin level may be found in infections, malignancy, tissue damage, Hodgkin's disease, rheumatoid arthritis, and systemic lupus erythematosus.

## ACID HEMOLYSINS FOR PAROXYSMAL
## NOCTURNAL HEMOGLOBINURIA

### Ham's Test[9] (Modified)

*Principle.* The patient's red cells are exposed at 37°C to the action of normal or the patients own serum, acidified to a pH of 6.5 to 7.0.

### Reagents and Apparatus
1. 0.2 N Hydrochloric acid
2. 0.85% Sodium chloride
3. Graduated pipets—0.1 ml, 1.0 ml
4. 37°C Waterbath
5. 20 ml Patient's defibrinated blood. Place 2 bent paper clips in the bottom of a 50-ml Erlenmeyer flask, and swirl it continuously for 10 to 15 minutes.
6. 10 ml Normal defibrinated blood of the same blood group (ABO) as the patient.
7. Centrifuge (GLC-1 Sorval)
8. Test tubes—12 x 75 mm

### Method
1. Centrifuge the defibrinated blood samples by spinning at 2,000 rpm for 5 minutes. The serum from each tube is saved and labeled.
2. Wash the cells 3 times with an equal volume of saline. Centrifuge the last washing at 3,000 rpm for 10 minutes to achieve adequate cell packing.
3. A 5% suspension of both patient's and normal red cells are prepared by adding 0.5 ml of packed cells to 9.5 ml saline.
4. Acidified serum is prepared by adding 0.05 ml 0.2 N hydrochloric acid to 0.95 ml of both the patient's and normal serum.
5. 0.5 ml samples of the 5% red cell suspension are introduced into 12 × 75 mm tubes and centrifuged at 2,000 rpm for 2 to 3 minutes. The saline-serum supernatant is completely removed with a Pasteur pipet.
6. Six 12 x 75 mm tubes are set up as in Table 4-5.
7. All the tubes are well shaken to mix, incubated at 37°C for 1 hour, and centrifuged at 2,000 rpm for 5 minutes. Examine the supernatants for hemolysis.

*Normal.* A positive test is indicated by hemolysis in the tubes containing the patient's cells with acidified serum (tubes 2 and 4), the other tubes being unaffected.

### Notes
1. The patient's serum is best obtained by defibrination. If it is obtained from blood that was allowed to clot at 37°C, it will often be hemolyzed.

TABLE 4-5. Ham's Test Methodology.

| TUBE | 1 | 2 | 3 | 4 | 5 | 6 |
|---|---|---|---|---|---|---|
| Cells (0.05 ml) | Patient's | Patient's | Patient's | Patient's | Normal | Normal |
| Serum (0.5 ml) | Patient's | | Normal | | Patient's | |
| Acid serum (0.5 ml) | | Patient's | | Normal | | Patient's |

2. Heating the serum at 56°C for 30 minutes destroys the complement activity needed for the hemolytic systems.

3. A positive test is usually diagnostic of paroxysmal nocturnal hemoglobinuria. False-positive tests are occasionally seen in congenital spherocytosis. If this is suspected, the test should be repeated using inactivated acidified serum (56°C for 30 minutes). In paroxysmal nocturnal hemoglobinuria, the inactivated modification produces negative results but remains positive in spherocytosis.

4. From 10 to 50% lysis is usually obtained in a positive test, when lysis is measured quantitatively on the basis of liberated hemoglobin. The test can be made more sensitive by using a young red cell population (reticulocytes) such as the upper red cell layer obtained by centrifugation.

5. Paroxysmal nocturnal hemoglobinuria (PNH) cells are *not* sensitive to acidification per se. The addition of the acid adjusts the pH of the serum to the optimum for the activity of the hemolytic system. The factor in normal serum which lyses PNH cells is complement. The fluid-phase-activated C3 component of the complement system is adsorbed on red cells without the necessity of amboceptor.[10] The role of properdin is unknown, but it is believed to act as a subcomponent of the C3 complex. Reduction in pH to 6.5 to 7.0 appears to facilitate the adsorption of C3.

### Crosby's Test[11]

*Principle:* Patient's red cells are added to a thrombin-acidified serum mixture. Thrombin has the ability to activate the hemolytic component in the test, but not in normal serum.

### *Reagents and Apparatus*
1. N/3 Hydrochloric acid
2. Topical thrombin*

---

* Parke, Davis

3. Defibrinated patient's cells
4. Normal serum compatible with the patient's cells
5. 0.85% Saline
6. 0.2-ml Graduated pipets—0.2 ml
7. Graduated pipets—2 ml
8. 37°C Waterbath

*Method*
1. The patient's cells are washed 3 times in normal saline.
2. 2 ml of normal serum, 0.1 ml of N/3 hydrochloric acid, and 0.2 ml of washed patient's cells are added to a tube and mixed.
3. 1 ml of the contents of the tube is removed and 50 units of thrombin (reconstituted as in the manufacturer's instructions) is added to it.
4. The tubes in 2 and 3 above are incubated at 37°C for 15 minutes and centrifuged at 2,000 rpm. for 15 minutes.

*Results.* A positive test for paroxysmal nocturnal hemoglobinuria is indicated if there is hemolysis in both the incubated tubes, the hemolysis being greater in the tube containing the thrombin.

*Note.* The test can be made quantitative by estimating the amount of hemoglobin liberated.

## SUGAR WATER TEST[12]

*Principle.* PNH red cells hemolyse when incubated with compatible normal serum in a sucrose solution of low ionic strength. The test depends on the fact that red cells adsorb complement components when suspended in a medium of low ionic strength, even in the absence of antibody. PNH cells, undergo lysis in these conditions by virtue of their increased sensitivity to complement.

*Reagents and Apparatus*
1. Clotted blood from both patient and ABO compatible donor.
2. Buffer (pH 6.1) 0.005M sodium dihydrogen phosphate ($NaH_2PO_4H_2O$): 690 mg of monobasic sodium phosphate is dissolved in 1 liter of distilled water.

0.005 M Disodium hydrogen phosphate ($Na_2HPO_47H_2O$): 135 mg of dibasic sodium phosphate is dissolved in 1 liter of distilled water.

910 ml of 0.005 M sodium dihydrogen phosphate is mixed with 90 ml of disodium hydrogen phosphate. The buffer can be stored indefinitely at 4°C.

3. Isotonic sucrose solution: 924 mg of sucrose (0.27M) is dissolved in 10 ml of double phosphate buffer. The pH is adjusted to 6.1 with 0.75 N sodium hydroxide or with 0.75 N hydrochloric acid.

4. 0.75 N Sodium hydroxide: Dissolve 3.0 g sodium hydroxide in 100 ml of distilled water.

5. 0.75 N Hydrochloric acid: 6.25 ml of 12 N (concentrated) hydrochloric acid is added to 100 ml of distilled water.

6. Centrifuge (GLC-1 Sorval)

*Method*

1. Separate the serum from the clotted blood samples of both patient and control.

2. A 50% saline suspension of cells is prepared from each sample from the residual clots.

3. Add to each of these tubes

0.85 ml sucrose solution

0.05 ml unacidified autologous serum

4. Add 0.1 ml of the 50% suspension of patient's red cells to one tube.

5. Add 0.1 ml of the control cells to the second tube.

6. Both the tubes are mixed and incubated at 37°C for 30 minutes.

7. Centrifuge both tubes at 2,000 rpm for 1 to 2 minutes and examine the supernatant for hemolysis.

*Results.* A positive test for PNH is indicated when the patient's cells are hemolyzed. The control cells should show no more than a trace of lysis.

*Notes*

1. Blood collected in EDTA or heparin is unsuitable for this test.

2. No hemolysis is found in other types of hemolytic anemia.

## DETECTION OF PAROXYSMAL COLD HEMOGLOBINURIA (PCH)

### Donath-Landsteiner Test

*Principle.* The Donath-Landsteiner antibody of PCH differs from normal cold antibodies in that it is more hemolytic toward normal cells. An autohemolysin in the patient's blood combines with the red cells only at low temperatures; on warming the blood to 37°C, these cells hemolyze if complement is present.

*Reagents and Apparatus*
1. Crushed ice
2. Tubes—10 x 77 mm
3. 37°C Waterbath

*Qualitative Method*
1. 5 ml of the patient's whole blood is added to each of 2 previously warmed tubes.

2. One tube is left at 37°C while the other is immersed in a bath of crushed ice for 30 minutes.

3. Remove the tube from the ice and place it at 37°. Leave both tubes at 37°C until their clots retract (approximately 1 hour).

*Results.* In PCH, the fluid exuded by the clot which was cooled will show hemolysis. The serum kept at 37°C will be free of hemolysis.

### Sanford's Method[13]

#### Reagents and Apparatus

1. 10% Saline dilution of guinea pig complement
2. 5% Patient's washed red cells
3. Patient's serum
4. 37°C Waterbath
5. Graduated pipets—1 ml
6. Refrigerator

#### Method

1. 5-ml Samples of test blood are added to oxalated and plain tubes.

2. The serum is expressed from the clot by incubating the plain tube at 37°C for 1 hour.

3. The cells from the oxalated blood are washed 3 times with saline and made up to a 5% suspension in saline.

4. Tubes are set up as in Table 4-6.

5. Place tubes 1 and 2 (Table 4-6) in the refrigerator for 30 minutes and incubate all 4 at 37°C for 2 hours.

*Results.* In PCH, hemolysis occurs in tube 1 and occasionally in tube 2. Tubes 3 and 4 should be free of hemolysis.

#### Notes

1. The highest temperature at which Donath-Landsteiner antibodies are absorbed onto red cells is 18°C. Therefore, no lysis is found unless the cell-serum suspension is cooled below this temperature.

2. Chilling in ice results in maximal absorption of the antibody, which is fixed on the cells. In the presence of sufficient complement, the

TABLE 4-6. Formulations for Sanford's Method of Detecting PCH.

| TUBE | 1 | 2 | 3 | 4 |
|---|---|---|---|---|
| 5% Red Cell Suspension (ml) | 0.2 | 0.2 | 0.2 | 0.2 |
| Patient's Serum (ml) | 0.5 | 0.5 | 0.5 | 0.5 |
| 10% Guinea Pig Complement (ml) | 0.2 | — | 0.2 | — |
| Normal Saline (ml) | 0.1 | 0.3 | 0.1 | 0.3 |

antibody lyses the cells when the suspension is warmed to body temperature.

## INDIRECT ANTIGLOBULIN TEST FOR THE DETECTION OF THE DONATH-LANDSTEINER ANTIBODIES

***Principle.*** The Donath-Landsteiner (DL) antibody can be detected by the indirect antiglobulin test using an IgG serum if the cells are washed in cold buffered saline. If cold saline is used, the DL antibody will remain on the cells during washing and will not be eluted. False-positive results due to red cell absorption of anti-H is avoided by the addition of an anticomplementary agent such as EDTA, which removes the calcium ions and so preventing C1 formation.

### Reagents and Apparatus
1. Buffered EDTA (pH 7,0). Dissolve 8.9 g of EDTA in 15 ml N sodium hydroxide, and make up the volume to 200 ml.
2. 0.85% Sodium chloride
3. Group O P-positive red cells
4. Centrifuge (GLC-1 Sorval)
5. 37°C Waterbath
6. "Broad-spectrum" antihuman globulin serum

### Note
1. The titer of the antihuman globulin sera used is critical. If negative results are found, the test should be repeated using titrations of the antihuman serum from 1:1 to 1:4096.
2. This technique is the most sensitive method of detecting the DL antibody present in an amount insufficient to cause lysis. It is also an excellent method to detect the DL antibody in old serum samples.

### Method
1. 0.1 ml of buffered EDTA is added to 5 ml of patient's serum.
2. Two sets of doubling dilutions of the buffered EDTA-patient's serum mixture from 1:1 to 1:128 are then made in 0.85% sodium chloride.
3. 1 volume of a 50% saline suspension of normal group O P-positive red cells is then added to 10 volumes of each dilution.
4. The tubes are mixed and one set incubated at 4°C for 1 hour; the second set at 37°C for 1 hour.
5. The cells from the dilutions at 4°C are washed 4 times using large volumes of cold saline, 1 drop of broad spectrum antihuman globulin is added.

6. The tubes are centrifuged for 15 seconds and inspected for agglutination using a hand lens.

7. The cells from the dilution at 37°C are also washed, using room temperature or warm saline, and the antihuman globulin test carried out as previously described. The incubation at 37°C is the negative control.

## DETECTION OF ANTIBODIES OF UNKNOWN THERMAL OPTIMUM

### Method 1

*Principle.* Patient's serum is titrated and exposed to group O red cells at two different temperatures.

*Reagents and Apparatus*
1. Graduated pipets—0.1 ml
2. Graduated pipets—1 ml
3. Normal saline
4. Group O $R_1R_2$ cells
5. 37°C Waterbath
6. Tubes—10 x 75 mm

*Method*
1. Duplicate doubling dilutions of patient's serum are made up in saline to a titer of 1:1024, and an equal volume of washed 20% group O $R_1R_2$ (CDe/cDE) cells is added to each set of tubes.

2. One group is incubated at room temperature; the other is placed in a 37°C waterbath.

3. Both dilutions are read microscopically for agglutination after 2 hours of incubation. Direct Coombs' tests are then carried out on all negative readings (p. 392).

*Results.* The highest dilution producing a positive result is recorded as the titer.

### Method 2

*Principle.* Acidified patient's serum is used in place of unacidified serum to enhance the titer of any cold antibody present.

*Reagents and Apparatus*
1. As in Method 1
2. 0.2 N Hydrochloric acid

*Method*
1. One volume of 0.2 N hydrochloric acid is added to 9 volumes of patient's serum.

2. Steps 1 to 3 of Method 1 are performed.

*Notes.* By acidifying the serum, the titer of any incomplete cold antibody is normally increased in relation to its titer when unacidified. No change is found if the antibody is of the warm type.

## Method 3

*Principle.* Complement needed for cold antibodies is destroyed by heat.

### Reagents and Apparatus
1. As in Method 1
2. 56°C Waterbath

### Method
1. Inactivate the patient's serum at 56°C for 30 minutes. This destroys normal complement.
2. Repeat the procedures of Method 1.

*Note.* Cold antibodies usually fail to sensitize red cells to antihuman globulin if the serum used for this sensitization has been heated to 56°C.

### Precautions
1. When setting up titrations that are to be incubated at 37°C, the cells and serum are first warmed to this temperature before mixing.
2. It is best to use at least 5 volumes of serum to 1 volume of cells for every titration.
3. Incubations should be carried out for at least 2 hours and all results read microscopically.

If the unknown antibody appears to be of the warm type, its specificity should be determined. The first step, if a Rhesus antibody is suspected, is to test its ability to react with group O $R_1R_2$ (CDe/cDE), group O $R_2R_2$ (cDE/cDE) and group O rr (cde/cde) cells, respectively. By using this panel, the range can be narrowed, and the antibodies can be determined by testing against O $R_1r$ (CDe/cde), O $R_1R_2$ (CDe/cDE), O $R_2r$ (cDE/cde) O R''r (cdE/cde), O R'r (Cde/cde), O R''R'' (cdE/cdE), and O R'R' (Cde/Cde) cells.

## DETECTION OF HEMOLYSINS

### Warm Type

*Principle.* Patient's serum is titrated in fresh normal serum to provide complement. The dilutions are incubated at 37°C with group O cells and read macroscopically for signs of hemolysis.

*Reagents and Apparatus.* As in the detection of antibodies (Method 1).

### Method

1. Warm hemolysins can be excluded in cases of acquired hemolytic anemia by making doubling dilutions of patient's serum in fresh normal serum.

2. The titrations are incubated with an equal volume of 2% group O Rhesus positive cells at 37°C for 2 hours and read macroscopically.

*Results.* The highest dilution producing hemolysis is recorded as the titer.

## Cold Type

*Principle.* Patient's serum is titrated in fresh acidified normal serum to enhance cold hemolysin activity in the presence of complement.

*Reagents and Apparatus.* As in the detection of antibodies (Method 2).

### Method

1. Cold hemolysins can be titrated by making doubling dilutions of patient's serum in fresh normal acidified serum.

2. The titrations are incubated with an equal volume of 2% group O Rhesus positive cells at room temperature for 2 hours and read macroscopically.

*Results.* The highest dilution producing hemolysis is recorded as the titer.

## DETECTION OF HEINZ BODIES

### Beutler's Method[14] (Method 1)

*Principle.* Acetylphenylhydrazine is added to the blood and the solution is incubated at 37°C for 4 hours. The red cells are then stained and examined for the presence of Heinz bodies.

### Reagents and Apparatus

1. Heparinized or EDTA blood

2. Buffer solution pH 7.6: M/15 potassium dihydrogen phosphate: dissolve 9.08 g of the anhydrous salt in 1 liter of distilled water. M/15 disodium hydrogen phosphate: dissolve 9.47 g of the anhydrous salt in 1 liter of distilled water. Add 13 ml of the M/15 potassium dihydrogen phosphate to 87 ml of the M/15 disodium hydrogen phosphate.

3. Crystal violet: 2 g of the stain is added to 100 ml of 0.73% sodium chloride. The mixture is shaken for 5 minutes and filtered.

4. 0.1 g of acetylphenylhydrazine is dissolved in 100 ml of the buffer solution.

5. Graduated pipets—0.1 ml

6. Graduated pipets—2 ml

7. 37°C Waterbath

*Method*

1. 0.1 ml of fresh heparinized blood is added to 2 ml of the acetylphenylhydrazine solution. The resulting solution is aerated by blowing air into it with a pipet.

2. Leaving the pipet in the tube, incubate at 37°C for 2 hours, reaerate and leave for another 2 hours.

3. A small drop of the treated blood is placed on a coverslip and inverted onto a glass slide on which has been placed a large drop of crystal violet stain.

4. The preparation is left for 10 minutes at room temperature for the cells to stain and is examined under the 97× oil immersion objective.

*Results.* The patient has a glutathione deficiency if more than 40% of the cells have 5 or more Heinz bodies.

## Method 2

1. 0.5% Methyl violet in normal saline
2. Heparinized blood

*Method*

1. Equal volumes of heparinized blood and methyl violet solution are mixed and the red cells allowed to stain for 10 minutes at room temperature.

2. The wet preparation is examined under a coverslip with the 97× oil immersion objective.

*Notes*

1. Heinz bodies are manifestations that probably represent areas of denatured hemoglobin and damaged red cell stroma. They are best seen in unstained wet preparations as highly refractile bodies on or near the periphery of the red cell. They also stain well with 1% brilliant cresyl blue in normal saline or with a 0.5% saline dilution of methyl violet. They are *not* stained with the Romanowsky dyes.

2. The size of the bodies ranges from 1 to 3 $\mu$ in diameter. They are formed in large numbers in cases of chronic drug intoxication, especially from many benzene derivatives. These organic chemicals are thought to cause oxidation damage to areas of the red cell stroma and hemoglobin.

3. In the normal red cell, glucose-6-phosphate dehydrogenase catalyzes the reduction of triphosphopyridine nucleotide. This helps in the synthesis of reduced glutathione, which protects the red cell stroma and hemoglobin from damage.

4. Red cells of patients, who either lack glucose-6-phosphate dehydrogenase or have a reduced level, are susceptible to hemolysis by many drugs, the most common being primaquine, naphthalene, phenacetin and fava bean products.

Heinz bodies are also seen in patients with polycythemia who are under treatment with phenylhydrazine. Other drugs associated with Heinz body formation are chlorates, naphthalene, phenacetin, resorcinol and sulfonamides.

## GLUTATHIONE ASSAY[15]

*Principle.* The method depends on the development of a stable yellow colored couplex with 5,5'-dithiobis-(2-nitrobenzoic acid) (DTNB). The test is read in 19 mm cuvets on a Coleman Junior Spectrophometer at a wavelength of 412 nm.

### Reagents and Apparatus
1. Precipitating solution: 1.67 g glacial metaphosphoric acid, 0.2 g disodium or dipotassium EDTA, and 30 g sodium chloride are dissolved in 100 ml distilled water. The solution is stable approximately 3 weeks at 4°C.
2. Phosphate solution: 0.3 g disodium hydrogen phosphate; 89.3 g of the salt are dissolved in 1 liter of distilled water. This solution is stable indefinitely unless molds form. If crystals develop during storage at 4°C they may be dissolved by heating.
3. DTNB Reagent: 40 mg 5,5-dithiobis-(2 nitrobenzoic acid) is dissolved in 100 ml of a 1% sodium citrate solution. The reagent is stable for at least 13 weeks at 4°C.
4. Stock standard glutathione solution: 2 mg metaphosphoric acid and 0.0625 g glutathione are dissolved in 100 ml of saturated aqueous sodium chloride. The solution is buffered and stored at −20°C in 2 ml aliquots (the standard does not freeze solid at this temperature).
5. Heparinized whole blood, patient and normal
6. Graduated pipets—2 ml
7. "Prothrombin time" pipets—0.2 ml
8. Graduated pipets—5 ml
9. Whatman No. 1 filter paper

### Method
1. Carry out the procedure on a normal blood in parallel with the test sample.
2. Determine the hematocrit of the heparinized whole blood sample. Add 0.2 ml of well-mixed blood to 1.8 ml distilled water. Allow the blood to hemolyze, and add 3.0 ml of precipitating solution.
3. Allow to stand for 5 minutes and filter through a Whatman No. 1 filter paper.
4. As soon as possible after the filtrates have been made, set up 4 tubes as in Table 4-7.

TABLE 4-7. Glutathione Assay Test Procedure.

|  | TEST | CONTROL | STANDARD | BLANK |
|---|---|---|---|---|
| Filtrate patient | 2.0 ml | — | — | — |
| Filtrate control | — | 2.0 ml | — | — |
| Stock standard 1:25 dilution | — | — | 2.0 ml | — |
| Phosphate solution | 3.0 ml | 3.0 ml | 3.0 ml | 5.0 ml |
| DTNB | 1.0 ml | 1.0 ml | 1.0 ml | 1.0 ml |

5. The tubes are mixed by inversion and their optical density read in a Spectrophotometer at 402 nm, using 19 mm cuvets.

### Calculation

$$\frac{\text{Optical density of the test}}{\text{Optical density of the standard}} \times \frac{62.5}{\text{hematocrit}} \times 100$$

$$= \text{mg\% glutathione in the red cells}$$

### Normal. >45 mg%

### Notes

1. Glutathione is a tripeptide of glycine, glutamic acid and cysteine. In the blood, almost all of the reduced glutathione (GSH) is found within the red cells. In individuals who are sensitive to the hemolytic action of drugs, the quantity of intracellular GSH is reduced, and it is unstable when the red cells are exposed to drugs such as acetylphenylhydrazine.

2. Using the above procedure, the optical density of the standard approximates 0.29 to 0.31.

## GLUTATHIONE STABILITY TEST[15]

**Principle.** When normal red cells are incubated with acetylphenylhydrazine there is little effect on the glutathione content, but in enzyme deficient red cells, a reduction of glutathione is found.

### Reagents and Apparatus

1. Acetylphenylhydrazine
2. As for the glutathione assay

### Method

1. 5 mg Acetylphenylhydrazine is placed in a plastic "Coulter" vial and 1 ml heparinized blood, less than 3 hours old added.

2. The blood is mixed well and incubated for 1 hour at 37°C.

3. The sample is remixed and reincubated for an additional hour at 37°C.

4. A glutathione assay is carried out on the treated blood as previously described (p. 154).

*Normal.* The glutathione level is reduced by less than 20% by incubation with acetylphenylhydrazine in normal blood. In cells that are enzyme deficient, the reduction is frequently in the order of 50%.

## QUALITATIVE ESTIMATION OF GLUCOSE-6-PHOSPHATE DEHYDROGENASE (MODIFIED)[16]

*Principle.* Red cells are hemolyzed and incubated with glucose-6-phosphate and triphosphopyridine nucleotide. If glucose-6-phosphate dehydrogenase is present in the cells, it removes hydrogen from the glucose-6-phosphate, being converted to the lactone by the hydrogen ions. Brilliant cresyl blue acts as the indicator.

### Reagents and Apparatus

1. Glucose-6-phosphate (G-6-P): 16.5 mg of G-6P disodium is dissolved in 1 ml of distilled water. The reagent is prepared fresh.

2. TRIS buffer pH 8.5 0.74 M: 17.9 g of trishydroxymethylaminomethane is dissolved in 50 ml of distilled water; 14.4 ml of 2.96 M hydrochloric acid is added. The buffer is adjusted to a pH of 8.5 with the acid.

3. Triphosphopyridine nucleotide 0.1% (TPN): 5 mg TPN is dissolved in 5 ml of distilled water. This reagent is prepared fresh.

4. Brilliant cresyl blue: 0.32 g of the stain is dissolved in 1 liter of distilled water.

5. Heparinized blood, packed cells, unknown

6. Heparinized blood, packed cells, normal control

7. Mineral oil

8. Graduated pipets—10 ml

9. Graduated pipets—1 ml

10. Micropipets—0.05 ml

11. 37°C Waterbath

### Method

1. Add 1 ml of distilled water and 0.2 ml of TRIS buffer to each of 2 tubes.

2. Mix well, add 0.1 ml of the unknown packed cells to one tube and 0.1 ml of the normal control cells to the other tube.

3. Add the following to both test and control:

|  | *ml* |
|---|---|
| G-6-P solution | 0.05 |
| 0.1% TPN | 0.05 |
| Brilliant cresyl blue | 0.25 |

4. The contents of the tubes are mixed and carefully overlaid with sufficient mineral oil to cover their surfaces.

5. Both tubes are incubated at 37°C for 6 hours, the tubes being examined at regular intervals for signs of decolorization.

*Normal.* A normal blood will show complete decolorization within 100 minutes.

### Notes

1. Blood with hematocrits below 25% should not be used. If anemic bloods are to be tested, the hematocrit should be adjusted to between 40 to 45% before the test is carried out.

2. Bloods having high reticulocyte counts can give false results, because these cells possess a higher G-6-PD level than mature red cells.

3. Utilizing radioactive labeling methods (Cr[51]), it is possible to show that the red cells deficient in glucose-6-phosphate dehydrogenase survive a shorter time in vivo, even when they are not stressed by the presence of drugs.

## QUANTITATIVE ESTIMATION OF GLUCOSE-6-PHOSPHATE DEHYDROGENASE[17]

*Principle.* EDTA blood is hemolyzed in a solution of NADP and distilled water. After lysis is complete, buffered substrate is added and the sample transferred to a cuvet and the optical density read at 340 nm. During lysis, other endogenous substances that could contribute to measured activity are exhausted; the enzyme 6-phosphogluconate dehydrogenase is almost completely inactivated during this lysis step and if present would contribute to the measured rate.

$$G\text{-}6\text{-}P = NADP \rightarrow 6\text{-phosphogluconate} + NADPH$$
$$G\text{-}6\text{-}PD$$

### Reagents and Apparatus

1. UV range spectrophotometer

2. Triethanolamine buffer (0.5 M; pH 7.5) 0.93 g triethanolamine hydrochloride and 0.2 g disodium ethylenediaminotetraacetic acid (EDTA) are dissolved in 50 ml distilled water. The pH is adjusted to 7.5 with 0.1 N sodium hydroxide and the total volume diluted to 100 ml with distilled water.

3. Triphosphopyridine nucleotide (0.01M): 25 mg of triphosphopyridine are dissolved in 1.0 ml of 1% sodium bicarbonate solution.

4. Glucose-6-phosphate; (0.031M): 130 mg of glucose-6-phosphate are dissolved in 10 ml distilled water.

The triphosphorpyridine nucleotide and glucose-6-phosphate should be stored stoppered in a refrigerator to 0 to 4°C. Both of these reagents are stable for 2 to 3 weeks under these conditions, but in the frozen state they may be kept for up to 3 months.

5. Digitoxins solution (saturated): 1 g digotixin is added to 100 ml distilled water, shaken to dissolve, and filtered.

6. EDTA blood sample

7. 0.85% Saline

**Method**

1. Wash 0.5 ml of EDTA whole blood twice with 5 ml physiological saline.

2. Suspend the sedimented cells in 1 ml of saline, mix well, and calculate the total red cell count by a conventional method (p. 000). The count should approximate $2 \times 10^3$/mm.

3. Add together:

|  | *ml* |
|---|---|
| Red cell suspension | 1.0 |
| Distilled water | 1.0 |
| Triethanolamine buffer | 0.7 |
| Digitonin solution | 0.3 |

4. Allow this mixture to stand for 15 minutes in a refrigerator, centrifuge at 1,000 g for 15 minutes and discard the insoluble material.

5. Pipet successively into the spectrophotometer cuvet

|  | *ml* |
|---|---|
| Triethanolamine buffer | 2.85 |
| Red cell hemolysate (from 3 above). | 0.05 |
| Triphosphopyridine nucleotide | 0.05 |

6. Set up a blank cuvet. Add:

|  | *ml* |
|---|---|
| Triethanolamine buffer | 2.90 |
| Red cell hemolysate (from 3 above) | 0.05 |

7. Mix the contents of both tubes with a glass rod flattened at one end. Keep at 25°C for 5 minutes and add 0.05 ml glucose-6-phosphate solution to both cuvets.

8. Read the test cuvet against the blank at a wavelength of 340 nm. Spectrophotometric measurements are: Light path 1 cm temperature 25°C (constant temperature cuvet chamber). The optical density increase should not be more than 0.030/minute. If greater, dilute the sample accordingly.

9. Wait for an optical density of about 0.020. Start a stopwatch and read the optical density at 2-minute intervals for 10 minutes. Calculate the mean optical density change/minute.

*Calculations*

0.05 ml Hemolysate is taken for the determination of G6-PD activity in the red cells, which on hemolysis is diluted threefold. Therefore, the total dilution factor is $3 \times 20 = 60$. Then $\Delta E_{340}$/minute $\times$ 60,000 = G6-PD units/ml red cell suspension.

$$\text{Therefore } \frac{\text{Units/ml red cell suspension} \times 10^9}{\text{Red cell count/ml}}$$

$$= \text{G-D-PD activity in units}/10^9 \text{ red cells.}$$

*Normal.* 6.5 to 7.9 Bücher units/$10^9$ cells

*Notes*

1. G6-PD is inhibited by primaquine and other 8-aminoquinalines in millimolar concentrations, as well as by phenylhydrazine.

2. A deficiency of the enzyme in the red cells is a major cause of congenital nonspherocytic hemolytic anemia. In this condition, the enzyme content of older red cells is decreased, resulting in a sensitivity to certain drugs including primaquine, chloramphenicol, the sulfonamides, and the nitrofurans.

3. The optimum pH of the G6 PD reaction is 8.3. Between pH 7.4 and 8.6 there is little change in the enzyme activity. The measurements are made at pH 7.5 because this is nearest to physiological conditions and allows a comparison to be made with other enzyme activities which are usually measured at this pH.

4. The use of phosphate buffer should be avoided because 0.1 M phosphate completely inhibits the enzymes.

5. Blood samples having high reticulocyte counts can produce false results, since these cells possess a higher G6-PD level than mature red cells.

6. Using radioactive methods ($C^{51}$) it has been shown that red cells deficient in G6-PD survive a shorter time in vivo, even when they are not stressed by the presence of drugs.

## SCREENING TESTS FOR GLUCOSE-6-PHOSPHATE DEHYDROGENASE DEFICIENCY

### Method 1[18] (Ascorbate-Cyanide)

*Principles.* When sodium cyanide and sodium ascorbate are added to blood, catalase is inhibited by the cyanide. This allows hydrogen peroxide to be produced from the coupled oxidation of ascorbate and hemoglobin. Glucose-6-phosphate dehydrogenase deficient cells are quickly oxidized by the hydrogen peroxide and brown methemoglobin develops.

### Reagents and Apparatus

1. 10 mg of sodium ascorbate and 5 mg of glucose are added into a series of tubes. (This mixture can be stored stoppered at $-20°C$ indefinitely.)

2. Iso-osmotic phosphate buffer (pH 7.4) (0.15M):

2.34 g of sodium dihydrogen phosphate ($NaH_2PO_3$. $2H_2O$) is dissolved in 100 ml of distilled water.

21.3 g of disodium hydrogen phosphate ($Na_2H,PO_4$ $2H_2O$) is dissolved in 100 ml of distilled water.

18 ml of the sodium dihydrogen phosphate is added to 82 ml of the disodium hydrogen phosphate.

3. 500 mg of sodium cyanide are dissolved in 50 ml of distilled water and 20 ml of iso-osmotic phosphate buffer (pH 7.4) are added.

5. EDTA anticoagulated blood

### Method

1. Aerate the blood by blowing air or oxygen through the sample until it turns a bright red color.

2. Add 2 ml of the aerated blood to a tube containing the prepared sodium ascorbate and glucose.

3. Add 2 drops of the sodium cyanide solution and incubate unstoppered at 37°C.

4. Remix the suspension after 2 hours' incubation and again after 3 to 4 hours.

5. Note the color of the suspension after each mixing.

### Results

Glucose-6-phosphate dihydrogenase deficient blood becomes brown within 1 to 2 hours while normal blood only darkens slowly over several hours. Heterozygotes with intermediate levels of enzyme activity also become brown within 2 hours.

### Note

The test is positive when there is a deficiency of G6-PD and of other enzymes of the hexosemonophosphate shunt, or when glutathione synthesis is defective.

## Method 2[19]

*Principle.* Glucose-6-phosphate is oxidized to 6-phosphogluconate, and triphosphopyridine nucleotide (TPN) is reduced to TPNH in the presence of G6-PD from the red cell homolysate. The red cells also contain 6-phosphogluconate which reduces more TPN. The TPNH when activated by ultraviolet light, produces a vivid fluorescence.

### Results and Apparatus
1. Glucose-6-phosphate (0.01M):
42 mg of glucose-6-phosphate are dissolved in 10 ml distilled water.
2. Triphosphopyridine nucleotide (0.0075M):
18.75 mg triphosphopyridine nucleotide are dissolved in 1.0 ml of 1% sodium bicarbonate solution.
3. Digotonin solution (saturated):
1 g digitonin is added to 100 ml distilled water. The mixture is shaken and filtered.
4. Potassium phosphate buffer (0.25 M, pH 7.4):
8.25 ml of 1 M stock dipotassium hydrogen phosphate and 1.75 ml of potassium dihydrogen phosphate are added together and made up to 100 ml with distilled water.
5. Reaction mixture
   The following reagents are added together:

|  | ml |
|---|---|
| 0.01M Glucose-6-phosphate | 0.10 |
| 0.0075M Triphosphopyridine nucleotide | 0.10 |
| Saturated digitonin | 0.20 |
| Potassium phosphate buffer | 0.30 |
| Distilled water | 0.30 |

6. EDTA anticoagulated blood
7. Ultraviolet light (Wood's lamp)
8. Whatman No. 1 filter paper

### Method
1. 1 volume of whole blood is added to 10 volumes of the reaction mixture and incubated 5 to 10 minutes at 37°C.
2. A drop of the blood reaction mixture is placed on a Whatman No. 1 filter paper and viewed under an ultraviolet lamp.
*Normal.* If normal G6-PD activity is present, the spot will fluoresce brightly. If the blood is G6-PD deficient, no fluorescence is seen.

## QUANTITATIVE ESTIMATION OF RED CELL PYRUVATE KINASE ACTIVITY[20]

*Principles.* Phosphoenolpyruvate (PEP) is converted by pyruvate kinase to pyruvate in the presence of adenosine diphosphate (ADP). The pyruvate is then converted to lactate by lactate dehydrogenase in the presence of nicotinamide-adenine dinucleotide phosphate (NADH). The conversion of NADH to $NAD^+$ is followed by measuring the changes in optical density at 340 nm.

### Reagents and Apparatus

1. Triethanolanine buffer:

4.62 g triethanolanine hydrochloride, 16.79 g potassium chloride, and 5.92 g magnesium sulfate ($MgSO_4$. $7H_2O$) are dissolved in approximately 900 ml of distilled water. The pH is adjusted to 7.4 with either hydrochloric acid or potassium hydroxide and the volume made up to 1 liter with distilled water.

The buffer can be aliquoted in small volumes and stored frozen at $-20°C$.

2. Adenosine diphosphate (ADP):

6.45 g of adenosine diphosphate are dissolved in 1 ml distilled water. This reagent is kept on ice during use.

3. Nicotinamide-adenine dinucleotide phosphate (NADH):

3.5 mg of NADH are dissolved in 1 ml distilled water. This reagent should be freshly prepared and kept on ice during use.

4. Lactic dehydrogenase (60 $\mu$/ml):

This reagent is obtained from Boehringer Corp. and is used in the suspension provided.

5. Phosphoenol pyruvate (Trisodium salt—PEP):

7.3 mg of PEP is dissolved in 1 ml distilled water. This reagent should be freshly prepared and kept on ice during use.

6. Fresh EDTA or heparinized blood (blood stored at 4°C for 24 hours can be used provided a control stored under the same conditions is assayed)

7. 6% Dextran

8. Preparation of hemolysate:

1 ml of 6% dextran is added to 3.5 ml of anticoagulated blood. A test tube is filled with this mixture and allowed to stand for 30 minutes at room temperature. The red cell free plasma is removed, 1 ml of dextran is added, and the volume made up to its original level of 4.5 ml with 0.9% saline. The tube is inverted to mix and the procedure repeated 6 times to ensure that the red cell suspension is leukocyte free.

The packed red cell volume is adjusted to 90% and the red cell concentration stored in an ice bath. (The packed cell volume is determined by the procedure on p. 75.)

Immediately prior to use, 0.1 ml of the leukocyte-free red cell mass is added to 4.0 ml of ice-cold distilled water and the resulting hemolysate stored frozen until tested.

9. UV range spectrophotometer (1 cm optical path)

*Method*

1. The following reagents are added in 3 silica cuvets:

|  | Test (ml) | Blank (ml) | Control (ml) |
|---|---|---|---|
| Triethanolamine buffer solution | 1.00 | 1.00 | 1.00 |
| Distilled water | 1.48 | 1.58 | 1.48 |
| NADH | 0.10 | — | 0.10 |
| ADP | 0.10 | 0.10 | 0.10 |
| LDH | 0.02 | 0.02 | 0.02 |
| PEP | 0.20 | 0.20 | 0.20 |

2. The test and blank reagent cuvets are placed at 37°C in a double-beam spectrophotometer and allowed to warm up for 2 to 3 minutes

3. The reaction is then started by adding 0.1 ml of the hemolysate to the test cuvet.

4. Read the optical density of the reaction at 340 nm at 30-second intervals for 5 minutes.

5. Repeat the procedure by adding 0.1 ml of the hemolysate to the blank cuvet and recording the optical densities.

6. Add 0.1 ml of 0.85% saline to the control cuvet, and record the optical densities over a 5-minute time span as above. (This checks for absorbance due to the oxidation of NADH in the absence of hemolysate.)

*Calculation*

$$\text{Pyruvate Kinase Activity} = \frac{\Delta_D/\text{min} \times 10^3}{6.22 \times \text{volume of red cells/cuvet } (\mu l)}$$

$$= \frac{\Delta_D/\text{min} \times 10^3}{6.22 \times \frac{0.1}{4.1} \times \text{packed cell volume of cell suspension units}}$$

*Normal.* 1.2 to 2.2 units

*Notes*

1. The pyruvate kinase unit is expressed as the $\mu$ mols of NADH oxidized/ml red cells/minute at 37°C.

2. A deficiency of the glycolytic enzyme pyruvate kinase is probably the most common cause of congenital nonsphenocytic hemolytic anemias.

3. Leukocytes are a rich source of pyruvate kinase. The leukocyte

activity of the enzyme is normal in Type II hemolytic anemias and consequently care should be taken to ensure that the red cell hemolysate is completely free of white cell contamination.

## SCREENING METHOD FOR THE DETECTION OF RED CELL PYRUVATE KINASE[19]

*Principle.* A phosphate group (phosphoenol-pyruvate) is transferred to ADP forming pyruvate and ADP in the presence of red cell pyruvate kinase. Lactic dehydrogenase in the red cell hemolysate, catalyzes the reduction of pyruvate to lactate with the resulting oxidation of diphosphopyridine nucleotide (DPNH) to diphosphopyridine (DPN). DPNH has the property of fluoresence, while DPH does not fluoresce under ultraviolet light.

### Reagents and Apparatus
1. Phosphoenolpyruvate (trisodium salt) PEP:
0.584 g of PEP is dissolved in 1 ml distilled water. This reagent should be freshly prepared and kept on ice during use
2. Adenosine diphosphate (ADP):
48.37 mg of ADP are dissolved in 1 ml distilled water. This reagent is kept on ice during use.
3. Nicotinamide-adenosine dinucleotide phosphate (NADH):
26.25 mg of NADH are dissolved in 1 ml distilled water. This reagent should be freshly prepared and kept on ice during use.
4. Magnesium chloride ($MgCl_26H_2O$):
16.24 mg of this salt are dissolved in 1 ml distilled water.
5. Potassium phosphate buffer (0.25M, pH 7.4):
8.25 ml of 1M stock dipotassium hydrogen phosphate and 1.75 ml of potassium dihydrogen phosphate are added together and made up to 100 ml with distilled water.
6. Reaction mixture: The following reagents are added together
 Phosphoenolpyruvate (PEP) ........................ 0.03
 ADP .............................................. 0.10
 NADH ............................................. 0.10
 Magnesium chloride ............................... 0.10
 Potassium phosphate buffer ....................... 0.05
 Distilled water .................................. 0.62
7. EDTA anticoagulated blood
8. Ultraviolet light (Wood's lamp)
9. Whatman No. 1 filter paper
10. 0.85% Sodium chloride

*Method*

1. The anticoagulated blood is centrifuged at 2,000 rpm for 5 minutes and the buffy coat removed.

2. One volume of the red cell mass is removed using a Pasteur pipet and added to 4 volumes of saline.

3. Approximately 0.02 ml of this cell suspension is then added to 0.20 ml of the reaction mixture.

A portion of this mixture is spotted on the filter paper immediately, and the remainder is incubated at 37°C for 30 minutes.

4. After the incubation, a second spot is made. After drying on the paper, the spots are examined under ultraviolet light.

*Normal.* The first spot from normal blood sample will fluoresce brightly, but the second spot will not fluoresce. Red cells, deficient in pyruvate kinase, fluoresce in both spots.

*Notes*

1. By making spots every 10 minutes it is possible to provisionally identify heterozygotes for pyruvate kinase deficiency.

## DETECTION OF SICKLE CELLS

*Principle.* Red cells homozygous for HbS can be induced to take on characteristic sickle shapes when exposed to reduced oxygen tension. Cells heterozygous for HbS are not normally detected by this test.

### Method 1

*Reagents and Apparatus*
1. Petroleum jelly
2. Slides and coverslips
3. 37°C Incubator

*Method*

1. A small drop of capillary blood is placed on a slide and covered with a coverslip. The perimeter of the coverslip is sealed with a ring of petroleum jelly.

2. The preparation is allowed to stand at room temperature for 4 to 6 hours. An alternative method is to place the preparation is a moist chamber composed of an inverted Petri dish enclosing a pledge of wet wool. Leave at 37°C for 4 to 6 hours. With either procedure examine under the 43× objective.

*Results.* Positive results show definite morphological changes in red cells, which take on elongated, flattened, holly leaf and occasionally sickle appearances. The cells at the periphery of the preparation usually exhibit marked changes more quickly.

**Method 2**

*Reagents and Apparatus*
1. 2% Aqueous sodium bisulfite, prepared fresh
2. Petroleum jelly
3. Slides and coverslips
4. 37°C Incubator

*Method*
1. A rubber band is secured around the end of the patient's finger and left for 4 to 5 minutes.
2. Obtain a small drop of capillary blood from the constricted finger and place on a slide with a drop of 2% sodium bisulfite. Mix the blood and reducing agent with an applicator stick. Place a coverslip over the preparation and seal with petroleum jelly as in the previous method.
3. Proceed as in step 2 in the preceding technique.

**Method 3**

*Reagents and Apparatus*
1. 10% Formol saline: add 10 ml of 40% formalin to 90 ml of normal saline.
2. Sterile mineral oil
3. Sterile syringe
4. Petroleum jelly
5. Slides and coverslips
6. 37°C Incubator

*Method*
1. The barrel of a sterile syringe is coated with sterile mineral oil.
2. 5 ml of formol saline is placed in a small beaker and overlaid with the mineral oil.
3. Obtain 5 ml of blood by venipuncture.
4. Gently dispense 1 to 2 ml of blood from the syringe into the formol saline and leave for 15 minutes at room temperature. Place a coverslip over the preparation and seal as in the preceding methods.
*Results.* The sickling observed in this preparation is present mostly on the periphery of the coverslip.

*Notes*
1. If the cells are heterozygous for HbS, the tests described do not normally provide positive results. However, incubated slides that are allowed to stand overnight occasionally produce 1 to 2% of the cells in sickle form.
2. Beside indicating sickle cell disease, a positive test can sometimes be found in hemoglobin S thalassemia (genetically, hemoglobin S hemoglobin F disease), when the blood is incubated overnight.

## FERROHEMOGLOBIN SOLUBILITY TEST[21]

***Principle.*** Several hemoglobin variants (HbD, HbG, etc) show an electrophoretic mobility similar to that of sickle cell hemoglobin. Reduced hemoglobin in strong phosphate buffer solution at a slightly acid pH is insoluble and forms crystal-like birefringent tactoids that obstruct and deflect light rays passing through the mixture, producing turbidity. The solubility of normal reduced hemoglobin is about one-half that of oxyhemoglobin, and the solubility of sickle reduced hemoglobin is no more than one-hundredth of that of the oxyhemoglobin.

### Reagents and Apparatus
1. Phosphate buffer pH 6.5, 2.87M:
289.2 g of dipotassium hydrogen phosphate and 164.7 g of potassium dihydrogen phosphate are dissolved in distilled water and the volume made up to 1 liter.
2. Phosphate buffer 2.49 M:
86.7 ml of the 2.87M phosphate buffer is diluted to 100 ml with distilled water.
3. Phosphate buffer 1.10M:
3.83 ml of the 2.87M phosphate buffer is diluted to 100 ml with distilled water.
4. Sodium dithionite
5. EDTA Anticoagulated blood
6. Spectrophotometer

### Method
1. Add 50 mg of sodium dithionite to 4.5 ml of the phosphate buffer and to 0.5 ml of a 5% hemoglobin solution.
2. The mixture is kept overnight at room temperature, filtered, and the optical density read at 540 nm.

### Results

TABLE 4-8. Percentages of Reduced Hemoglobin in Phosphate Buffer Solutions of Different Concentrations.

| Hemoglobin Type | 1.10M (%) | 2.49M (%) | 2.87M (%) |
|---|---|---|---|
| AA | 100 | 90–95 | 13–20 |
| AD | 100 | 90–95 | 13–20 |
| AS | 100 | 25–35 | 5–20 |
| SS | 100 | 3–10 | 2–4 |

*Note.* Some other hemoglobin variants (Hb-C-Georgetown and Hb-C-Harlem) will also precipitate when subjected to acidified phosphate buffer.

## DETECTION OF FETAL CELLS IN MATERNAL BLOOD (KLEINHAUER)[22]

*Principle.* Hemoglobin A is eluted from the red cells by an acid phosphate buffer; fetal hemoglobin resists this elution.

### Reagents and Apparatus
1. Fixative: 80% ethyl alcohol
2. Acid buffer solution: (pH 3.5)
   Citric acid monohydrate ....................... 1.46 g
   Disodium hydrogen phosphate ................. 0.86 g
   Distilled water ........................... to 100 ml
3. EDTA blood
4. Normal saline
5. 0.5% Aqueous erythrosin B
6. Coplin jar

### Controls
Positive:
1. 10 volumes adult blood
      1 volume ABO compatible cord blood
2. Cord blood
Negative:
Adult blood (from male donor)

### Method
1. One volume of blood is diluted with 1 volume of normal saline and placed in a clean stoppered tube.
2. Thin blood smears are made from this dilution by the method described under differential white cell counts. The smears are allowed to dry in air and are fixed for 2 to 5 minutes in 80% ethyl alcohol.
3. The buffer is warmed to 37°C in a Coplin jar and the fixed smears are immersed in it for 10 minutes. Agitate the slides continuously.

If the preparation is successful, the buffer becomes slightly tinged with hemoglobin (whether fetal cells are present or not).
4. Wash smears with distilled water for 10 to 20 seconds.
5. Stain with erythrosin-B for 5 minutes.
6. Wash smears in running tap water for 1 minute.
7. Examine using 40× magnification.

**Results.** Normal adult cells appear as pale gray-pink "ghosts" in the background, whereas fetal cells stand out as dark refractile structures which appear to have numerous layers.

## Clayton Modification of the Kleinhauer-Betke Method[23]

### Reagents and Apparatus

1. Buffer: McIlvaine's buffer. pH 3.2

Stock solution A: 0.1 M citric acid (19.2 g citric acid) is dissolved in 1 liter distilled water.

Stock solution B: 0.2 M sodium phosphate (28.4 g disodium hydrogen phosphate dihydrate) is dissolved in 1 liter distilled water.

Add 40 ml of stock solution B to 160 ml of stock solution A. Store at 4°C.

2. Stains:

*Biebrich Scarlet*

Biebrich scarlet (water soluble) . . . . . . . . . . . . . . . . . . . 2 g
Phosphotungstic acid . . . . . . . . . . . . . . . . . . . . . . . . . . . . 0.6 g
Glacial acetic acid . . . . . . . . . . . . . . . . . . . . . . . . . . . . . 10 ml
50% Ethyl alcohol . . . . . . . . . . . . . . . . . . . . . . . . . . . . 200 ml

(This stain tends to loose staining ability on standing).

*Aniline Blue*

Add a small quantity of aniline blue to distilled water so that a royal blue color develops.

3. Fixative: 80% ethyl alcohol
4. EDTA blood
5. Normal saline
6. Coplin jar

**Controls.** As in the Kleinhauer-Betke method.

### Method

1. Dilute the blood with an equal volume of saline.
2. Prepare very thin blood smears.
3. Fix smears in 80% ethyl alcohol for 5 minutes.
4. Rinse smears with distilled water.
5. Immerse in McIlvaine's buffer (pH 3.2) for 5 minutes keeping the smears continuously agitated.
6. Rinse in distilled water.
7. Stain with Biebrich scarlet in Coplin jar for 2 minutes.
8. Wash smears in distilled water to remove excess stain, and repeat a second time to complete the wash.
9. Stain with aniline blue for 1 minute.
10. Wash smears in running tap water for 1 minute.
11. Examine under 40× magnification.

**Results.** Normal adult cells are well laked. Reticulocytes are colorless except the cell membrane and reticulum which are gray-blue. Incompletely laked adult cells have a distinctive pale blue-pink appearance.

*Notes*

1. Interpretation of the acid-elution methods for the assay of transplacental hemorrhage must be made in light of the limitations of the test. Under both normal and pathological conditions, adult red cells may contain small amounts of fetal hemoglobin.

2. Fetal hemoglobin may be present in normal adult blood up to 1 per cent of the total hemoglobin. Therefore, occasional stained cells may be seen. Usually these have "intermediate" staining properties, lacking the highly refractile and deeply stained appearance of the characteristic fetal cell.

3. Increased levels of fetal hemoglobin can be found in adult blood in some pathological states.

a. Very high levels are found in hereditary persistence of fetal hemoglobin. This is a genetically acquired characteristic in which the heterozygotes possess approximately 15 to 30 per cent fetal hemoglobin.

Using acid-elution methods, fetal hemoglobin is evenly distributed throughout the red cell population.

b. Increased levels of fetal hemoglobin are also found in hemolytic anemia, acquired aplastic anemia, acute leukemia, and other conditions in which the bone marrow is under stress. The levels found, however, do not usually exceed 4 per cent.

c. There is a tendency for the fetal hemoglobin level to rise a little during the first trimester of pregnancy and then to fall to slightly below normal by the time of delivery.

Fetal cells appear as smooth homogeneous cells with a scarlet red color.

## ESTIMATION OF SERUM BILIRUBIN[24]

**Principle.** Serum is treated with diazotized sulfanilic acid to produce a red color that is compared with a known standard. The proteins are precipitated with methyl alcohol.

*Reagents and Apparatus*

1. Van den Bergh diazo reagent A: 1 g of sulfanilic acid is added to a 1-liter flask with 500 ml of distilled water and 15 ml of concentrated hydrochloric acid.

2. Van den Bergh diazo reagent B: 0.5 g of sodium nitrite is added to 100 ml of distilled water.

3. Working diazo reagent: 10 ml of diazo A is added to 0.3 ml of diazo B.

4. Absolutely methyl alcohol
5. Diazo blank: 15 ml of concentrated hydrochloric acid is made up to 1 liter with distilled water.
6. Fresh serum from unhemolyzed blood
7. Oswald-Folin pipets—0.5 ml
8. Graduated pipets—10 ml
9. Graduated pipets—1 ml
10. Spectrophotometer

*Method*

1. 0.5 ml of serum is added to 9.5 ml of distilled water. Draw 5 ml of the serum dilution into a tube and label as the "test." Label the remainder of the dilution as the "blank."

2. 1 ml of diazo blank is added to the blank tube and 1 ml of freshly made diazo reagent to the test. Leave both tubes for exactly 2 minutes, and read the optical densities spectrophotometrically at a wavelength of 540 nm, zeroing the galvanometer with the blank tube. This is the direct bilirubin. Calculate the total direct bilirubin from the calibration curve.

3. 6 ml of methyl alcohol is added to both the "blank" and the "test" tubes. Mix by inversion and allow to stand for 30 minutes at room temperature.

4. Repeat the reading as in step 2. This is the total bilirubin—direct and indirect.

*Calibration*

*Reagents and Apparatus:*
1. 30% Human serum albumin*
2. Phosphate buffer pH 7.4
   M/15 potassium dihydrogen phosphate ............ 19.2 ml
   M/15 disodium hydrogen phosphate ............... 80.8 ml
3. Pure bilirubin standard†
4. 0.01 N Sodium hydroxide
5. Graduated pipet—10 ml
6. Volumetric flasks—10 ml
7. Analytical balance

*Method*

1. 10 ml of 30% human serum albumin is added to 90 ml of phosphate buffer.

2. 20 mg of pure bilirubin† is accurately weighed and ground using a mortar and pestle, with 4 ml of 0.01 N sodium hydroxide.

3. When the bilirubin is completely in solution, it is added to a

---

* Available from Dade Reagents
† Available from Matheson, Coleman and Bell

volumetric flask and made up to a total volume of 100 ml with the diluted albumin prepared in step 1. This is a 20 mg per 100 ml stock standard.

4. Set up tubes as shown in Table 4-9.

5. Determine bilirubin estimations on these dilutions, using the same technique as for the serum in the test procedure.

6. Plot the optical densities of the standards against the bilirubin values (mg%).

*Note.* Commercially prepared standards are freely available from many laboratory supply houses.

### Normal Values

Adult . . . . . . . . . . . . . . . . . . . . . . . . 0.3–0.8 mg% total bilirubin
Infants . . . . . . . . . . . . . . . . . . . . . . 0.5–2.5 mg% total bilirubin

## ESTIMATION OF ACETYLCHOLINESTERASE[25]

*Principle.* Red cells in a buffered solution are incubated with an acetylcholine substrate. The red cell cholinesterase catalyzes the formation of acetic acid from the acetylcholine, with a corresponding fall in pH.

### Reagents and Apparatus

1. Buffer pH 8.1:
   Sodium barbitol . . . . . . . . . . . . . . . . . . . . . . . . . . . . . . 4.12 g
   Anhydrous potassium dihydrogen phosphate . . . . . . . . 0.54 g
   Potassium chloride . . . . . . . . . . . . . . . . . . . . . . . . . . . . 44.73 g
   Distilled water . . . . . . . . . . . . . . . . . . . . . . . . . . . . . . . 900 ml

The pH is adjusted with approximately 28 ml of 0.1 N hydrochloric acid. The total volume is then made up to 1 liter with distilled water.

2. Substrate: 2% acetylcholine. Keep at 4°C in small aliquots in sealed tubes. 2 drops of toluene is added as a preservative.

3. 0.01% Aqueous saponin

4. Red cell hemolysate: 5 ml of heparinized or defibrinated blood is centrifuged at 2,500 rpm for 10 minutes. The plasma is discarded and the cells washed twice in normal saline. The supernatant is discarded and an

TABLE 4-9. Composition of Bilirubin Standards.

| TUBE | 1 | 2 | 3 | 4 | 5 | 6 |
|---|---|---|---|---|---|---|
| Diluted albumin (ml) | — | 1.25 | 2.5 | 3.75 | 4.5 | 4.75 |
| Stock standard (ml) | 5 | 3.75 | 2.5 | 1.25 | 0.5 | 0.25 |
| Final bilirubin Standard (mg%) | 20 | 15 | 10 | 5 | 2 | 1 |

equal volume of saline added to the red cell deposit. The cells are resuspended and 0.4 ml of the cell suspension is added to 9.6 ml of the saponin solution. This hemolysate can be kept in the freezer for up to 6 hours.

5. Volumetric pipets—3 ml

6. pH Meter

*Method*

1. 3 ml of the buffer is placed in each of the 2 tubes labeled "test" and "blank," and 3 ml of the red cell hemolysate is added to the test.

2. Using any pH meter standardized at 25°C, the pH of both the test and the blank tubes are recorded.

3. 0.6 ml of the substrate is added to both the test and blank tubes, the contents mixed well and the exact time of addition of the substrate recorded. This is the initial time.

4. Leave the tubes for 1 hour and determine the pH of the samples, recording the time. This is the final time

*Calculation.* The results are expressed as the change of pH per hour.

$$\text{Change of pH per hour} = \frac{\text{initial pH} - \text{final pH}}{\text{initial time (in hr)} - \text{final time (in hr)}}$$

*Normal.* 0.5 to 1 pH unit per hour

*Notes*

1. If the pH of the blank falls more than 0.01 pH unit, a fresh substrate should be prepared and the test repeated.

2. Reduced red cell acetylcholinesterase activity, which is located in the red cell stroma, has been demonstrated in patients with paroxysmal nocturnal hemoglobinuria. A similar reduction in the activity is found in ABO hemolytic disease of the newborn.

3. Actylcholinesterase content of reticulocytes and young red cells is increased, and measurement of the enzyme in the red cells can aid in the evaluation of bone marrow activity.

## RED CELL SURVIVAL

### Radioactive Chromium (CR$^{51}$) Method

*Principle.* $Cr^{51}$ has a half-life of 27.8 days. The chromium salts used for labeling red cells is hexavalent sodium chromate ($Na_2Cr^{51}O_4$). This salt passes through the red cell membrane, and the chromium$^{51}$ becomes reduced to the trivalent form, which binds with the cellular protein. Trivalent chromium does not pass into the red cells and thus cannot be easily used to label them.

**Reagents and Apparatus**
1. 50 μc Sterile amounts of hexavalent sodium chromate ($Cr^{51}$)
2. ACD solution (p. 147)
3. Scintillation counter
4. Sterile saline
5. Centrifuge
6. Sterile graduated pipets—10 ml
7. Sterile syringes

**Method**
1. 15 ml of patient's whole blood is added to 5 ml of sterile ACD solution in a sterile screw-cap bottle.
2. The blood is centrifuged at 2,500 rpm for 5 minutes and the plasma discarded.
3. 50 μc of sterile hexavalent sodium chromate is added to the blood and the solution mixed by inversion.
4. The blood is allowed to stand at room temperature for 30 minutes and the red cells are washed 3 times in sterile saline by centrifuging at 2,500 rpm for 5 minutes. This removes the unattached $Cr^{51}$.
5. Sufficient saline is added to the red cell button to make up the volume to 25 ml; 20 ml of this suspension is immediately injected intravenously into the patient.
6. The labeled red cells are allowed to equilibrate throughout the recipient's circulation for 10 minutes, and 6 ml of the blood is collected from a vein in the other arm. This is added to 2 ml of ACD solution.
7. The radioactivity of this blood sample is determined and used as a baseline.
8. Additional blood samples are taken in the same way 24 hours later and at subsequent intervals (depending on the rate of red cell destruction) up to 25 days.

*Calculation.* The percentage red cell survival on any one day is calculated from the following:

$$Cr^{51} \text{ survival on day T } \% = \frac{\text{Counts per minute per ml blood day T}}{\text{Counts per minute per ml blood day O}} \times 100$$

where day O is the baseline reading and day T the day the survival is estimated.

*Notes*
1. Radioactive counts are carried out in a scintillation counter containing a thallium-activated sodium iodide crystal.
2. The loss of radioactivity from the circulation is caused by two factors, the loss due to hemolysis and hemorrhage, and a leakage of the

sodium chromate from the cells. The leakage or elution occurs in two phases, a short period of rapid elution with a half-life of up to 2 days, and a slow component in which the half-life is between 44 and 77 days.

3. The $Cr^{51}$ method for red cell survival time is not easily carried out in routine laboratories; for this reason, Ashby's differential agglutination test is sometimes used.

*Normal.* Red cell half-life 28 to 38 days

## Ashby's Method[26]

*Principle.* Red cells of different but compatible blood groups are transfused into the patient. Blood samples are taken at regular intervals and the patient's red cells agglutinated, using avid antisera. The rate of disappearance of the donor's cells is then determined.

### Reagents and Apparatus
1. Antisera of high avidity
2. Compatible donor's cells
3. ACD plastic blood bag
4. Apparatus described for red cell counts (p. 41)
5. Sahli pipets—0.02 ml
6. Graduated pipets—1 ml

### Method
1. 500 ml of compatible donor's cells is collected and packed by centrifugation and the plasma discarded.

2. A sample of whole blood from the patient is obtained and centrifuged. The avidity of the antiserum is checked by adding 1 volume of cells to 1 volume of antiserum. Leave at room temperature for 1 hour and examine microscopically to ensure that at least 90% of the cells are agglutinated.

3. Transfuse the donor's packed cells to the patient.

4. One hour after the transfusion, a second specimen of blood is taken and a red cell count determined. This represents the 100% standard.

5. Blood samples are taken at daily intervals for the first week and then at 3-day intervals for 2 months. The percentage of surviving cells is estimated as shown in the following steps.

6. 0.02 ml of blood is added to 1 ml of saline.

7. 1 volume of this suspension is added to 1 volume of antiserum and the cell-serum mixture stoppered, mixed and allowed to stand at room temperature for 1 hour. The mixture is centrifuged at 1,500 rpm for 1 minute, and the button of cells is *gently* agitated to break up the sediment and free the agglutinates.

8. The suspension is then recentrifuged at the same speed and *gently* shaken. The larger agglutinates are allowed to settle to the bottom of the tube for 1 minute.

9. A Neubauer hemocytometer is charged with the supernatant of free cells and the total number of *free* cells counted and expressed as a total per cubic millimeter.

10. The number of free cells present is expressed as a percentage of the number present immediately after the transfusion (in 4 above).

*Calculation.* A graph can be constructed, using the cell count at 1 hour as the 100% standard, with time plotted as abscissa against the percentage cell survival as ordinate.

*Normal.* Red cell half-life 40 to 60 days

*Notes*

1. The usual combinations of patient and donor cells are given in Table 4-10.

2. The disadvantages of the Ashby method are that it is impossible to study the survival of the patient's cells in his own circulation, that large volumes of blood have to be used in transfusion, and that it is of such importance to use an avid antiserum against the patient's cells.

## ESTIMATION OF URINARY FORMIMINOGLUTAMIC ACID[27]

*Principle.* In patients with folic acid deficiencies, an intermediate product of histidine metabolism appears in increased amounts in the urine instead of being metabolized to glutamic acid.

The presence of this product can be demonstrated by urinary electrophoretic techniques, using cellulose acetate strips.

*Reagents and Apparatus*
1. L-histidine monohydrochloride
2. Concentrated hydrochloric acid
3. FIGLU (formiminoglutamic acid)
4. Cellulose acetate electrophoresis

TABLE 4-10. Usual Combinations of Patient and Donor Cells.

| PATIENT | DONOR | ANTISERUM |
|---------|-------|-----------|
| A | O | Anti A |
| B | O | Anti B |
| AB | O | Anti A and Anti B |
| M | N | Anti M |
| MN | N | Anti M |
| N | M | Anti N |

5. Ninhydrin solution: dissolve 0.2 g of ninhydrin in 6 ml of ethyl alcohol, and make up the total volume to 100 ml, using diethyl ether.

6. Petri dish

7. Pyridine-acetic acid buffer:
Pyridine . . . . . . . . . . . . . . . . . . . . . . . . . . . . . . . . . . . . . . . . . . . . . . . 50 ml
Glacial acetic acid . . . . . . . . . . . . . . . . . . . . . . . . . . . . . . . . . . . . 20 ml
Distilled water . . . . . . . . . . . . . . . . . . . . . . . . . . . . . . . . . . . to 4 liters

8. Pipets—10 $\mu$l

9. Oven

10. Concentrated ammonia

### Method

1. 15 g of L-histidine monohydrochloride is mixed in a glass of water and given orally to the patient, who is in a fasting state.

2. Exactly 3 hours after taking the histidine, the patient is instructed to empty his bladder; this urine is discarded. All the urine voided in the next 5 hours is collected and preserved with 1 ml of concentrated hydrochloric acid.

3. Measure the total urinary output and separate an aliquot for analysis.

4. Prepare a FIGLU marker by adding a known amount of FIGLU to acidified normal urine, or use a FIGLU-positive urine from a patient with a folic acid deficiency.

5. Float the cellulose acetate strips on the surface of the pyridine-acetic acid buffer to ensure even impregnation of the strips. Blot lightly between 2 sheets of filter paper and mount in any suitable electrophoretic horizontal tank.

6. Set the distance between the shoulder pieces of the tank so that there is approximately a 1-cm overlap of the strips.

7. Mark 4 application sites so that 6.5 ml of the test urine are applied to the 2 inner sites, and 6.5 ml of FIGLU marker to the 2 outer sites.

8. Apply a constant current of 200 volts for 30 minutes.

9. Remove the strips and dry them in a 90°C oven for 10 to 15 minutes.

10. Cut the strips lengthwise into 2 identical halves, expose 1 half to concentrated ammonia vapor for 30 minutes, and dry for a few minutes in the oven.

11. Both strips are stained by passing slowly through the ninhydrin solution in a Petri dish.

12. To stop the strips from curling, they are laid flat between 2 sheets of filter paper lying between cardboard. This is clipped together and placed in an oven at 100°C for 5 minutes. Full color develops about 30 minutes later and is inspected, using a bright transmitted light.

*Results*. Three migrations are seen on each strip: glycine near the application point, histidine near the cathode and glutamic acid toward the anode.

FIGLU merges with glutamic acid and is seen only on the strip exposed to the concentrated ammonia. By comparing the intensity of the color of the test FIGLU with that of the marker, a semiquantitative estimate of the amount of FIGLU present can be made.


## HEMOGLOBIN BREAKDOWN PRODUCTS IN THE URINE AND FECES

### *Qualitative Urinary Porphobilinogen*[28]

*Principle*. Porphobilinogen condenses with Ehrlich's reagent in acid solution to produce a red color which is not extractable with amyl alcohol containing 25% benzyl alcohol. Urobilinogen forms a similar dye, but this is completely extracted by the organic solvent mixture.

#### *Reagents and Apparatus*
1. Ehrlich's reagent: 0.7 g of p-dimethylaminobenzaldehyde is dissolved in 150 ml of concentrated hydrochloric acid and made up to 250 ml with distilled water.
2. Saturated aqueous sodium acetate
3. Amyl alcohol-benzyl alcohol mixture: 3 volumes of pure amyl alcohol is added to 1 volume of pure benzyl alcohol.
4. Freshly voided urine
5. Graduated pipets—1 ml
6. Graduated pipets—5 ml
7. Centrifuge

#### *Method*
1. 1 ml of the urine is added to 1 ml of Ehrlich's reagent and mixed well. The urine is left for 2 minutes at room temperature and 2 ml of saturated aqueous sodium acetate is then added and mixed.
2. 2 ml of amyl alcohol-benzyl mixture is added to the contents of the tube, which is stoppered and gently shaken by inversion for 1 minute.
3. The tube is centrifuged at 2,000 rpm for 5 minutes and the supernatant is examined.

*Result*. A red color in the upper layer of the supernatant denotes the presence of urobilinogen, and a pink color in the lower layer indicates the presence of porphobilinogen.

## Qualitative Detection of Coproporphyrin[29]

*Principle.* Spectroscopic examination of urine at a wavelength of 405 nm shows a pink to red fluorescence when either coproporphyrin or uroporphyrin is present. Uroporphyrin can be distinguished from coproporphyrin by the different solubilities of the two substances in acid solution.

### Reagents and Apparatus
1. Glacial acetic acid
2. Diethyl ether
3. Wood's light (ultraviolet)
4. 5% Hydrochloric acid
5. Freshly voided urine
6. Graduated pipets—10 ml
7. Volumetric flask—25 ml
8. Separatory funnel—100 ml

### Method
1. 10 ml of glacial acetic acid is added to 25 ml of freshly voided urine in a separatory funnel; 50 ml of ether is added to the mixture and the funnel is shaken vigorously for 2 to 3 minutes. The solvents are allowed to separate and the urine is drawn off. The separation is repeated on the same urine with 50 ml of fresh ether. The urine is again separated and the organic solvent is examined under ultraviolet light.

2. The two ether extracts are combined and washed in 10 ml of 5% hydrochloric acid. The washings are examined under ultraviolet light.

*Results:* A strong red fluorescence in the ether extract before the acid wash indicates the presence of uroporphyrin. If the fluorescence persists after the acid wash, it indicates the presence of coproporphyrin.

### Notes
1. A small amount of coproporphyrin is normally excreted in the urine. The range is from 100 to 250 $\mu$g per day.
2. The excretion of coproporphyrin is increased when erythropoiesis is hyperactive in hemolytic anemias, polycythemia, pernicious anemia and aplastic anemia. It is very high in lead poisoning and in liver disease, but is reduced in kidney disease.
3. The increase in urinary coproporphyrin is known as porphyrinuria. There is no increase in uroporphyrin excretion. Normally there is no porphobilinogen found in the urine and only small amounts of uroporphyrin are present.

## Qualitative Urobilinogen Estimation

*Principle.* Urobilinogen reacts with Ehrlich's reagent to form a red color.

### Reagents and Apparatus
1. Ehrlich's reagent:
   p-Dimethylaminobenzaldehyde ....................... 2 g
   Concentrated hydrochloric acid ................... 50 ml
   Distilled water ................................. 50 ml
2. Freshly voided urine
3. Graduated pipets—10 ml
4. Pipets graduated in 0.1 ml— 1 ml
5. Pipets graduated in 0.01 ml—0.1 ml

### Method
1. Set up dilutions of the patient's urine as shown in Table 4-11.
2. 1 ml of Ehrlich's reagent is added to each of the tubes and allowed to stand at room temperature for 5 minutes for the color to develop.
3. Normal urine shows no more than a faint red color, which is intensified by heating. The highest dilution of urine giving a positive Ehrlich's test is taken as a result.
*Normal.* No color is given by normal urine diluted more than 1:20.

## Quantitative Urobilinogen Estimation[30]

*Principle.* Urobilin is reduced to urobilinogen by alkaline ferrous sulfate. The total urobilinogen is extracted in acid solution and determined colorimetrically by Ehrlich's reagent.

### Reagents and Apparatus
1. Modified Ehrlich's reagent: 0.7 g of p-dimethylaminobenzaldehyde is dissolved in 150 ml of concentrated hydrochloric acid; 100 ml of distilled water is added slowly.
2. 20% Ferrous sulfate: 20 g of powdered ferrous sulfate septahydrate is added to 92 ml of distilled water and shaken until dissolved.

TABLE 4-11. Dilutions of Urine for Urobilinogen Estimation.

| TUBE | 1 | 2 | 3 | 4 | 5 | 6 | 7 |
|---|---|---|---|---|---|---|---|
| Urine (ml) | 10.0 | 1.0 | 0.5 | 0.3 | 0.25 | 0.2 | 0.1 |
| Distilled water (ml) | — | 9.0 | 9.5 | 9.7 | 9.75 | 9.8 | 9.9 |
| Final dilution | — | 1:10 | 1:20 | 1:30 | 1:40 | 1:50 | 1:100 |

3. 10% Sodium hydroxide
4. Glacial acetic acid
5. Saturated aqueous sodium acetate
6. Light petroleum BP 40–60°C
7. Standard: 1 ml of alcoholic 0.05% phenolphthalein is added to 5 ml of aqueous sodium carbonate, and the total volume is made up to 100 ml with distilled water. This solution is equivalent to a urobilinogen level of 0.387 mg per 100 ml.
8. 24-Hour urine specimen: The urine is collected in a brown jar containing 5 g of anhydrous sodium carbonate and 100 ml of light petroleum.
9. Volumetric flask/100 ml
10. Measuring cylinders 100 ml
11. Filter funnel and paper
12. Graduated pipets—10 ml
13. Graduated pipets—5 ml
14. Spectrophotometer

*Method*
1. The total 24-hour urine volume is measured and an aliquot of 50 ml is placed in a flask with 25 ml of ferrous sulfate.
2. 25 ml of 10% sodium hydroxide is added to the flask and the mixture is allowed to stand for 30 minutes at room temperature and filtered; 50 ml of the filtrate is acidified with 5 ml of glacial acetic acid in a separatory funnel.
3. 30 ml of light petroleum is added and the mixture is vigorously shaken. The extraction is repeated with fresh petroleum at least 3 times.
4. The combined extracts are washed with distilled water and the urobilinogen extracted by shaking thoroughly with 2 ml of Ehrlich's reagent; 4 ml of saturated sodium acetate is added and the total volume shaken.
5. The color intensity of the aqueous layer is immediately compared against that of a standard spectrophotometrically at a wavelength of 540 nm. The galvanometer is zeroed with a blank composed of 4 ml of sodium acetate and 2 ml of Ehrlich's reagent.

*Calculation*

$$\frac{0.093 \times \text{optical density of the unknown}}{\text{Optical density of the standard}} \times \frac{\text{volume of 24-hour urine}}{100}$$

$$= \text{mg of urobilinogen per 24 hours.}$$

*Normal.* 0.4 to 1.0 mg per 24 hours

### Qualitative Estimation of Urinary Urobilin

**Schlesinger's Test**

*Principle.* Urobilinogen is converted to urobilin by iodine. The urobilin produces a green fluorescence due to the formation of zinc urobilin with alcoholic zinc acetate.

*Reagents and Apparatus*
1. 10% Aqueous barium chloride
2. Lugol's iodine:
   Iodine . . . . . . . . . . . . . . . . . . . . . . . . . . . . . . . . . . . . . . . . . . . . . . 1 g
   Potassium iodide . . . . . . . . . . . . . . . . . . . . . . . . . . . . . . . . . 2 g
   Distilled water . . . . . . . . . . . . . . . . . . . . . . . . . . . . . . . . . 100 ml
3. Saturated alcoholic zinc acetate
4. Graduated pipets—10 ml
5. Filter funnel and paper
6. Hand spectroscope

*Method*
1. 10 ml of urine is added to 5 ml of 10% barium chloride.
2. The solution is filtered and 2 to 3 drops of iodine and 5 ml of saturated alcoholic zinc acetate are added to the filtrate and mixed well by constant inversion.
3. The supernatant is examined with a hand spectroscope. Zinc urobilin shows an absorption band at the junction of the blue and green regions of the spectrum.

**Alternative Method**

*Reagents and Apparatus*
1. Ammonium persulfate crystals
2. Chloroform
3. Saturated alcoholic zinc acetate
4. Ethyl alcohol
5. Graduated pipets—10 ml
6. Separatory funnel—25 ml

*Method*
1. A few crystals of ammonium persulfate are added to 5 ml of urine in a small separatory funnel. The mixture is shaken well and 5 ml of the saturated alcoholic zinc acetate added.
2. The contents are again mixed well, 10 ml of chloroform is added and the contents mixed again.
3. The solvents are allowed to separate out and the chloroform is

extracted and clarified by adding 1 to 2 drops of ethyl alcohol. The resulting solution is examined in ultraviolet light.

**Results.** A golden yellow fluorescence in the chloroform indicates the presence of urobilin.

### Estimation of Stercobilinogen (Fecal Urobilinogen)[31]

**Principle.** As described under urinary urobilinogen (p. 180).

**Reagents and Apparatus.** As described under urinary urobilinogen (p. 180).

**Method**

1. 1.5 g of fresh stool is weighed and emulsified in 9 ml of distilled water.

2. 10 ml of 20% ferrous sulfate and 10 ml of 10% sodium hydroxide are added and the emulsion is mixed well.

3. The emulsion is allowed to stand for 2 hours in the dark and filtered through a No. 1 Whatman filter paper.

4. 2 ml of the filtrate is then pipeted into a dry 250-ml cylinder, 2 ml of Ehrlich's reagent is added and the mixture allowed to stand for 10 minutes at room temperature.

5. 6 ml of saturated sodium acetate is added to the cylinder, and the resulting color is compared spectrophotometrically with that of the standard at a wavelength of 540 nm. The blank used to zero the galvanometer is composed of 2 ml of filtrate, 2 ml of hydrochloric acid (150 ml of concentrated acid and 100 ml of distilled water) and 6 ml of sodium acetate.

**Calculation**

$$\frac{\text{Optical density of the test} \times 3.87}{\text{Optical density of the standard}} \times \text{volume of the final colored solution}$$

$$= \text{mg urobilinogen per 100 g of feces}$$

**Normal.** 30 to 220 mg %

**Notes**

1. The amount of fecal urobilinogen depends on the amount of bilirubin entering the intestine in the liver bile. Fecal urobilinogen is increased in conditions in which there is an increased breakdown of hemoglobin to bilirubin, as in the hemolytic anemias. Fecal urobilinogen is decreased if there is any obstruction of bile flow into the intestine. The most complete degree of obstruction is found in obstructive jaundice due to a tumor.

2. Urinary urobilinogen is derived from that part of the urobilinogen absorbed from the intestine and carried by the blood to the kidneys. The

remaining absorbed urobilinogen returns to the liver and is excreted again in the bile. The amount present depends both on the amount of bilirubin entering the intestine and on the ability of the liver to excrete the urobilinogen coming to it from the intestine.

3. The excretion of urobilin in the urine is not a reliable index of hemolysis, because excessive urobilinuria is as much an indication of liver dysfunction as a sign of increased red cell destruction.

## CLINICAL CONSIDERATIONS

### Hemolytic Anemia

The hemolytic anemias cover a wide range of blood dyscrasias caused by the abnormal destruction of red cells in vivo. Normally, as the cells increase in age, they become poikilocytic and are fragmented and engulfed by the reticuloendothelial system. Hemoglobin is broken down to hemosiderin and bilirubin, the hemosiderin being stored in the liver and the spleen, and the bilirubin being taken by the liver and excreted as bile pigments in the urine and feces.

The erythrocytes break down more easily, due to inherent deformities. Two main types of anemias exist, congenital and acquired.

### Congenital Hemolytic Anemia

Abnormalities in the morphology of the red cells is a feature of the disease.

#### Hereditary Spherocytosis

This disease is characterized by the presence of jaundice without urinary bile pigments. Spherocytes, ulceration of the legs and an increased osmotic fragility are often present, the disease sometimes affecting families, inasmuch as it is inherited by simple mendelian laws. The patient has mild jaundice and sometimes a large spleen. Due to the abnormal blood destruction, nucleated red cells and reticulocytes are often present, and other red cell regenerative and degenerative inclusions are seen. The direct anti-human globulin test is normally negative, unless a secondary sensitization is present.

The anemia is very variable in degree, rarely being severe. The jaundice follows a similar pattern, in that the degree of bilirubinemia is also mild. The erythrocytes tend to be spherical, their mean diameter being less than normal, whereas their thickness is usually greatly increased. The osmotic fragility is increased, as is the mechanical fragility. The red cell indices show a normal or slightly reduced mean cell volume and normal mean cell hemoglobin and mean cell hemoglobin concentration values.

### Sickle Cell Anemia

This disease, transmitted by mendelian inheritance, is confined to Negroes. The disease takes two distinct forms—the sickle cell trait and sickle anemia.

*Sickle Cell Trait.* This is a heterozygous form in which there is one gene for sickle cell hemoglobin (HbS) and one for normal hemoglobin (HbA). This form of the disease is recessive, the blood picture and the clinical condition being normal, with the exception of the characteristic electrophoretic pattern.

*Primary Sickle Cell Anemia.* This is in the homozygous state, there being two genes carrying abnormal HbS. The symptoms include an enlarged liver and spleen; ulceration of the legs is also commonly found as are various other symptoms.

The blood picture shows a moderate anemia with a normal MCV and MCHC. In stained smears, anisocytosis is present with some incidence of abnormally elongated cells, some of which may be crenated, oat-shaped or sickle-shaped. Even during quiescent periods there is a reticulocytosis of between 5 and 10 per cent, and a moderate degree of polychromasia is seen.

The osmotic fragility is moderately decreased and small numbers of siderocytes are usually found in the blood. In a hemolytic crisis, a mild leukocytosis is present along with a granulocytosis. Under reduced oxygen tension, the blood undergoes sickling and bizarre forms are also present when incubated. The diagnostic test is the separation of HbS by electrophoretic techniques. Occasionally, HbF may be demonstrated to levels of 20% of the total hemoglobin. The bone marrow shows a marked erythroid hyperplasia, but when in an aplastic crisis, there is a maturation arrest of the red cell precursors.

### Mediterranean Anemia or Thalassemia

These diseases are prevalent in countries in the Mediterranean area or in patients whose ancestors originated from this geographic area. However, thalassemic syndromes have been reported in a wide band extending over northern Africa and southern Europe to Thailand and the Philippines, including Spain, Portugal, Italy, Greece, Syria, Turkey, Iran, Iraq, Egypt, Israel, Armenia, Indonesia, Ceylon, Burma, Malaya, Vietnam, China, Belgium, Congo and South Africa.

The classical thalassemic patient is deficient in normal adult hemoglobin. The disease is characterized by a failure to synthesis normal hemoglobin chains which leads to the production of red cells that do not survive circulatory stresses. The abnormal synthesis is due to an inability to produce either of the two normal polypeptide chains ($\alpha$ or $\beta$). The disease manifests itself as the $\alpha$ or $\beta$ type, both of these varieties being theoretically possible in the homozygous and heterozygous forms.

Homozygous $\alpha$-thalassemia (major) is believed to be incompatible with life.

Homozygous $\beta$-thalassemia (major) is often fatal during infancy. The syndrome shows a severe anemia and the patient frequently has a large spleen and liver. New bone formation produces a "hair-on-end" appearance of the skull. Active erythropoietic marrow is also found in the spinal vertebrae, ribs, and pelvis.

The laboratory results show a marked anemia with nucleated red cells and a reticulocytosis. A transient leukocytosis is also present, but the platelet count is within normal limits. Other manifestations of anemia are poikilocytosis and increased numbers of stippled cells. Many target cells are seen together with hypochromic red cells.

The serum iron is normal or increased and the iron-binding capacity may be totally saturated. Red cell survival is diminished and hemosiderin deposits are present in the spleen, liver, and other organs.

Hemoglobin electrophoresis may show 15 to 90 per cent HbF together with varying amounts of HbA and $HbA_2$. Starch gel electrophoresis is diagnostic of the disease, especially for the detection of $HbA_2$ and can be supported by the alkali-denaturation method for HbF.

Heterzygous $\beta$-thalassemia (minor) shows a variable degree of anemia, with increases in the numbers of target cells, stippled cells, poikilocytes, and polychromatic red cells. Hemoglobin F ranges from 2 to 5% and $HbA_2$ is occasionally increased.

Heterozygous $\alpha$-thalassemia (minor) is usually mild in severity and asymptomatic. Small quantities of HbF are found in infants, but in its place is found Barts' hemoglobin ($\alpha_4$). This hemoglobin moves faster than HbA and slower than HbH on cellulose acetate electrophoresis at pH 8.6 and is alkali-resistant like HbF. The diagnosis of this form of thalassemia is best made on genetic family studies.

Hemoglobin H disease is a form of $\alpha$-thalassemia. The abnormality results from a deficiency in $\alpha$-peptide chain production which affects all three normal hemoglobins A, $A_2$ and F. Hemoglobin H can be detected as an extremely fast moving moiety using cellulose acetate electrophoresis, and by the presence of intracellular HbH inclusion bodies in the red cells (p. 34).

### Hemoglobin C Disease

This disease, found mostly in Negroes, is characterized by splenomegaly, and a hemolytic anemia. The peripheral blood is remarkable for the presence of numerous target cells. Occasionally HbC crystals may be seen intracellularly in moist red cell preparations. The osmotic fragility is decreased (increased red cell resistance) and there is often a mild reticulocytosis. The diagnostic test is hemoglobin electrophoresis which shows characteristic HbC migration.

## Miscellaneous Conditions

Other congenital hemolytic anemias have been described, most of which show similar laboratory findings. Sickle cell hemoglobin C disease, hemoglobin D disease, hemoglobin E-thalassemia, and others have all been variably described in the literature. The differentiation between the hemoglobinopathies is made electrophoretically, differences in the isoelectric points of the various hemoglobins allowing their ionic mobilities to be studied (pp. 24-30).

## Acquired Hemolytic Anemia

### Sensitization

The transfusion of incompatible blood is the best example of an acquired hemolytic anemia. The severity of the crisis produced depends upon the avidity of the patient's serum to react with the incompatible donor's cells. The crisis shows three distinct phases:

1. The patient may complain of pain in the back and arms, show urticarial reactions, rigors, elevated pulse and temperature, circulatory collapse, hemoglobinuria, hemoglobinemia and jaundice.

2. The second stage takes place approximately 24 hours later. There is usually complete or partial kidney failure and jaundice becomes more apparent. Kidney function tests are all abnormal.

3. The third stage, that of diuresis, lasts as long as the period of anuria of the preceding stage. The patient voids large volumes of urine; this is accompanied by a corresponding depletion of body electrolytes. The laboratory findings include an increased serum bilirubin, reduced serum haptoglobin, increased plasma hemoglobin (immediate postreaction) and increases in hemoglobin breakdown products in the urine.

### Hemolytic Disease of the Newborn

This is a disorder of variable severity. The incompatibility is normally found in the Rhesus blood groups of the mother and father, the usual circumstance being that the mother is Rhesus negative (d.d) whereas the father is Rhesus positive (D.d) or (D.D.). During the course of gestation, blood from the Rhesus-positive infant crosses the placenta, producing antibodies (i.e., anti-D) in the maternal circulation. These antibodies find their way back to the fetal circulation, destroying fetal cells and causing the syndrome. Although there is little damage with the first pregnancy, the disease increases in severity with successive pregnancies.

Hemolytic disease of the newborn can also be produced by other blood group antigens and antibodies, including the ABO and Kell blood groups (see pp. 407, 433).

The blood picture at birth follows a familiar pattern. The hemoglobin is often low in parallel with the red count, there also being present marked macrocytosis and polychromasia. The characteristic feature of the disease is the presence of rubricytes in the peripheral blood. Reticulocyte levels, as well as the leukocyte count, are often increased and platelets are usually reduced in number.

The direct anti-human globulin test on cord blood is always positive when Rhesus sensitization has occurred. Usually the reaction is strong, its speed being proportional to the degree of sensitization; mildly affected infants show only a weak antiglobulin reaction.

The osmotic fragility produces variable results. In cases due to anti-Rhesus incompatibility, the fragility is found to be normal, whereas in cases produced by antibodies from the ABO system, an increased fragility is found. The serum bilirubin level of the cord blood varies from 1 to 9 mg % and sometimes increases to over 25 mg % in untreated cases.

### Paroxysmal Nocturnal Hemoglobinuria

This chronic disease produces moderately severe anemia. Hemoglobinuria is always found and the patient is deeply jaundiced, the attacks occurring without apparent cause. The factors which can precipitate an attack include infections, transfusions and surgery. The urine contains increased amounts of urobilinogen, hemosiderin and albumin. The blood picture is macrocytic, with reticulocytes, stippled cells, anisocytosis, poikilocytosis and scanty rubricytes present. Mild leukopenia and thrombocytopenia are present, with normal osmotic fragility. Oxyhemoglobin and free hemoglobin are sometimes detected in the plasma. Serum bilirubin levels are not excessively raised, the highest level being 4 mg%. The bone marrow shows an erythroid hyperplasia, no megaloblasts being present. The anti-human globulin and Donath-Landsteiner tests are both negative, the diagnostic tests being the demonstration of acid hemolysins in Ham's test. Crosby's test is also a sensitive diagnostic tool.

### Paroxysmal Cold Hemoglobinuria

This disease is precipitated by a variation in temperature and is due to a specific hemolysin that combines with and destroys the red cells when the temperature is lowered. The disease is frequently found in acquired or congenital syphilis. Investigations show a raised serum bilirubin level with hemoglobinuria, a negative Coombs' test and a positive and diagnostic Donath-Landsteiner test.

### Idiopathic Autoimmune Hemolytic Anemia

This is an acute anemia of unknown cause, normally associated with pyrexia and leukocytosis. The form of the disease is similar to other hemolytic breakdowns. The direct anti-human globulin test is positive and autoagglutination is commonly present, making reliable blood grouping difficult. Normal results are found in the Donath-Landsteiner test, Ham's test, Crosby's test and the osmotic fragility test. The clinical symptoms are fever, vomiting, headache and backache. The antibody responsible for this condition is difficult to isolate, although its thermal optimum can be determined. Such sensitization can be due to allergic substances, bacteria and drugs

Warm antibodies are occasionally the result of immunization against the patient's cellular antigens or can be produced as a result of an incompatible blood transfusion reaction. Cold reacting antibodies, once thought to be nonspecific, are frequently specific in nature, and are occasionally reactive against the I antigens on adult red cells.

## REFERENCES

1. Parpart, A. K., Lorenz, P. B., Parpart, P. B., Gregg, J. R., and Chase, A. M.: The osmotic resistance (fragility) of human red cells. J. Clin. Invest., 26: 636, 1947.
2. Dacie, J. V., and Lewis, S. M.: Practical Hematology. ed. 4, p. 171. New York, Grune & Stratton, 1968.
3. Ham, T. H., and Castle, W. B.: Studies on destruction of red blood cells. Proc. Am. Philos. Soc., 82: 411, 1940.
4. Murphy, J. R.: Erythrocyte metabolism III. Relationship of energy metabolism and serum factors to the osmotic fragility following incubation. J. Lab. Clin. Med., 60: 86, 1962.
5. Shen, S. C., Castle, W. B., and Fleming, E. M.: Experimental and clinical observations on increased mechanical fragility of erythrocytes. Science, 100: 387, 1944.
6. Cartwright, G. E.: Diagnostic Laboratory Hematology. p. 292. New York, Grune & Stratton, 1968.
7. Brus, I, and Lewis, S. M.: The haptoglobin content of serum in hemolytic anemias. Br. J. Haematol., 5: 348, 1959.
8. Wenk, R. E.,: Haptoglobin Estimation (Semi-Quantitative Electrophoresis) in Haptoglobin. p. 32. Crique CC 49. Commission on Continuing Education. A.S.C.P., 1968.
9. Ham, T. H.: Studies in destruction of red blood cells. I. Chronic hemolytic anemia with paroxysmal nocturnal hemoglobinuria: an investigation of the

mechanism of hemolysis, with observations on five cases. Arch Intern. Med., *64*: 1271, 1939.

10. Yachnin, S., and Ruthenberg, J. M.: The initiation and enhancement of human red cell lysis by activation of the first component of complement and by first component esterase; studies using normal red cells and red cells from patients with paroxysmal nocturnal hemoglobinuria. J. Clin. Invest., *44*: 518, 1965.

11. Crosby, W. H.: Paroxysmal nocturnal hemoglobinuria. A specific test for the disease based on the ability of thrombin to activate the hemolytic factor. Blood, *5*: 843, 1950.

12. Hartmann, J. R., Jenkins, D. E., and Arnold, A. B.: Diagnostic specificity of sucrose hemolysis test for paroxysmal nocturnal hemoglobinuria. Blood, *35*: 462, 1970.

13. Sanford, A. H.: Discussion: Recurring acute hemolytic crises with hemoglobinuria. Proc. Mayo Clin., *8*: 115, 1933.

14. Beutler, E., Deru, R. J., and Alving, A. S.: The hemolytic effect of primaquine VI. An in vitro test for sensitivity of erythrocytes to primaquine. J. Lab. Clin. Med., *45*: 40, 1955.

15. Beutler, E., Duron, O., and Kelly, B. M.: Improved method for the determination of blood glutathione. J. Lab. Clin. Med., *61*: 882, 1963.

16. Motulsky, A. G., Kraut, J. M., Thieme, W. T. L., and Musto, D. F.: Biochemical genetics of glucose-6-phosphate dehydrogenase deficiency. Clin. Res., *7*: 89, 1959.

17. Lohr, G. W., and Waller, H. D.: Glucose-6-phosphate dehydrogenase. *In* Bergmeyer, H. U.: Methods of Enzymatic Analysis. New York, Academic Press, 1963.

18. Jacob, H. S., and Jandl, J. H.: A simple visual screening test for glucose-6-phosphate dehydrogenase deficiency employing ascorbate and cyanide. New Eng. J. Med., *274*: 1162, 1966.

19. Beutler, E.: A series of new screening procedures for pyruvate kinase deficiency, glucose-6-phosphate dehydrogenase deficiency and glutathione reductase deficiency. Blood, *28*: 533, 1966.

20. Valentine, W. N., Tanaka, K. R., and Miwas,: A specific erythrocyte glucolytic enzyme defect (pyruvate kinase) in three subjects with congenital non-spherocytic hemolytic anemia. Trans. Assoc. Am. Physicians, *74*: 100, 1961.

21. Jonxis, J. H. P., and Huisman, J. H. J.: A Laboratory Manual on Abnormal Hemoglobins. ed. 2, p. 37. Oxford, Blackwell Scientific Publications, 1968.

22. Kleinhauer, E., Hildegard, B., and Betke, K.: Demonstration of fetal hemoglobin in erythrocytes of a blood smear. Klin. W. Schr., *35*: 637, 1957.

23. Clayton, E. M., Jr., Foster, E. B., and Clayton, E. P.: New stain for fetal erythrocytes in peripheral blood smears. Obstet. Gynecol., *35*: 642, 1970.

24. Malloy, H. T., and Evelyn, K. A.: Determination of bilirubin with photoelectric colorimeter. J. Biol. Chem., *119*: 481, 1937.

25. Michel, H. O.: An electrometric method for the determination of red blood cell and plasma cholinesterase activity. J. Lab. Clin. Med., *34*: 1564, 1949.

26. Dacie, J. V., and Mollison, P. L.: Survival of normal erythrocytes after

transfusion to patients with familial hemolytic anemia (acholuric jaundice). Lancet, *1*: 550, 1943.

27. Kohn, J., Mollin, D. L., and Rosenbach, L. M.: J. Clin. Path., *14*: 345, 1961. As quoted by Dacie, J. V., and Lewis, S. M.: Practical Hematology. ed. 3, p. 328. New York, Grune & Stratton, 1963.

28. Rimington, C.: Qualitative determination of porphobilinogen and porphyrins in urine and feces. Association of Clinical Pathologists. Broadsheet No. 36. 1961.

29. Benson, P. F., and Chisholm, J. J.: A reliable qualitative urine coproporphyrin test for lead intoxication in young children. J. Pediatr., *56*: 759, 1960.

30. Watson, C. J.: Studies of urobilinogen; improved method for quantitative estimation of urobilinogen in urine and feces. Amer. J. Clin. Path., *6*: 458, 1936.

31. King, E. J., and Wootton, I. D. P.: Micro-Analysis in Medical Biochemistry, ed. 3, p. 136. London, J. & A. Churchill, 1956.

# 5

# *Hemostasis*

## THEORIES OF BLOOD COAGULATION

The theories of blood coagulation have altered substantially in the last sixty years. The classical theories proposed by Morawitz, Nolf, Bordet, Stuber and Howell had all merged into a more concise form in which the parts of the puzzle appeared to be in place. This was not destined to last, and more recent advances in coagulation research have been directed toward an intricate enzymatic system in which various inactive precursors are activated in a *cyclic* chain reaction.

Hemostasis is the result of a series of related and overlapping events. Damage to a vessel wall is followed by an immediate reflex vasoconstriction of the vessel and platelets, attracted to the site of injury, form a hemostatic mechanical plug.

### Morawitz's Theory

The basic mechanism of hemostasis can be divided into a biochemical phase in which an intricate enzymatic system produces the clot, and a vascular phase, in which the vessel constricts, thus slowing down the rate of blood loss. The original theory of Morawitz postulated a two-phase biochemical reaction.

Prothrombin + calcium ions + thromboplastin = thrombin
Thrombin + fibrinogen = fibrin

According to this theory, when blood is shed, the platelets come into contact with a water-wettable surface and disintegrate, liberating thromboplastin, which combines with calcium and prothrombin to form thrombin. Fibrinogen, in the presence of thrombin, forms fibrin. This simple explanation is now known to be more complex and is usually divided into three stages:

1. The formation of plasma thromboplastin by the extrinsic or intrinsic pathways.
2. The conversion of prothrombin to thrombin.
3. The conversion of fibrinogen to fibrin.

In addition, the following mechanisms play an important role in the control of bleeding and of hypercoagulation:

1. Autocatalytic mechanisms.
2. Inhibition of the coagulation process.

Thirteen blood factors are now thought to be involved in the coagulation process, and many new inhibitors are rapidly being discovered. Because of this and the various synonyms given to these factors, the student has been thoroughly confused in the past. The International Committee of Nomenclature of Blood Clotting Factors has now recommended that all the recognized plasma substances known to play a role in the processes of hemostasis be referred to as shown in Table 5-1.

## Cascade or Waterfall Theory

If a blood vessel is broken, the following changes take place in vivo:

Platelets are attracted to the site of the vessel injury, liberating adsorbed coagulation factors and platelet granules (platelet Factor 3, which is a

TABLE 5-1. Nomenclature for Blood Factors Devised by the International Committee of Nomenclature of Blood Clotting Factors.

| INTERNATIONAL COMMITTEE'S FACTOR | SYNONYMS |
| --- | --- |
| I | Fibrinogen |
| II | Prothrombin, Thrombogen, Plasmozyme, Serozyme |
| III | Thromboplastin (tissue), Thrombokinase, Cytozyme |
| IV | Calcium |
| V | Labile factor, Proaccelerin, Plasma Ac globulin, Prothrombin accelerator |
| VI* | Accelerin, Serum Ac globulin |
| VII | Stable Prothrombin conversion accelerator, Stable factor, Serum accelerator, Proconvertin-convertin, Autoprothrombin I, Cothromboplastin |
| VIII | Antihemophilic globulin, Antihemophilic factor, Thromboplastinogen, Platelet cofactor I |
| IX | Plasma thromboplastin component, Christmas factor, Platelet cofactor II, Autoprothrombin II |
| X | Stuart factor, Stuart-Prower factor |
| XI | Plasma thromboplastin antecedent |
| XII | Hageman factor |
| XIII | Fibrin stabilizing factor |

* It is doubtful whether Factor VI is a distinct entity.

thromboplastin-like substance), and aid in the mechanical sealing of the injury. Serotonin is released by the platelets, helping in spontaneous vaso-constriction.

The contact substances, Factors XI and XII, are present in the circula-tion in an inactive state. Factor XII becomes activated by foreign water-wettable surfaces in vitro. This activation is thought to be triggered by the broken surface of the endothelial lining of the blood vessel. Once in an active state, it commences an intricate chain reaction, resulting in the formation of intrinsic thromboplastin, which corresponds to Morawitz's thromboplastin.

Thromboplastin is also formed in vivo by a secondary but equally im-portant pathway. When body cells are broken, tissue juices containing a thromboplastin precursor are liberated. These juices activate a second thromboplastin cycle, ending with the formation of extrinsic thrombo-plastin.

Thromboplastin, in the presence of additional accelerator substances, converts prothrombin to thrombin, which in turn converts fibrinogen to fibrin. An important idea in this theory is that, as soon as a trace of thrombin has been formed, it acts as an autocatalyst, speeding up the liberation of platelet substances, the synthesis of thromboplastin, and the conversion of more prothrombin to thrombin, and that finally it cata-lyzes the conversion of fibrinogen (see Fig. 5-3).

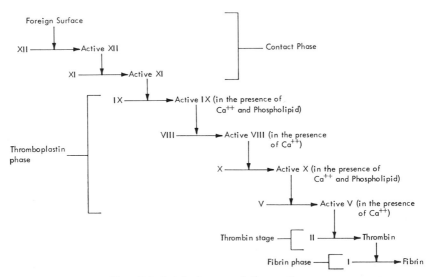

FIG. 5-1. Intrinsic coagulation pathway.

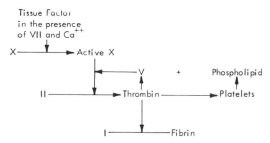

FIG. 5-2. Extrinsic coagulation pathway.

## Platelet Function in Coagulation

The main physiological function of platelets is to aid blood coagulation. This function can be broken down into two sections: (1) to act as a hemostatic seal, and (2) to transport coagulation factors and aid in the intrinsic and extrinsic thromboplastin pathways. As soon as the platelet contacts the foreign surface, a primary reaction takes place, which is thought to be between Factors VIII, IX and IV. This produces morphological changes, taking the form of platelet swelling, pseudopodial movement, agglutination and finally fusion of the platelets to each other. During this time, platelet granules move toward the outer surface of the cell and become liberated in the plasma. These granules are thought to be rich in a phospholipid substance similar to thromboplastin. Clot retraction in platelets is not completely understood. One hypothesis is that the phenomenon is a physiological ligature, drawing the edges of the injured vessels together, thus securing hemostasis. Another coagulation function lies in the absorption and transportation of coagulation factors to the sites of vessel injury, where they are then liberated to promote intrinsic thromboplastin formation.

## DISSOLUTION OF BLOOD CLOTS

The digestion of fibrin is carried out by an enzyme, plasmin. In normal situations, its precursor, plasminogen is converted to plasmin in the presence of activators associated with the vascular endothelium. Purified plasminogen is a glycoprotein possessing a molecular weight of 143,000. It undergoes slow spontaneous activation to plasmin, but the plasmin which results tends to be unstable. Plasmin lyses fibrin, fibrinogen, Factor V, Factor VIII, prothrombin, Factor XII, casein, and gelatin, and it hydrolyses various synthetic esters.

Activators of plasminogen include (beside the vascular endothelium) the adrenals, lymph nodes, prostate, thyroid, and lung tissues, urine,

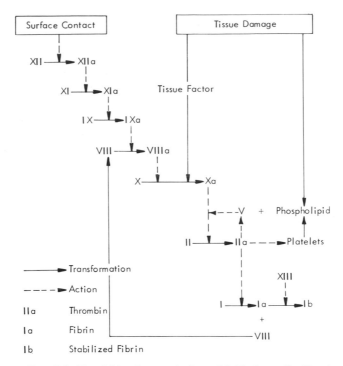

FIG. 5-3. Total blood coagulation. (McFarlane, R. G.: A clotting scheme for 1964. Genetics and the Interaction of Blood Clotting Factors. p. 50. Stuttgart, F. K. Schattauer-Verlag, 1964)

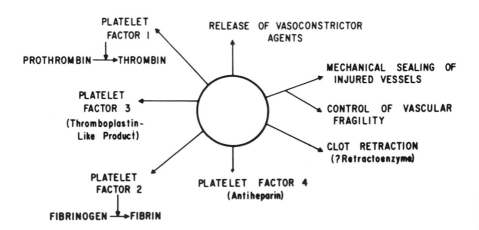

FIG. 5-4. Diagram of platelet function. (Stefanini, M., and Dameshek, W.: The Hemorrhagic Disorders. ed. 2, p. 17. New York, Grune & Stratton, 1962)

(urokinase) and streptokinase. Both plasmin and plasminogen are inhibited by epsilon-aminocaproic acid (EACA), and plasmin is also inhibited by soybean and pancreatic trypsin.

In the normal coagulation process, fibrinogen is attacked by the proteolytic enzyme thrombin, which cleaves small fragments (fibrinopeptides, A and B) from the fibrinogen molecule. The remaining portion is termed the fibrin monomer and is polymerized to form the fibrin clot.

In the normal fibrinolytic process, fibrin is attacked by the proteolytic enzyme plasmines which break fibrin and fibrinogen into several fragments, X, Y, D and E, (Fig. 5-5).

## TESTS OF THE HEMOSTATIC MECHANISM

*Laboratory Equipment and Glassware.* The equipment essential for carrying out hemorrhagic tests is very simple and limited in scope. The basic pieces of equipment are a thermostatically controlled, well-insulated waterbath and adequate timing devices. Stopwatches that operate by foot pedals are available, but, with practice, a technologist can easily manage to carry out procedures, using two stopwatches.

### Fibrometer

*Principle.* The Fibrometer Coagulation Timer is an electromechanical instrument designed to measure the coagulation properties of plasma or serum for diagnostic use and anticoagulant therapy control.

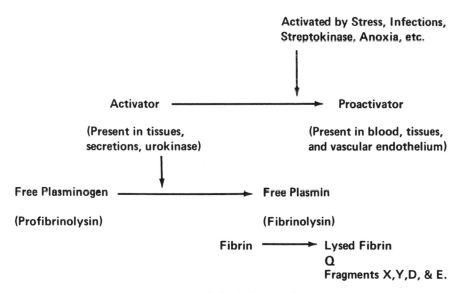

FIG. 5-5. Fibrinolytic activity.

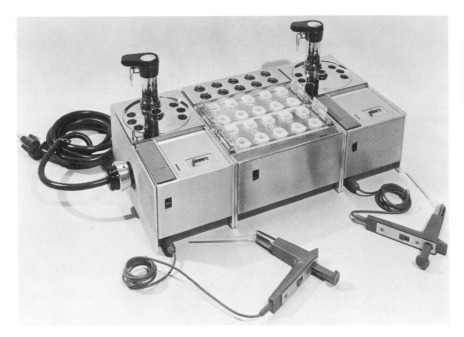

FIG. 5-6. Fibrometers with heating block and automatic pipet. Alternative automated and semi-automated equipment which can be used includes the Electra 600T,* the Fibrometer† and the Coagulyzer‡.

Plasma is added to reagents in a special Fibrotube cup, and the machine is activated either automatically with the automatic pipet or manually by depressing the timer bar. The probe arm, after a predetermined delay, drops into the reaction vessel and alternately descends and rises in a sweeping motion to seek and sense initial clot formation. When the end point occurs, the electrode and timer stop, the end point being registered on the digital readout in seconds and tenths of a second.

### Method

1. Plasma and coagulation reagents are pipeted into the reaction well, either manually or with the automatic pipet.

2. The timer is started, either by depressing the timer bar or by the activation of the automatic pipet.

3. When a clot has formed, the timer stops, the end point is recorded from the digital readout, and the probe arm is returned to its rest position by the technologist. The electrode probe is wiped clean with a lint-free

---

* Available from Scientific Prod. Division Amer. Hosp. Supply.

† Available from B.D. & Co. Rutherford, N.J.

‡ Available from Sherwood Medical Industries, St. Louis, Mo.

cloth and the readout button depressed to reset the timer after recording the reading.

*Notes*

1. The temperature of the warming and reaction wells is kept constant at 37 ± 0.5°C by means of a two-stage heating circuit. After turning the instrument on, operating temperature is reached within 10 minutes; this is indicated by the appearance of a *red light*. Tests *should not* be carried out if the indicator light is not on.

2. The automatic pipet is controlled by a plunger. When it is positioned with the two notches at the top, 0.2 ml will be delivered; by rotating the plunger 180°, the single notch will be on top and the delivery will be 0.1 ml. When the pipet is in the OFF position, it can be operated without activating the Fibrometer. By placing the switch in the ON position, the Fibrometer will be activated with the next discharge of the plunger.

Plastic disposable tips are inserted in the forward end of the pipet with a firm turning motion. A new disposable tip should be used with each new plasma.

## Electra 600

This apparatus detects the formation of a fibrin clot by the change in density of the reacting reagents. Such electro-optical methods can be

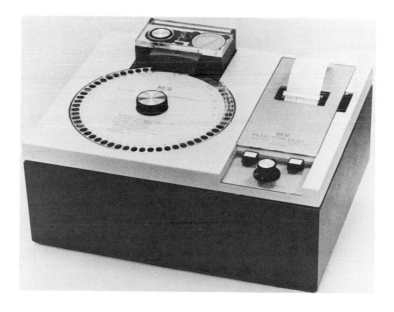

FIG. 5-7. The Electra 600. (Courtesy of M.L.A., Inc.)

easily adapted to fully automated methodologies, in that they detect the changes in optical density of a series of tests placed on an automatic turntable. All results are read from a printout tape. The Electra 600 can be used to find the "end point" of any coagulation test ending in a fibrin clot.

The Coagulyzer also employs the same principle in detecting the formation of a fibrin clot.

### Coagulyzer

*Principle.* The Coagulyzer is a fully automated apparatus designed to perform prothrombin times, activated partial thromboplastin times, prothrombin consumption tests and factor assays. The coagulation end point is read photo-optically and the results displayed on a printout tape. The instrument can be operated in any of three automated modes, or in a manual mode, as determined by particular test procedures.

#### Method (for prothrombin times)
1. Turn on the power switch 5 to 10 minutes before use to allow the temperature to reach 37°C.
2. Control and test plasmas are pipeted into a series of disposable plastic cuvets situated at the turntable.
3. Sufficient thromboplastin—calcium reagent needed for the tests is placed in the first reagent well.

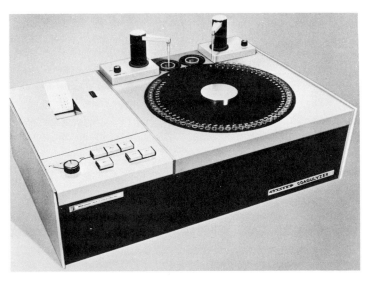

Fig. 5-8. The Coagulyzer. (Courtesy of Sherwood Medical Industries)

4. The Selector switch is turned to the PT-1 mode, and the pipet switch (for pipet 1) is turned to the 0.2 ml mode.

5. The Start switch is depressed, and the results read from a paper-tape printout after completion.

### Notes

1. To carry out coagulation tests requiring two pipeting steps (APTT etc.), a similar procedure is carried out, except that the mode selector is turned to the APTT position, and partial thromboplastin added to reagent reservoir 2 and calcium to reservoir 1. Both pipets are set to the 0.1 ml position, and test plasmas are added to the cuvets on the turntable.

2. The Coagulyzer accepts any reagent provided it is clear. Diatomaceous earth activated partial thromboplastin reagents are not suitable for photo-optical coagulation detectors and cannot be used.

### Glassware Cleaning

1. All glassware used for tests by hemostasis must be scrupulously clean. All tubes and pipets should be emptied of specimens and placed in physiological saline to prevent protein precipitation.

2. A hot soapy waterwash and individual brushing of the tubes should be carried out followed by copious rinsing in tap water and distilled water.

3. If the tubes are not yet clean enough, they should be immersed in chromic acid cleaning solution and left overnight. Pipets which have been used for kaolin or celite should be washed well in tap water first and immersed in the acid cleaning solution.

4. After the acid soaking, all glassware should be washed either by hand or in a pipet washer with copious volumes of tap water and rinsed at least 5 times in distilled water.

5. The pipets and tubes can be dried in a warm oven.

Chromic Acid Cleaning Solution:
    Potassium dichromate . . . . . . . . . . . . . . . . . . . . . . . . . . . . 10 g
    Concentrated sulfuric acid . . . . . . . . . . . . . . . . . . . . . . 25 ml
    Distilled water  . . . . . . . . . . . . . . . . . . . . . . . . . . . . . . . 75 ml

### Notes

1. Traces of detergent or acid-chromate mixture will inhibit many of the clotting mechanisms.

2. All scratched or etched glassware should be discarded, because this introduces increased foreign surface activation and produces unreliable results.

3. All coagulation studies should be carried out in a standard size tube.

### Collection of Blood Specimen

1. The method of collection of blood specimens greatly influences the final results of the tests. The following precautions should be observed when collecting blood for hemorrhagic tests:

a. The specimen must be free of tissue juice contamination.

b. The blood should not be hemolyzed, either from actual venipuncture or from delivering the sample through the needle of the syringe.

2. The two-syringe technique is recommended when carrying out critical hemorrhagic tests, but can be avoided for routine work. The method involves the use of siliconized syringes (Siliclad* or Desicote†), following the manufacturer's instructions in the preparation of the glassware. Lacking these instructions, glassware should be coated in the following way:

a. The glassware should be chemically cleaned and immersed in the silicon solution. Take care not to breathe the vapors, because the silicon is in a corrosive vehicle. Do not allow it to contact the skin; it can initiate a dermatitis. For maximal protection, it is advisable to wear rubber gloves and to siliconize all glassware in a hood.

b. After the glassware is air dried, it is quickly immersed in acetone to dissolve the silicon solvent, rinsed well in distilled water and allowed to dry in a 37°C incubator.

3. A clean venipuncture is made with a normal glass syringe.

4. A few millimeters of blood is withdrawn and the tourniquet released. The patient is instructed to open his hand and the syringe is disconnected from the needle hub.

5. A clean siliconized 20-ml syringe is quickly attached to the needle and the patient is instructed to clench his fist, thus helping to build up the blood pressure in the vein.

6. The plunger of the syringe is *slowly* withdrawn until 20 to 25 ml of blood is taken.

7. The blood is delivered into the following tubes for a full coagulation workup:

a. 4.5 ml of blood is added to either 0.5 ml of 1.34% sodium citrate or 0.5 ml of citric acid-sodium citrate buffer.

b. 10 ml of blood is added to a clean graduated centrifuge tube.

c. 7 ml of blood is added to dipotassium EDTA.

d. 1-ml samples are placed in each of three 10 × 75-mm tubes for the Lee-White coagulation time.

---

* Available from Clay-Adams, New York, N.Y.
† Available from Beckman Instruments Inc., Palo Alto, Calif.

### Sodium Citrate-Citric Acid Buffer

1. 0.1 M Sodium citrate: 29.4 g of sodium citrate dihydrate is dissolved in 1 liter of distilled water.

2. 0.1 M Citric acid: 19.2 g of citric acid is dissolved in 1 liter of distilled water.

3. 3 volumes of 0.1 M sodium citrate and 2 volumes of 0.1 M citric acid are mixed. This buffered anticoagulant is used in the proportion of 1 volume of anticoagulant to 9 volumes of blood.

### Variables in Testing

1. Because the processes of blood coagulation are enzymatic, the environmental pH of the solution is of prime importance. All coagulation tests should be carried out at a pH of 7 to 7.5.

2. Most tests are also determined at the in vivo blood temperature of 37°C. It is important that the in vitro temperature not vary from this figure by more than ±0.5°C.

3. When preparing or reconstituting reagents, distilled water lacking heavy trace metals should be used, although deionized water can be used.

4. A large microscope lamp, fitted with a blue filter, offers an excellent light source for observing fibrin formation.

Table 5-2 gives the storage time of plasma when used for coagulation tests.[2]

## TESTS OF HEMOSTATIC FUNCTION

### Determination of the Bleeding Time

*Ivy Method*[3]

*Principle.* The duration of bleeding from a standard cut is measured. The bleeding depends upon the elasticity of the blood vessel wall and upon the quantity and functional ability of platelets.

TABLE 5-2. Maximal Storage Time at 5°C of Plasma Specimen When Used with Various Anticoagulants.

|  | POTASSIUM OR SODIUM OXALATE 0.1M | SODIUM CITRATE 0.1M | SODIUM CITRATE-CITRIC ACID BUFFER 0.1M |
|---|---|---|---|
| 1-Stage Prothrombin | 4 hours | 4 hours | 4 hours |
| PTT | 2 hours | 2 hours | 4 hours |
| TGT | 2 hours | 2 hours | 4 hours |

### Reagents and Apparatus
1. Stopwatch
2. Sphygmomanometer cuff
3. Filter paper
4. Disposable lancet

### Method
1. A sphygmomanometer cuff is placed around the patient's arm above the elbow and the pressure maintained at 40 mm of mercury.
2. Three punctures are made with a disposable lancet to the full depth of the needle on the flexor surface of the forearm, with care taken to avoid visible veins.
3. Blot the drops of blood at 15- to 30-second intervals, with care taken *not* to touch the skin with the filter paper. Continue until the bleeding ceases.
4. Average the bleeding times of the three punctures.
*Normal.* 2 to 7 minutes

### Notes
1. The normal range for this test should be determined in each laboratory. The skin puncture severs small arterioles and venules as well as capillaries. Unless a standardized incision is made, the bleeding time will vary. The important technical aspect of the test is that the bleeding time depends on the *surface area* of the incision more than on the depth of the incision.
2. The test, however carried out, is a comparatively crude one and not suitable for detecting minor bleeding variations.

## Duke's Method[4]

*Principle.* As in the Ivy technique.

### Reagents and Apparatus
1. Stopwatch
2. Disposable lancet
3. Filter paper

### Method
1. Towels are draped over the patient's shoulder and the ear is punctured in a manner similar to that of the Ivy method. A stopwatch is started as soon as the puncture is made.
2. At 15- to 30-second intervals, the blood is carefully absorbed with filter paper, with care taken *not* to touch the skin surface with the paper. Continue until the bleeding ceases.
*Normal.* 0 to 5 minutes

*Notes.* It is essential that the ear be warm and that the flow of blood should be spontaneous.

## Secondary Bleeding Time (Borchgrevink and Waaler)[5]

*Principle.* A long incision is made on the forearm and the primary bleeding time is determined as in the Ivy method. The wound is allowed to heal, the clot is carefully freed from the incision and the bleeding time of the wound is measured again. This is the secondary bleeding time.

### Reagents and Apparatus
1. Metal shield, 1 mm thick, having a perforation 14 mm in length (This can be made in the hospital workshop.)
2. Adjustable guard to allow exactly 2 mm of scalpel blade to protrude
3. Scalpel blades
4. Filter papers
5. Stopwatch

### Method
1. A 14-mm incision, 1 mm deep, is made on the volar surface of the forearm with a new scalpel blade, using the shield to guide the blade.
2. The wound is allowed to bleed freely and the blood blotted away with filter paper at 30-second intervals. Care should be taken to avoid touching the wound or the skin with the paper.
3. The primary bleeding time is the time taken for this bleeding to stop.
4. Exactly 24 hours after the incision had been made, renewed bleeding is provoked in the same cut by gently removing the crust with a surgical blade. Care must be taken not to cut new vessels or cause new tissue damage. After the initiation of bleeding, the test is carried out as described for the primary time.

### Normal
Primary bleeding time 3 to 11 minutes
Secondary bleeding time 0 to 9 minutes

*Note.* The secondary bleeding time is prolonged when the intrinsic clotting system is disturbed, as in hemophilia. In these conditions, the primary bleeding time is often normal. In thrombocytopenia, both the primary and secondary bleeding times are abnormal.

## Template Bleeding Time[6]

*Principle.* This method is similar in principle to the secondary bleeding time, except that the incision is smaller.

### Reagents and Apparatus
1. The Template System* consists of 3 components.

---

* Manufactured by the Machine Shop, University of Washington, School of Medicine, Seattle, Wash.

a. Blade handle. This is a rectangular block of polystyrene 4.5 cm × 2.5 cm × 0.6 cm. A rectangular slot, 6 mm wide by 1 mm deep is cut in the upper longitudinal face of the block to accommodate a Bard-Parker blade No. 11. Within this slot, to one side of the center, 5 holes are placed 2 mm apart for the insertion of stainless steel screws. Only 2 screws are needed to secure the blade; the 5 holes are made to accommodate the various types of blade available.

b. Aluminum measuring gauge. This gauge is 4.5 cm × 3.5 cm × 0.6 cm thick. Along one longitudinal edge an L-shaped groove is cut measuring 2.5 mm wide and 1 mm deep. A central slot measuring 1.1 cm wide and 2.5 mm deep is also cut along the entire upper longitudinal face. The blade handle and gauge permit one to standardize the depth of the incision as follows:

The blade is placed in the handle with the sharp end protruding, and 2 screws are loosely set in place. With both the blade handle and measuring gauge as a flat surface, the protruding blade is placed at a right angle to the L-shaped groove of the gauge. The opposing surfaces of the gauge and handle are pushed flush against one another and the blade tip is pushed forward until it touches the inner wall of the L-shaped groove. The screws are tightened. To confirm that the blade still protrudes the proper distance after the screws are tightened, stand the handle upon the gauge with the blade protruding into the central slot.

c. Polystyrene template. This measures 5.5 cm × 2.5 cm × 1.5 mm thick. It is used to standardize the length of the incision. The template has a central slit measuring 11 mm long and 1 mm wide. When the blade is secured in the handle and placed through the slit, an incision will be made that is 9 mm long and 1 mm deep.

2. Filter paper
3. Stopwatch

### *Method*

1. A sphygmomanometer cuff is placed around the patient's arm above the elbow and the pressure maintained at 40 mm of mercury.

2. After waiting 30 seconds, the template is placed on the forearm about 5 cm distal to the antecubital crease and pressed firmly against the skin to flatten the skin surface.

3. Three incisions are made with a smooth rapid movement along the entire length of the slit, approximately 1.5 cm apart, with care taken to avoid superficial veins.

4. Start a stopwatch immediately after the incisions are made.

5. Blot the blood resulting from the incision with Whatman No. 1 filter paper without touching the wound edges, every 30 seconds, until blood no longer stains the paper.

6. The mean of the times for the individual cuts is the bleeding time.
*Normal*. 2½ to 10 minutes

*Note*
1. The measuring gauge and template are cleaned by washing in warm soapy water after each use and stored in 70% alcohol.
2. The blade is discarded after each use. Since the wound does not begin to bleed until between 5 or 10 seconds after the cut is made, blood should not contaminate the template or blade holder.


## ASPIRIN TOLERANCE TEST

*Principle*. It has been postulated that blood contains an undetermined factor that can be measured by the bleeding time. Aspirin is thought to be an antagonist to this factor, its action depending on its acetyl linkage.

*Reagents and Apparatus*
1. As in the Ivy bleeding time (p. 203)
2. Aspirin

*Method*
1. The Ivy bleeding time is determined as described on page 203.
2. The patient is allowed to ingest 10 gr of aspirin. If the patient is a child, 5 gr are given.
3. The Ivy bleeding time is repeated 2 hours after the ingestion of the aspirin.
*Normal*. The bleeding time becomes moderately prolonged after ingestion of 10 gr of aspirin. The degree of prolongation should be estimated by carrying out the test on a sufficient number of normal subjects to obtain a valid normal range for each laboratory.
*Note*. In patients with a functional platelet defect, or with abnormal morphology of capillary vessels (as frequently found in von Willebrand's disease), the ingestion of a standard dose of aspirin often produces bleeding times in excess of twice the normal.


## CLOT RETRACTION (MODIFIED TOCANTINS' METHOD)[8]

### Quantitative Technique

*Principle*. Blood is allowed to clot in a clean tube and is left for 1 hour at 37°C to allow the clot to retract from the glass walls. The clot is removed, and the free red cells and serum are measured and expressed as a percentage of the total plasma available.

### Reagents and Apparatus
1. Graduated centrifuge tube
2. Wooden applicator stick
3. 37°C Waterbath

### Method
1. 10 ml of whole blood is placed in a clean graduated conical centrifuge tube. An applicator stick is placed in the blood before it clots.
2. The blood is allowed to clot and is placed in a 37°C waterbath for exactly 1 hour.
3. At the end of this time, the clot is withdrawn by gently removing the applicator stick and draining the free cells and serum from the clot.
4. The characteristics of the clot are noted and reported as either complete or poor retraction and firm or friable clot.
5. The volume of the free cells and serum produced by the clot is measured and a hematocrit is determined by the method described on page 67.

### Calculation

$$\frac{\text{Volume of serum and cells expressed from the clot} \times 100}{(100 - \text{hematocrit})} = \text{clot retraction}$$

For example, if the hematocrit is 46% and 4 ml of free cells and serum is expressed from 10 ml of blood:

100 to 46 the percentage of plasma present in the whole blood of the patient. But 40% of the cells and serum were expressed, the maximum being 100 to 46 or 54%; thus:

$$\frac{40}{54} \times 100 \text{ the percent of normal clot retraction} = 74\%$$

### Normal. 58 to 97%

### Notes
1. By this method, anemic bloods are corrected for increased plasma volume.
2. Friability runs parallel to clot retraction and may be determined by washing out the clot with water. If the clot is easily and cleanly washed away, it is not abnormally friable.
3. Clot retraction is influenced by the concentration of fibrinogen, by platelet numbers and by the glass surfaces.
4. The test is a useful index of platelet function and numbers and it is thought to measure the nondescript platelet "retractoenzyme." Retraction is impaired when the total platelet count falls to below 100,000 per cu mm.

**Qualitative Technique**

*Principle.* This is the same as in the method described on page 208, except that the serum and free red cells are not measured, the retraction being estimated quantitatively over a 24-hour period.

*Reagents and Apparatus*
1. Clean test tube
2. 37°C Waterbath

*Method*
1. 5 ml of whole blood is allowed to clot and the blood is placed in a 37°C waterbath for 24 hours.

After about 1 hour, the clot begins to pull away from the glass surface. In about 24 hours, a normal clot will show maximal retraction.

## PLATELET COUNTS

### *Manual Methods*

**Direct Technique**

*Principle.* The number of platelets in a sample of diluted blood is counted in a hemocytometer of known dimensions. From the number of cells seen, the total platelet count of the undiluted sample is calculated.

*Reagents and Apparatus*
1. Diluting fluids:
   a. *Brecher-Cronkite fluid.*[9] 1 g of ammonium oxalate is dissolved in 100 ml of distilled water. The solution is filtered and stored in the refrigerator at 4°C.
   b. *Dacie's fluid*[10]
   Sodium citrate .................................. 5.0 g
   40% Formaldehyde............................. 1 ml
   Distilled water ............................. to 100 ml
1 ml of 0.2% brilliant cresyl blue is added to 19 ml of the above fluid just prior to use. The counting fluid should be filtered before use.
   c. *Rees-Ecker fluid*[11]
   Brilliant cresyl blue........................... 0.1 g
   Sodium citrate ................................. 3.8 g
   40% Formaldehyde ........................... 0.2 ml
   Distilled water ............................. to 100 ml
   d. *Lempert's modification of Kristenson's fluid*[12]
   Solution A—Sodium citrate ...................... 1 g
                Mercuric chloride................. 0.002 g
                Brilliant cresyl blue ............. 0.2 g

Dissolve the above salts in 100 ml of distilled water warmed to 45°C.

Solution B—Urea .............................. 20 g
            Buffered distilled water pH 7.2 ...... 100 ml
This solution should be stored in the refrigerator. Equal volumes of solutions A and B are mixed before use and centrifuged. The supernatant is decanted and used to dilute the blood.

   e. *Oettle's-Spring's fluid*[13]
Cocaine hydrochloride .......................... 0.3 g
Sodium chloride .............................. 0.02 g
Distilled water ................................ 10 ml
*Caution—This fluid is highly poisonous.*
2. Hemocytometer
3. Thoma red cell pipet

### Method
1. Pipet the diluting fluid to the 0.5 mark on the Thoma pipet and carefully draw up EDTA blood so that the level of the diluting fluid is at the 1 mark and that of the blood at the 0.5 mark.
2. Wipe the external surface of the pipet free of blood and complete the dilution by pipeting diluting fluid to the 101 mark, with care taken to avoid the introduction of air bubbles.
3. Shake the pipet to mix the dilution and expel the first few drops of the dilution from the pipet.
4. Proceed to set up the hemocytometer as in the red and white cell counts and fill the hemocytometer in the same manner.
5. Allow the platelets to settle in a moist chamber for 15 to 30 minutes at room temperature.
6. Using the 43× high dry objective of the microscope, count all the cells seen in the total center square (1 mm × 1 mm) of both sides of the chamber. The platelets will be more readily recognized by carefully altering the focus of the microscope with a fine adjustment, and by reducing the illumination by closing the iris diaphragm. Platelets appear as highly refractile bodies.

### Calculation
1. The volume of one center square is 1 mm × 1 mm × 0.1 mm = 0.1 cu mm. The total volume counted (both sides of the chamber) is: 0.1 cu mm × 2 = 0.2 cu mm.
2. If 400 platelets are counted in the total volume, there are 400 platelets in 0.2 cu mm. Because the dilution was 1:200, there are 400 × 200 platelets in 0.2 cu mm of undiluted blood. In 1 cu mm of undiluted blood, there are 400 × 200/0.2 platelets = 400,000 platelets per cu mm of blood.

3. An abbreviated form of calculation is to multiply the number of platelets counted by 1,000.

## Indirect Technique

### Cramer's and Bannerman's Method[14]

#### Reagents and Apparatus
1. Diluting fluid:

Sodium citrate ................................. 0.2 g
Sodium chloride .............................. 0.8 g
1% Aqueous brilliant cresyl blue ................. 1 ml
Formalin ...................................... 2 ml
Distilled water ........................... to 100 ml

2. Siliconized tube—10 × 75 mm
3. Grease-free slides
4. Coverslips
5. Laboratory stopcock grease
6. Moist chamber composed of an inverted Petri dish with a pledge of wet wool

#### Method
1. 2 to 3 drops of EDTA blood is added to 3 ml of the diluting fluid in a siliconized tube.

2. The fluid and blood are mixed and 1 drop is placed on a grease-free slide and covered with a clean coverslip.

3. The preparation is sealed with wax to prevent evaporation and is kept in a moist chamber for 30 minutes. The ratio of platelets to red cells is determined. Count at least 1,000 red cells.

4. Determine the total red cell count by either manual or automatic methods.

*Calculation.* If the red cell count is 5,000,000 per cu mm and there are 50 platelets counted per 1,000 red cells, there are

$$\frac{5,000,000 \times 50}{1,000} = 250,000 \text{ platelets in 1 cu mm of blood.}$$

### Dameshek's Method[15]

#### Reagents and Apparatus
1. Diluting fluid:

Sodium citrate ............................. 0.4 g
Glucose .................................... 8.0 g
Brilliant cresyl blue ...................... 0.15 g
40% Formalin .......................... 3 drops
Distilled water .......................... 100 ml

Filter the fluid prior to use.
2. Grease-free slides
3. Coverslips
4. Laboratory stopcock grease
5. Moist chamber as in the method described on page 210.

### Method
1. A finger puncture is made through a drop of the diluting fluid, the mixture of blood and fluid is transferred to a slide, and a wet sealed preparation is set up as in the preceding technique.
2. The slide is left for 30 minutes in a moist chamber and the ratio of red cells to platelets is counted.
*Calculation.* As in the preceding method.

### Fonio's Method

### Reagents and Apparatus
1. Diluting fluid: 14% aqueous magnesium sulfate
2. As in the preceding technique
*Method.* As in the preceding technique.

### Direct Slide Method

### Reagents and Apparatus
1. Grease-free slides
2. Wright's stain

### Method
1. A thinly spread blood smear is stained with Wright's stain and examined under the $97\times$ oil immersion lens of the microscope.
2. 1,000 red cells are counted and the number of platelets seen is noted.
*Calculation.* As in the previous indirect methods.
*Normal.* 150,000 to 500,000 per cu mm

### Notes
1. The use of the EDTA blood as an anticoagulant has removed the one major difficulty in platelet counting, the clumping of the platelets after short in vitro exposure.
2. Accurate counting can be achieved only by the most careful regard to detail, especially in the cleanliness of the apparatus and the diluting fluids.
3. The use of the phase contrast microscope has improved the accuracy of manual methods by aiding in the recognition and differentiation of platelets from extraneous debris.

## Automatic Methods

### Coulter Model B

*Principle.* The basic principle employed by all the Coulter counters is found on page 51. The Model B is equipped with a 70 $\mu$m aperture tube and offers the advantage over the Model F and Model FN in that both upper and lower thresholds can be set.

Red cells are lightly centrifuged and a platelet count determined on the supernatant plasma. The final result is corrected for the hematocrit to produce a whole blood platelet count.

### Reagents and Apparatus
1. Coulter Counter—Model B equipped with a 70 $\mu$ aperture tube
2. Glass or plastic vials—15 ml capacity*
3. Capillary pipets—5 $\mu$l
4. Filtered normal saline or Isoton*
5. Centrifuge, Sorvall RC3
6. Microhematocrit centrifuge
7. EDTA anticoagulated blood

### Method[16]
1. The Coulter is set up as in the manufacturer's instructions. Using platelet-rich plasma, the amplification and aperture controls are set so that the platelet population peaks at one-third of the height of the oscilloscope screen. Platelet counts are taken at all threshold settings between 1 and 10, and a curve of the count against the threshold is plotted. The plateau of this curve should occur between 5 and 10; if it does not, the amplification and aperture controls must be changed until the plateau is between these limits. The midpoint of this plateau is chosen as the lower threshold setting and 10 times this setting is taken as the upper threshold.

2. The following instrument settings have been used successfully:

   Thresholds 4 and 50
   Aperture ½
   Amplification ¼
   Gain 50
   Matching switch L64

3. The blood is mixed and the hematocrit determined by the procedure on page 73.

4. The remainder of the blood is centrifuged in the RC-3 centrifuge at 650 rpm for 5 minutes (125 g).

5. 5 $\mu$l of the resulting plasma from the *middle* of the plasma layer is

---

* Available from Scientific Products, Evanston, Ill.

added to 15 ml of diluent, capped and the mixture gently inverted to mix. Do not shake the vial vigorously to mix.

6. The plasma platelet dilution is counted in duplicate on the Model B. The oscilloscope should be carefully observed for large platelets, plugging by extraneous material, or electrical interference.

7. The whole blood platelet count is determined from the raw plasma platelet count, and corrections made for coincidence, dilution, hematocrit, and trapped plasma, from the correction tables supplied by the manufacturer.

8. Platelet counts over 600,000/cu mm blood are rediluted by adding 5 ml of diluent to 5 ml of the original diluent and doubling the resulting count.

9. Platelet counts under 50,000/cu mm blood are rediluted by adding 15 $\mu$l of plasma to 15 $\mu$l of diluent. The resulting count is then divided by 3 to produce the count/cu mm blood.

### Autocounter

***Principle.*** The Autocounter* is a fully automated system for quantitating platelet counts in whole blood. The components of the counter are a sampler, proportioning pump, manifold, counting module, and recorder. The sampler holds 40 disposable cups which are aspirated at a rate of 60 per hour. The samples are held in suspension by a rotating mixer, and are aspirated by the proportioning pump which propels diluting fluids and samples at a uniform rate through the manifold. This is a closed system consisting of both glass and plastic tubing in which both samples, refer-

---

\* Available from Technicon Instrument Corp., Tarrytown, N.Y.

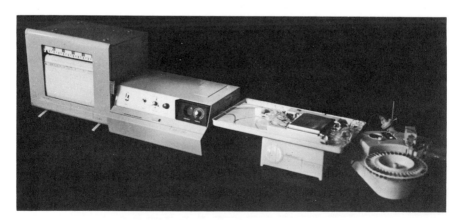

FIG. 5-9. The Autocounter. (*Right to left*): Sampler, pump and manifold, counter, recorder. (Courtesy of Technicon Instrument Corp.)

ence material, and reagents are brought together under the same conditions.

The diluted sample is passed to the counting module, an optical-electronic device, which senses the number of optical disturbances per time unit created by the passage of individual particles through the focal point of a light beam.

The results are presented as analog signals to a single-pen chart recorder which plots a continuous tracing of peaks, the height of which is proportional to the number of cells in each sample. Comparison to a series of standard peaks provides an accurate particle count.

The optical system is shown in Figure 5-9. Light from the lamp passes through a condensing lens, uniformly illuminating the primary aperture, which has a small rectangular opening in its center. A projection lens picks up the light coming through this aperture and forms a reduced image of the aperture in the center of the flow cell. This results in a small, brightly illuminated view volume, sharply defined by the reduced aperture image and the size of the flow passage in the flow cell. The light emerges from the flow cell and is blocked by a dark-field disc, which prevents any direct light from entering the photomultiplier tube.

If a clear liquid passes through the flow cell, the light rays are blocked by the dark-field disc and no light energy reaches the photomultiplier tube. However, if particles such as platelets, are dispersed in the liquid stream, they are illuminated as they pass through the view volume. When this occurs, the particles become secondary sources of illumination, scattering light in the forward direction, beyond the dark-field disc. The objective lens collects this light and focuses it through a small aperture in front of the photomultiplier tube. The aperture blocks out stray light, allowing only the scattered light from the particles to enter the photomultiplier tube. As each particle passes through the view volume, an electrical pulse is generated.

### Reagents and Apparatus

1. Filtered 2M urea

2. Wash solution: 8 g of sodium hydroxide is added to 500 ml of distilled water in a 1-liter volumetric flask. Mix until dissolved and then slowly add 10 ml of Tergitol NPX, mixing continuously. Allow the mixture to cool to room temperature.

3. Platelet standard*

Alternatively, fresh normal EDTA anticoagulated blood is diluted and phase contrast platelet counts carefully determined by two different observers in quadruplicate. The results are averaged and the sample

---

* Available as Platelet Reference N Product T03-0418 from Technicon Instrument Corp., Tarrytown, N.Y.

stored at 4°C until ready to use. It has been found that such bloods have platelet counts which are reduced approximately 4% per day over a 5-day period.

4. Autocounter

*Method*[17]

1. The apparatus is set up as in the manufacturer's instructions.

2. The electrical power is turned on to all modules except the sampler; distilled water is run through all lines in the manifold for 5 minutes prior to running reagents.

3. Whole blood samples and platelet references are loaded on the sampler tray in accordance with the following protocol:

| Position | Cup Contents |
| --- | --- |
| 1-2 | Reference standard |
| 3-20 | Unknowns |
| 21 | Reference standard |
| 22-39 | Unknowns |
| 40 | Reference standard |

4. The sample tray is mounted in position and the Autocounter wash timer set to the OFF position.

5. The wash timer is rotated until it is in the top SET position against the mechanical stop.

6. The threshold knob is adjusted to 40 and the recorder zero control is set so that it traces a zero baseline on the recorder.

7. The threshold knob is adjusted for the value obtained from the threshold curve plotted prior to setting up (below).

8. Turn the sampler power on. After 3 minutes the first peak will appear on the recorder. As soon as the first curve has passed through its crest, the wash timer switch is set on the counting module to position 60. This actuates the wash timer in synchronization with the sampler.

9. When the second reference standard arrives at a steady-state, the sensitivity control on the counting module is adjusted to set the recorder pen to the level of the reference. When the twentieth sample is read, and the reference standard appears as the tracing, it should be readjusted by means of the sensitivity control if necessary.

*Notes*

1. For samples whose values exceed the limitations of the chart paper, it is necessary to make a 1:3 dilution of the sample, in filtered 0.85% saline.

2. The final dilution of the module as described is 1:1500.

3. If capillary bloods are desired to be counted, the manifold can be adjusted as in the operating manual, and blood samples collected in Unopettes* having a 1:40 dilution. The set-up and standardization is the same as previously described, and the results are divided by 5 to give the platelet count.

### Threshold Curve Adjustment

1. The determination of an accurate threshold curve is important in adjusting the threshold setting on the counter. Incorrect adjustment too low can mean that extraneous particles and electrical noise will be counted, producing a falsely raised count. Too high a threshold setting results in white cells being counted.

2. With reagents pumping through the manifold, a vial of reference standard is sampled in the steady-state, care being taken to agitate the sample to keep the cells in suspension.

3. Turn the Autocounter wash timer switch off, and rotate the wash timer to a sample position.

4. Adjust the threshold control to 14, and as the particles arrive at the counter, adjust the sensitivity control so that the recorder is plotting a steady-state plateau at the reference value.

5. Turn the threshold knob to 0, and advance the dial 2 digits every 30 seconds. Continue advancing the threshold until the recorder reaches 0 on the chart paper.

6. The apparatus is switched to WASH and the sample probe placed in a wash solution.

7. Steps 2 to 5 are repeated, using fresh EDTA anticoagulated blood. *Do not* readjust the sensitivity control in step 4.

8. The values of the threshold settings are plotted against the chart platelet values on linear graph paper.

9. The slopes of the reference standard and the blood should be similar. The slope between the threshold of 8 and 24 should drop approximately 75,000 cells, and never more than 97,500 or less than 37,500.

Pick a point on the curve in which the line is as near to parallel as possible and set the threshold at this reading.

## Coulter Thrombocounter

*Principle.* When suspended in an electrolyte, platelets can be sized and counted by passing them through an aperture with a specific path of current flow for a given length of time. As particles pass through the aperture and displace an equal volume of electrolyte, the resistance in the path of current changes. This results in corresponding current and voltage

---

* Becton, Dickinson, and Co., Rutherford, N.J.

changes. The magnitude of each change is directly proportional to the volumetric size of the particle producing the change.

### Reagents and Apparatus

1. Thrombocounter*
2. Platelet kit* (plastic tubing from blood bank donor set, capillary pipet, pipet adaptor)
3. Isoton* (buffered saline)
4. Pipet—3.3 λ
5. EDTA anticoagulated blood

### Method[18]

1. Set up the apparatus as in the manufacturer's instructions.
2. EDTA blood is aspirated into the plastic sedimentation tubes and allowed to settle for 30 to 60 minutes.
3. Once a plasma layer is formed, it can be diluted at any convenient time during the next three hours. When ready for dilution, the tube is held in the inverted position and the red cell portion cut off with scissors, leaving a portion of the tube with only platelet-rich plasma.
3. Dilute 3.3 λ plasma in 10 ml Isoton and gently mix, avoiding bubbles.
4. An auxiliary beaker filled with Isoton is placed behind the apparatus and the rubber hose leading to the auxiliary inlet inserted into the electrolyte.
5. Place the diluted plasma sample on the sample stand with the aperture and external electrode fully immersed.
6. Open the control stopcock. When the manometer mercury has been drawn past the start electrode, clear the numeric readout by quickly pressing the Reset switch. Close the control stopcock.
7. Read the platelet count from the readout.
8. The readout count is then matched and converted to the plasma platelet count by connecting the dilution and coincidence factors (table supplied by the manufacturer).
9. The whole blood platelet count is obtained by finding the hematocrit for the blood sample and matching it to a conversion table supplied by the manufacturer. This factor is multiplied by the plasma platelet count to give the whole blood platelet count (e.g., if the machine count is 20,000 and the hematocrit is 30%, the plasma platelet count is 655,500; the conversion factor is 0.63 and the whole blood platelet count is then 0.63 × 655,500 or 412,965).

### Note

1. If the machine count exceeds 30,000, the sample dilution should be doubled from 1:3,000 to 1:6,000. Rerun this rediluted sample and multiply

---

* Available from Coulter Electronics, Inc., Hialeah, Fla.

the final plasma platelet by two. Multiply this result by the hematocrit conversion factor to give the total platelet count.

## ESTIMATION OF PLATELET ADHESIVENESS IN VITRO

### Hellem's Technique[19]

*Principle.* Platelets are counted in whole blood, exposed to a standard foreign surface and recounted. The difference in the count is expressed as the adhesive index.

#### Reagents and Apparatus
1. Glass beads—0.5 mm in diameter*
2. Plastic disposable blood bank donor set
3. Platelet count apparatus

#### Method
1. Routine platelet counts are carried out on EDTA blood by the method described on page 209.
2. 9 volumes of blood is anticoagulated with 1 volume of 3.8% sodium citrate and allowed to drip through a plastic tube containing 5 g of the glass beads.
3. The contact time for the blood to pass entirely through the glass filter is approximately 30 minutes. A platelet count is carried out on the filtered sample.

*Calculation.* The results are expressed as the number of platelets adhering to the beads as a percentage of the normal venous count.

*Normal.* 28 to 68%

### Salzman's Method[20] (Modified)

*Principle.* A platelet count is carried out on EDTA anticoagulated blood and is passed through a plastic tube containing glass beads. A second platelet count is determined on the sample after exposure to the beads. The difference between the two counts is expressed as a percentage of the venous count.

#### Reagents and Apparatus
1. Plastic tube—7 inches long, ID 0.116 inches
2. Glass beads—type 070 Superbrite†
3. Harvard Pump—Model 975
4. Column. 1.3 g of the beads are added into the plastic tube so that it is filled to a length of 4 ⅝ inches. A ML/ML Adapter‡ is fitted at each end of the tube.
5. 20 ml Plastic syringe

---

* Available from 3M Company, St. Paul, Minn., as "Superbrite" beads.
† Available from 3M Company, St. Paul, Minn.
‡ Available from Becton, Dickinson & Co., Rutherford, N.J.

*Method*

1. 10 ml of blood is drawn into the syringe and immediately placed in the infusion pump.

2. The tubing filled with beads is attached to the syringe tip and the pump run for 1 minute (the infusion pump should deliver 4 ml of blood).

3. Run the blood through the tubing into a tube containing EDTA anti-coagulant (1).

4. Quickly stop the pump, disconnect the tube with glass beads, and reconnect a plain tube without beads.

5. Run blood through this tube in the same way for 1 minute and collect into a second tube containing EDTA (2).

6. Determine the platelet counts in duplicate on each tube of blood collected (p. 209).

*Calculation*

$$\text{Platelet adhesiveness} = \frac{\text{Count tube 2—Count tube 1} \times 100}{\text{Count tube 2}}$$

*Normal.* 20 to 60%

*Notes*

1. A decreased tendency of the platelets to adhere to foreign surfaces is seen in von Willebrand's disease, Glanzmann's thrombasthenia, Waldenström's macroglobulinemia, myelofibrosis, and in some case of uremia.

2. Large doses of bishydroxycoumarin decreases platelet adhesion, while inadequate doses enhance adhesiveness.

3. It is important that each laboratory determine its own normal range for the technique, since much depends on the size and makeup of the beaded column.

## ESTIMATION OF PLATELET ADHESIVENESS IN VIVO

### Borchgrevink's Technique[21]

*Principle.* A standard cut, 1 mm deep and 10 mm long, is made in the flexor surface of the forearm. The platelets are counted in the blood issuing from the wound and also counted in blood from a standard venipuncture. The difference in the two counts represents the platelets retained on the wound.

*Reagents and Apparatus*

1. Metal shield 1 mm deep, having a perforation 10 mm in length

2. Scalpel blade with adjustable guard as used in the Secondary Bleeding Time (p. 205).

3. Platelet count apparatus

*Method*

1. The venous platelet count is determined by the method described on page 209.

2. An incision, 1 mm deep and 10 mm in length, is made on the volar surface of the forearm.

3. The capillary platelet count is determined by the blood issuing from the wound.

*Calculation.* The number of platelets adhering to the cut surface of the wound is expressed as a percentage of the normal venous platelet count.

*Normal.* 24 to 58%

*Notes*

1. In fresh citrated blood, adhesion is low but increases during a few hours' storage at 4°C. Storage at room temperature does not increase adhesion.

2. Adhesion is reduced by increasing the concentration of sodium citrate, of sodium oxalate and of EDTA, but not by increasing the concentration of heparin.

3. The presence of red cells increases platelet adhesion, and the existence of a specific factor in the red cells (Factor R of Hellem) is postulated, this factor aiding in the promotion of platelet adhesion to foreign surfaces.

4. Methods of estimating the adhesion of platelets have two serious disadvantages. First, they depend on differences between the results of two platelet counts, a technique that has a wide range of normal and is open to multiple technical errors.

Secondly, it is assumed that the platelets lost as a result of passing the blood over a particular surface are those that have adhered to that surface. Contact with such surfaces may have stimulated platelet disintegration without adhesion, thus reducing the number available for counting.

## PLATELET AGGREGATION TEST[22]

*Principle.* Platelet aggregation denotes the adhesion of one platelet to another. The phenomenon can be induced by adding aggregating agents to platelet-rich plasma which is being continually stirred. The rate and degree of aggregation can be measured spectrophotometrically and recorded. Aggregation depends on the presence of calcium and other aggregating agents.

When adenosine diphosphate (ADP) is added to platelet-rich plasma, platelet aggregation commences immediately. When the concentration of ADP is varied, a second phase of aggregation is seen which is believed to correspond to the release reaction. The ADP concentration which demonstrates this second phase varies from subject to subject and is best demonstrated at 37°C.

A two-phase response is also seen with epinephrine and thrombin.

### Reagents and Apparatus

1. Platelet Aggregometer* fitted with a Bausch and Lomb VOM5 Recorder
2. Disposable cuvets* with siliconized stir bars—0.5 ml
3. Centrifuge with tachometer
4. Ice bath
5. Siliconized:
    Conical centrifuge tubes—10 ml
    Pasteur pipets
    Serological pipets—10, 0.5, and 0.1 ml
6. Tubes—12 × 75 mm and 15 × 100 ml
7. Plastic syringes—20G needles

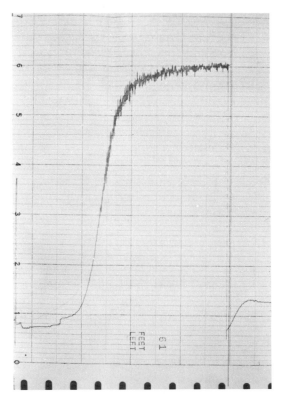

FIG. 5-10. Platelet aggregation of platelet-rich-plasma following addition of collagen.

---

* Available from Payton Associates, Inc., Buffalo, N.Y.

Fig. 5-11. Platelet aggregation of platelet-rich-plasma following addition of 1:500 ADP.

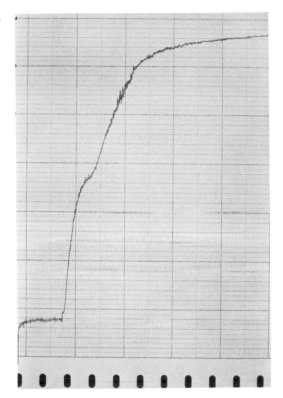

8. Parafilm
9. Stopwatch
10. Preparations of siliconized apparatus

Siliconize all glassware, using the technique described on page 000. Siliconization of the stir bars should be carried out using a similar method *except* that the bars are *not* rinsed in distilled water but are dried either in a hot-air oven or a 37°C incubator.

11. Tyrode's buffer: (pH 7.35)

Stock I: Use when preparing stock collagen suspension and diluting stock for working suspensions.

160 g sodium chloride, 4 g potassium chloride, 20 g sodium bicarbonate, and 1 g of sodium dihydrogen phosphate are dissolved in distilled water and made up to 1 liter. The pH is adjusted using 0.1 N hydrochloric acid.

Stock II: 0.1 M magnesium chloride ($MgCl_2 6H_2O$)

20.33 g of the salt are dissolved in 900 ml of distilled water and the volume made up to 1 liter.

Stock III: 0.1 M calcium chloride ($CaCl_2 6H_2O$)

21.99 g of the salt are dissolved in 900 ml of distilled water and the volume made up to 1 liter. Both Stock II and III are stable for 2 to 3 months when stored at 4°C.

12. Washing fluid 1. Calcium-free Tyrode's with heparin.

50 ml of Stock I, 20 ml of Stock II, 1 g of dextrose and 3.5 g of bovine albumin Faction V (Pentax) are added to 800 ml of di-ionized water. The reagents are mixed, made up to 1 liter, and the pH adjusted to 6.2.

5 units of heparin/ml washing fluid are added just before use.

13. Washing fluid 2. Calcium-free Tyrode's with heparin. Prepare as above, omitting the heparin.

14. Tyrode's albumin. Suspending medium.

50 ml of Stock I, 10 ml Stock II, 20 ml Stock III, 3.5 g bovine albumin Faction V (Pentax) and 1 g of dextrose are added to deionized water and made up to 1 liter. The pH is adjusted to 7.35. This reagent should be prepared daily.

15. ACD formula A (pH 5.0)

0.8 g of citric acid (anhydrous) 2.2 g sodium citrate (anhydrous) and 2.45 g dextrose are dissolved in 100 ml of distilled water.

16. ADP Stock (adenosine 5-dihydrogen phosphate)

100 mg ADP is dissolved in 10 ml of distilled water. The resulting dilutions are aliquoted in small volumes (0.2 ml), sealed with parafilm, and stored at −20°C immediately. This reagent should be renewed every 2 to 3 months.

17. Owren's buffer (pH 7.35)

11.75 g of sodium diethyl barbitone, 14.67 g of sodium chloride, and 430 ml of 0.1 N hydrochloric acid are added to distilled water and the volume made up to 2 liters.

18. Working concentrations of ADP

a. 0.01 ml of Stock ADP is added to 10 ml of Owren's buffer to produce 1.0 $\mu$g/ml concentration.

b. 1 ml of solution (a) is added to 1 ml of Owren's buffer to produce 0.5 $\mu$g/ml concentration.

c. 0.6 ml of solution (a) is added to 1.4 ml of Owren's buffer to produce 0.3 $\mu$g/ml concentrations.

d. 0.2 ml of solution (a) is added to 1.8 ml of Owren's buffer to produce 0.1 $\mu$g/ml concentrations.

19. 0.1 ml of epinephrine chloride solution (1 mg/ml; Parke, Davis & Co.) is diluted with 1.82 ml Owren's buffer.

20. Collagen reagent

a. 40 mg of bovine collagen (Sigma) is added to 2 ml saline, vortexed 5 minutes and centrifuged; 0.05 ml of the supernatant is added to 0.5 ml plasma. Alternatively, collagen may be prepared as follows.

b. Achilles tendon obtained from the autopsy room is used. Fat, muscle and blood vessels are removed from the tendon, cut into small pieces and washed in saline; 1 g of the tendon is placed in a blender and emulsified with 30 ml of Tyrode's buffer; alternately blending for 30-second intervals for 10 minutes.

The supernatant is centrifuged at 40 g and filtered through 3 layers of surgical gauze. The resulting supernatant contains only very fine particles and is stored frozen in 0.2 ml aliquots for up to 6 months. For use dilutions are made from 1:2 to 1:256 in Tyrode's solution.

21. Thrombin* (Fibrindex)

Bovine thrombin is reconstituted according to the manufacturer's instructions. Additional dilutions of this stock are made with Tyrode's solution to produce final concentrations of 0.1, 0.25, 0.5, 1.0, 2.5, and 5.0 units/ml plasma.

22. Collection and preparation of test sample

6 volumes of blood are collected and added to 1 volume of ACD. All the glassware should be either siliconized or plastic.

The blood is centrifuged in a Sorval RC2-B centrifuge using a HB-4 head at 750 rpm for 10 minutes (164 g).

The platelet-rich plasma (PRP) is separated into centrifuge tubes, the total volume measured, and a platelet count determined by a standard technique. The PRP is recentrifuged at 5,000 rpm for 6 minutes (4080 g) and the plasma removed. The platelet volume is recorded.

23. 10 volumes of washing fluid are added to 1 volume of the platelet mass and centrifuged at 5,000 rpm for 6 minutes. The platelets are rewashed twice using the same procedure but substituting washing fluid II

---

\* Available from Ortho Diagnostics, Raritan, N.J.

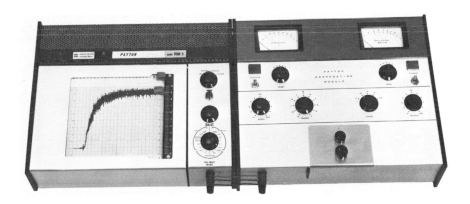

FIG. 5-12. Payton Aggregometer, showing typical normal platelet response to collagen. (Courtesy of Payton Associates, Inc.)

and finally resuspended in a small volume of Tyrode's albumin so that the platelet count approximates 250,000/cu mm.

### Method

1. Switch on the Aggregometer and set the recorder to "Standby." Allow 15 minutes to warm up to 37°C.

2. The Aggregometer (0.470 cuvet) is set as follows.
   Stir bar speed: 900 rpm
   "Range": 3
   Level: 0.2
   "Output" and "Zero": 0

3. The recorder is set as follows.
   Full scale values: 0.01 volts
   Power: "Measure"

4. The pen is placed at 1 on the chart paper using the "Zero Set" control. The "Power" set is adjusted to the "Standby" setting.

5. Platelet-rich plasma, platelet-poor plasma, ADP working solutions, and dilute suspensions of collagen are prepared and kept on ice.

6. The Aggregometer is calibrated with both platelet-rich and platelet-poor plasma. Using siliconized pipets, 0.9 ml volumes of platelet-rich and platelet-poor plasma are respectively transferred to each of two cuvets. One stir bar is added to each.

7. The platelet-poor plasma is placed in the cuvet holder and the recorder power switch turned to "Measure."

8. The pen is set at 9 on the chart paper scale, using the Aggregometer "Output" control.

9. The recorder control is turned to "Standby" and the platelet-poor plasma removed from the apparatus and replaced with platelet-rich plasma.

10. The recorder switch is turned to "Measure", and using the module "Zero" control, the pen is set to 1 on the chart paper scale.

11. The recorder control is returned to "Standby" and steps 7 and 8 are repeated, adjusting the pen to 9 if necessary.

12. 0.9 ml of the platelet-rich plasma is pipeted into a cuvet, the stir bar added, and the cuvet placed in the holder.

13. The recorder switch is set to "Measure," and using the Aggregometer "Zero" control, the pen is adjusted to 1 on the chart paper scale.

14. The recorder switch is set to "Record" and a stable baseline tracing is obtained for at least 1 minute.

15. 0.1 ml of the collagen is added to the platelet-rich plasma in the cuvet in turn, with care taken not to form any bubbles in the plasma.

16. The pen is allowed to run long enough for the reaction to reach the maximal level, and a characteristic curve is obtained with the pen returning to the baseline as the platelets deaggregate (Fig. 5-12).

17. The runs are repeated using the ADP dilutions.

*Notes*

1. The patient should be fasting and "nonsmoking" for at least 8 hours prior to the test.

2. No aspirin or aspirin compounds should be taken for 1 week before testing. Other drugs known to affect platelet aggregations should be avoided for 48 hours prior to testing and include phenylbutazone, antihistamines, antidepressants, atropine and sulfinpyrazone.

*Interpretation*

The interpretation of platelet aggregation tests is difficult. Aggregation is abnormal with a variety of aggregating agents in Glanzmann's thrombasthenia and in normal individuals who have ingested as little as 5 gr of aspirin. This drug will cause the second phase of the ADP-induced aggregation to disappear and will completely inhibit aggregation by collagen.

Aggregation by epinephrine is impaired in thrombocythemia and occasionally in other myeloproliferative diseases.

Bowie, et al[16] suggest that "patients with prolongation of bleeding time and abnormal platelet adhesiveness also should have platelet aggregation tests. Platelet aggregation with epinephrine might be the most appropriate screening procedure."

In normal individuals two phases of platelet aggregation are always seen when epinephrine is used. If the aggregation is monophasic or reduced in amplitude, aggregation tests using collagen and ADP are suggested.

## DETECTION OF PLATELET ANTIBODIES

### Method 1 (Modified Van de Wiel, et al.)[23]

*Principle.* After test serum has been incubated at 37°C for 24 hours, it is inactivated to destroy complement and mixed with platelet-rich plasma, mixed and examined for microscopic agglutination.

*Reagents and Apparatus*

1. Serum: Blood should be allowed to clot at 37°C and kept at 4°C for 12 to 24 hours before the serum is removed. The serum is inactivated by heating to 56°C for 30 minutes; 0.1 g of barium sulfate is added to 1 ml of serum and agitated for 15 minutes at room temperature. The mixture is centrifuged at 2,000 rpm for 5 minutes.

2. Platelets: Platelets from a Group O blood are used; 9 ml of blood is

collected, using a siliconized syringe, and added to 1 ml of 2% disodium EDTA in saline. The mixture is centrifuged at 1,000 rpm for 10 minutes to obtain a platelet-rich plasma, which is removed with a siliconized Pasteur pipet and placed in a siliconized tube. The platelets are centrifuged at 3,000 rpm for 15 minutes to obtain a platelet button, which is washed 3 times with 1% EDTA in saline. The platelets are resuspended in a volume of fluid to give a concentration of approximately 500,000 per cu mm.

3. Kline depression slide
4. Kahn shaker

*Method*

1. 0.05 ml of serum is added to 0.025 ml of platelet suspension on a nonsiliconized Kline depression slide.

2. The slide is agitated at 80 to 110 movements per minute for 30 minutes and examined, using the 10× objective of the microscope.

*Results.* Agglutination should be visible to the naked eye but can be confirmed under the low-power objective of the microscope.

*Notes*

1. A serum containing no platelet antibodies should be used as a negative control, and, if possible, one having antibodies should be used as a positive control.

2. The test can be repeated at 4°C and at 37°C, depending on whether cold or warm antibodies are to be detected.

**Method 2[24]**

*Principle.* Serum incubated for 24 hours is inactivated and mixed with platelet-rich plasma. The suspension is incubated at 56°C and the results read microscopically, using depressed glass slides.

*Reagents and Apparatus*

1. Siliconized glassware
2. EDTA blood
3. Refrigerated centrifuge
4. Kahn shaker
5. 37°C and 56°C Waterbaths
6. Microscope
7. Kline depression slides

*Method*

1. Patient's blood is collected aseptically in a sterile unsiliconized glass tube and allowed to clot and remain at 37°C for 24 hours.

2. The blood is centrifuged at 3,000 rpm for 15 minutes and the sterile serum transferred to a second tube and inactivated at 56°C for 30 minutes.

3. 10 ml of venous blood compatible with that of the patient is added to EDTA and mixed well. The blood is centrifuged at 1,000 rpm for 15 minutes in a refrigerated centrifuge at 4°C. The platelet-rich plasma can be refrigerated until used.

4. 0.3 ml of inactivated serum (from step 2) is added to 0.1 ml of platelet-rich plasma in a test tube (10 × 75-mm).

5. The tube is shaken and incubated overnight at 37°C. The following morning, the platelets are resuspended by *gently* tapping the tube and the suspension is decanted onto a depression (well) slide.

6. The slide is placed in a moist chamber for 30 minutes, agitated on a Kahn shaker and examined at 100× magnification for platelet clumping.

*Results.* The degree of platelet clumping is graded 0 to 4+.

*Notes*
1. The platelet suspension should be used on the day of preparation, preferably within 4 hours of preparation.

2. The platelet donors should be screened for platelet agglutinins and should have no history of blood transfusions or pregnancy.

3. If possible, positive and negative controls should be included in the test.

4. A minimum of four platelet donors should be used to make up the platelet pool.


## Platelet Antiglobulin Consumption Test (Modified Dausset et al.)[25]

*Principle.* The test is designed to demonstrate antibody globulin absorbed onto platelets by exposing antiglobulin serum to platelets and testing for a reduction in titer of the antiglobulin serum.

*Reagents and Apparatus*
1. Glassware: Siliconized glass tubes are prepared as described on page 202.

2. Platelet suspension: Normal or patient's platelets are obtained from 9 ml of venous blood, collected in 1 ml of 2% disodium EDTA in saline. The blood is separated in a refrigerated centrifuge at 1,000 rpm for 10 minutes to obtain platelet-rich plasma. This is recentrifuged at 3,000 rpm to obtain a platelet button. The button is washed 3 times in 1% disodium EDTA in saline and resuspended in 1 drop of the EDTA solution. 0.02-ml aliquots are transferred to two 8 × 75-mm tubes.

3. Coated red cells: 1 volume of a 50% suspension of washed Group O Rhesus-positive (D) cells is suspended in 9 volumes of albumin or slide test anti-D, previously diluted 1:16 with saline. The cells and antiserum are allowed to stand for 1 hour at 37°C.

4. Anti-human globulin serum (Coombs') 1:128

5. Patient's and control sera: Serum is obtained from blood allowed to clot at 37°C. After centrifugation, 1 volume of 2% disodium EDTA in saline is added to 9 volumes of serum and the solution is stored at −20°C until used.

6. Tubes—10 × 75 mm

7. Centrifuge

*Method*

1. 0.15 ml of anti-human globulin serum is added to the platelet button, which is resuspended in the serum and allowed to stand at room temperature for 15 minutes. It is centrifuged at 1,000 rpm for 5 minutes to obtain the serum that had been consumed.

2. The anti-human globulin serum obtained from the centrifuged specimen is titrated in saline in doubling dilutions to 1:1024. One volume of anti-D sensitized cells is added to each of the 10 tubes.

3. The highest dilution of the anti-human globulin which shows a positive reaction with the coated cells is recorded.

4. The anti-human globulin titration is repeated, using a sample of the serum which had not been exposed to the platelets.

*Results.* The test is considered positive if there is a 3-tube reduction in titer between the absorbed and unabsorbed serum.

*Notes*

1. The anti-human globulin consumption is reported to give between 50 and 60% positive results in idiopathic thrombocytopenic purpura and between 25 and 30% positive results in secondary thrombocytopenic purpura. The exact significance of positive tests is still in dispute. Reduction in the titer of an anti-human globulin serum can be brought about by globulin adsorbed to platelets, without this necessarily being an auto-antibody.

2. Platelet antibodies are known to be produced in patients receiving large quantities of whole blood, platelet-rich plasma or platelet concentrates. The incidence of antibodies increases with the length of exposure to foreign platelets. If a leukemic patient is treated with platelet concentrates and the platelet survival is followed by radioactive studies, the platelet response slowly diminishes and platelet antibody production increases in an inverse ratio.

## Complement Fixation Technique for the Detection of Platelet Antibodies[26]

*Principle.* Platelet antigen and antibody in the presence of complement do not hemolyse sensitized sheep cells. The antigen with complement, but not in the presence of antibody, hemolyses the sensitized sheep cells.

**Reagents and Apparatus**

All glassware used should be siliconized as on page 202.

1. Platelet preparation

Platelets from 3 Group 0 donors are collected and concentrated as described on page 227. The platelet concentrate is washed 3 times in 5 times its volume of saline, and resuspended in 1% ammonium oxalate.

2. The platelet buffer is then rewashed twice in saline and resuspended in 0.1% sodium azide in saline so that the concentration approximates 300,000/cu mm. This concentrate may be stored at 4°C, and is stable for one month.

3. Veronal buffer (pH 7.4)

   a. 4.6 g of 5.5-diethyl barbituric acid (M wt 184.2) is dissolved in 500 ml of hot deionized water.

   b. 83.3 g of sodium chloride, 2.25 g sodium bicarbonate, and 3.0 g 5.5-diethyl barbituric acid (M wt 306.18) are dissolved in 1 liter of deionized water at room temperature.

   c. 20.0 g of magnesium chloride ($MgCl_2 6H_2O$) and 4.0 g of calcium chloride are dissolved in 100 ml deionized water.

5.0 ml of reagent (c) is added to the total reagents (a) and (b) and the volume made up to 2 liters with deionized water. The pH is adjusted to 7.4 with sodium hydroxide or hydrochloric acid as necessary. Dilute this stock buffer 1:5 with deionized water before use.

4. 1:400 hemolysin: 1:100 hemolysin is diluted as follows:

   4 ml of 5% phenol is added to 94.0 ml of saline. The dilution is mixed and 2 ml of hemolysin stored in 5% glycerin. This dilution is further diluted 1:3 with buffer to produce a working 1:400 hemolysin dilution.

5. Preparation of sensitized sheep cells.

   3 ml of sheep cells are washed 3 times with saline and once with barbital buffer and made up to a 2% veronal buffered suspension (i.e., 0.2 ml of packed red cells added to 9.8 ml of 1/5 veronal buffer). An equal volume of hemolysin diluted 1:400 in buffer is added to the 2% sheep-cell suspension.

10 ml of the 2% sheep cell suspension is added to 10 ml of the 1:400 hemolysin and incubated at 37° for 30 minutes with occasional mixing. The sensitized sheep cells can be stored at 4°C for one hour.

6. Dilution of complement

   Fresh or reconstituted lyophilized guinea pig complement is diluted as shown in Table 5-3.

After the dilutions have been made, the complement is stable for one week at 4°C.

7. Patient's serum

Inactivate the patient's serum by heating at 56°C for 30 minutes.

TABLE 5-3.

| Dilution | 1:20 | 1:30 | 1:35 |
|---|---|---|---|
| Complement (ml) | 0.2 | 0.1 | 0.1 |
| Diluted 1:5 (ml) Veronal buffer | 3.8 | 2.9 | 3.4 |

Dilute the inactivated serum 1:8 by adding 2 volumes of the serum to 14 volumes of 1:5 diluted buffer.

8. Eleven siliconized tubes (10 × 75 mm) are set up in a 4-row rack in the following scheme (Tables 5-4 to 5-7):

TABLE 5-4.

| | TUBE | | |
|---|---|---|---|
| Row 1 | 1 | 2 | 3 |
| Undiluted patient's serum (vols) | — | 1 | — |
| 1:8 Patient's serum (vols) | 1 | — | — |
| 1:20 Complement (vols) | 1 | 1 | 1 |
| Platelet preparation (vols) | 1 | 1 | 1 |

TABLE 5-5.

| | TUBE | | |
|---|---|---|---|
| Row 2 | 4 | 5 | 6 |
| Undiluted patient's serum (vols) | — | 1 | — |
| 1:8 Patient's serum (vols) | 1 | — | — |
| 1:30 Complement (vols) | 1 | 1 | 1 |
| Platelet preparation (vols) | 1 | 1 | 1 |

TABLE 5-6.

| Row 3 | | TUBE 7 | 8 | 9 |
|---|---|---|---|---|
| | Undiluted patient's serum (vols) | — | 1 | — |
| 1:8 Patient's serum (vols) | | 1 | — | — |
| | 1:35 Complement (vols) | 1 | 1 | 1 |
| | Platelet preparation (vols) | 1 | 1 | 1 |

TABLE 5-7.

| Row 4 | | TUBE 10 | 11 | 12 |
|---|---|---|---|---|
| | Undiluted patient's serum (vols) | — | 1 | — |
| 1:8 Patient's serum (vols) | | 1 | — | — |
| | 1:20 Complement (vols) | 1 | 1 | — |

The tubes are incubated at 37°C for 1 hour.

9. 0.5 ml of 1:5 diluted buffer and 0.1 ml of sensitized sheep cells are added to all of the tubes. Set up tube 12 containing 0.5 ml of 1:5 diluted buffer and 0.1 ml of sensitized sheep cells, as the nonhemolyzing control tube.

10. Incubate all 12 tubes at 37°C for 40 minutes. Shake them occasionally.

11. Remove from the incubator and place at 4°C for at least 2 hours or leave overnight. Read for hemolysis.

### *Interpretation*

1. Tubes 3, 6, and 9 are the negative-antigen control tubes and should all show hemolysis.

2. Tubes 10 and 11 are the negative-antibody control tubes and should also show hemolysis.

3. Tube 12 is the sheep cell control and should not show lysis.

4. The 1:8 dilution of the patient's serum and the complement dilution are used to eliminate false results due to prozone effects.

5. Hemolysis in tubes 1, 2, 4, 5, 7, or 8 indicate a negative test for platelet antibody.

Positive results show hemolysis in one or more of these tubes.

### Notes

1. Tubes 1, 4 and 7 use the same dilution (1:8) of patient's serum with different dilutions of complement.

2. Tubes 2, 5 and 8 use undiluted patient's serum with different dilutions of complement.

### Factors Which Influence the Hemolytic Action of Complement[27]

1. Effect of hemolysin concentration

The hemolytic efficiency of complement depends upon the amount of hemolytic antibody used for sensitization of the cells. Generally, the hemolytic activity increases with the degree of sensitization, and it may be necessary to remove hemolysin from the patient's serum by absorption with red cells.

2. Effect of red cell concentration

The extent of lysis of sensitized red cells is independent of the concentration of the sensitized cells.

3. Effect of reaction volume

The hemolytic activity of complement varies inversely with the total reaction volume. If the quantities of sensitized cells and complement are kept constant, but the volume of the reaction system is increased by the addition of extra diluent, the degree of lysis diminishes. This is because the effectiveness of C2 and C3 depends upon concentration.

4. Effect of temperature

Temperatures of 37°C ± 0.2°C should be maintained for 90 minutes.

5. Effect of ionic strength

The hemolytic activity of complement varies inversely with the ionic strength of the diluent.

6. Effect of pH

The hemolytic activity of complement declines with an increase in pH. Optimal pH is 7.2 to 7.4.

7. Effect of calcium and magnesium ions

Both of these ions enhance the hemolytic activity of complement. Anions such as citrate, EDTA and pyrophosphate, bind magnesium and calcium cations, thus inhibiting the complement pathway.

**The Detection of Platelet Antibodies by Inhibition of Clot Retraction[28]**

*Principle.* Damage to 90% of the platelets in freshly collected blood prevents clot retraction. If this damage is due to the presence of platelet antibodies, the test will screen potential sera for their presence. The test can be made more sensitive by allowing an incubation period to precede clotting so that antibody and complement have additional time to affect platelets. It can also be modified for the detection of drug-dependent antibodies.

*Reagents and Apparatus*
1. Tubes—12 × 75 mm
2. Patient's and normal serum—ABO compatible
3. Applicator sticks
4. Drugs: Quinidine; 1 mg of the drug is dissolved in 1 ml of distilled water. Alternately a 200 mg tablet is crushed, and dissolved with mixing in 100 ml of warm distilled water. Mixing should continue for 20 to 30 minutes. The insoluble material is separated by centrifugation, and the supernatant kept for use.
5. 0.1 M Magnesium chloride
6. 0.1 M Calcium chloride
7. Centrifuge (GLC-1 Sorval)

**Method 1 (Immediate Test)**
1. The patient's blood is allowed to clot and is incubated at 37°C for 2 hours.
2. The serum is separated and 0.4 ml is placed in each of 2 tubes. 0.4 ml of normal serum is also placed in 2 tubes.
3. If a drug-associated antibody is suspected, 0.1 ml of the drug is added to 1 tube of each set and 0.1 ml of distilled water to the remaining 2 tubes.
4. 1 ml of fresh normal ABO compatible blood is added to each tube and a wooden applicator stick inserted into the tubes.
5. The tubes are incubated at 37°C for 2 hours. Make sure that once the clot has formed it is separated from the walls of the tube.
6. The clot is inspected and assessed for degree of retraction.
*Note.* This test can be modified to produce quantitative results by following the procedure on page 207.

**Method 2 (Delayed Test)**
1. The patient's blood is allowed to clot and is incubated at 37°C for 2 hours.

2. The following reagents are set up in 4 tubes as in Table 5-8:

TABLE 5-8.

| TUBE | 1 | 2 | 3 | 4 |
|---|---|---|---|---|
| Patient's serum (ml) | 0.1 | 0.1 | — | — |
| Normal Serum (ml) | — | — | 0.1 | 0.1 |
| 0.1 M Magnesium chloride | 0.02 | 0.02 | 0.02 | 0.02 |
| Drug solution | 0.02 | — | 0.02 | — |

3. 10 ml of fresh EDTA anticoagulated ABO compatible normal blood is centrifuged at 1,000 rpm for 5 minutes.

4. The resulting platelet-rich plasma is removed and adjusted approximately to a concentration of 200,000 platelets/mm$^3$.

5. 0.3 ml of the normal platelet suspension are added to all tubes and incubated at 37°C for 60 minutes.

6. 0.02 ml of 0.1 M calcium chloride is added to each tube to trigger coagulation. The tubes are reincubated at 37°C for 1 hour.

7. The clots are assessed quantitatively for their degree of retraction.

*Interpretation.* Failure of the clots exposed to the patient's serum, or the patient's serum plus drug, to retract as fully as clots exposed to normal serum suggests the presence of lytic platelet antibodies.

### Notes

1. 50 to 75% of potent complement-fixing antibodies found in quinidine-induced thrombocytopenia and in post-transfusion purpura inhibit clot retraction using the immediate test.

2. The delayed test is more sensitive. It is also capable of detecting some platelet isoantibodies reacting with histocompatibility antigens.

3. Complement fixation and lysis are the most sensitive tests for the detection of platelet antibodies. They are, however, time consuming and technically difficult to carry out in contrast to a modified clot-retraction method, which can be routinely performed in any laboratory.

## TOURNIQUET TEST

### Hess' Technique

*Principle.* A sphygmomanometer is placed around the patient's arm at a pressure midway between the systolic and diastolic blood pressures. At such a level, the blood is pumped to the arm and hand, but not allowed to easily return to the circulation. The net result is that the capillaries are subjected to an increased internal pressure.

### Reagents and Apparatus
1. Sphygmomanometer
2. Timer
3. Stethoscope

### Method
1. A sphygmomanometer cuff is placed around the patient's arm, inflated to a point midway between the systolic and diastolic pressures and left for 5 minutes.
2. The cuff is removed and the patient is instructed to lift his arm to shoulder height. The area immediately below the antecubital fossa is gently flicked with the hand and examined for the presence of multiple petechiae. Occasionally petechiae are also seen on the dorsal surface of the hand.

*Results.* More than 5 to 10 petechiae is abnormal.

## Semiquantitative Method

### Method
1. The test can be carried out so as to produce a semiquantitative estimation of the degree of capillary permeability. A circle, 6 cm in diameter, is marked out on the antecubital fossa and the skin examined for any blemishes resembling petechiae. If found, they are marked with ink.
2. The sphygmomanometer cuff is inflated to 50 mm of mercury and left for 15 minutes. On releasing the pressure, the number of petechiae are counted, using a 300-watt lamp 2 feet from the arm.

*Normal.* 0 to 8 petechiae

## Negative Pressure Method

*Method.* A suction cup termed a petechiometer* is placed on the volar surface of the forearm, 2 cm distal to the flexure of the elbow. A negative pressure of 200 mm is applied for 1 minute and the skin is then examined for the presence of petechiae.

*Normal.* The lowest negative pressure that causes formation of petechiae is 200 to 350 mm.

*Notes*
1. To properly evaluate capillary resistance, the student should be aware of the following:
Capillary resistance is subject to physiologic variations. It tends to

---

* Available from Rexall Drug Co., Los Angeles, Calif.

decrease as the day advances, apparently as the result of the diurnal rhythm of adrenocortical activity. It may fluctuate from day to day due to variations in the strain factor of everyday life, and it shows seasonal variations with a tendency to decrease in the late winter and early spring in the temperate zones.

2. Capillary resistance undergoes changes, lasting for a period of hours up to several days, from stressful stimuli, physical as well as emotional. In the immediate response, the underlying cause seems to be a sudden vasopressin discharge with an interplay between vasopressin and histamine. The late response appears to be due to an increase in the corticosteroid production and the sensitivity of the capillaries to the available corticosteroids.

3. 8% of healthy persons with no bleeding tendency have low capillary resistance levels.

## WHOLE BLOOD CLOTTING TIME

### Lee and White Method[29]

*Principle.* A trauma-free venipuncture is carried out, and the time interval between the drawing of the blood and its coagulation is recorded as the coagulation time.

#### Reagents and Apparatus
1. Clean—8 mm diameter
2. 37°C Waterbath
3. Stopwatch
4. Syringe rinsed with normal saline before use—5 ml

#### Method
1. 3 ml of blood is collected by a clean trauma-free venipuncture and the first 1 ml discarded. The stopwatch is started as soon as blood is seen in the syringe.

2. 1 ml of the blood is transferred to an 8-mm diameter tube and placed in a 37°C waterbath.

3. The tube is tilted at 30-second intervals through an angle of 90° until the blood has coagulated. The watch is stopped and the time taken for the blood to clot is recorded.

*Normal.* 6 to 10 minutes

1. Many variations of this original technique are used. A commn practice is to dispense blood into 3 tubes and average the coagulation time of all 3 samples. Another frequently used modification is the use of a *dry siliconized* syringe when performing the venipuncture.

2. Care should be taken to *always* tilt the tube in the same direction and through the same angle.

3. Temperature control of the waterbath and chemically clean tubes are essential to the accuracy of the test. Blood clots twice as fast as 37°C as at room temperature.

4. The size of the tubes used must be standardized, inasmuch as blood clots faster in narrower tubes because of the increased foreign surface area in contact with the blood.

## Silicon Tube Method[30]

*Principle.* The principle of this method is similar to that described for the Lee and White technique, except that all glassware used is siliconized.

### Reagents and Apparatus
1. Siliconized tubes—8 mm
2. Siliconized syringe and needle
3. 37°C Waterbath
4. Stopwatch

*Method.* Steps 1 to 3 of the Lee and White technique (p. 238) are carried out and the coagulation time recorded.

*Normal.* 18 to 25 minutes

## Dale and Laidlaw Technique[31]

*Principle.* Capillary blood is allowed to fill a narrow tube having a small lead bead in its lumen. The time taken for coagulation to occur is indicated by rotating the tube and observing when the bead is firmly held by fibrin threads.

### Reagents and Apparatus
1. Capillary tube, 1.5 to 2 mm in diameter and 15 mm in length with constricted ends, containing a small movable lead shot
2. Stopwatch

### Method
1. Capillary blood is obtained from the finger; the capillary tube is filled quickly and the stopwatch is started.

2. The tube is grasped at each end by forceps and immersed in a waterbath at 37°C. It is slowly tilted and the movement of the lead shot noted.

3. The coagulation time is the elapsed time between the moment of puncture and the arrest of the movement of the shot.

*Normal.* 1 to 3 minutes

*Note.* It is convenient to view the shot against a shielded light arranged behind the waterbath in which the tube is immersed.

### Significance of Coagulation Time

1. The in vitro estimation of a coagulation time is of limited value, even when detailed attention to technique is given. The Lee and White coagulation time, or modifications of it, are the most accurate techniques available. The test is sensitive only to severe bleeding disorders when the levels of specific coagulation factors fall to 1 to 2% of normal. This means that a hemophiliac would require 98% depletion of the normal anti-hemophilic globulin level before being diagnosed by the coagulation time.

2. The test is nonspecific in the sense that, in theory at least, deficiencies of any of the factors involved in the formation of a fibrin clot could led to an abnormal result.

3. The test is now used primarily as an index for controlling patients on heparin therapy and should not be routinely used as a mass screening test to detect hemorrhagic disorders.

4. The use of the siliconized adaptation of the Lee and White method is more sensitive when minor coagulation defects are present.


## RECALCIFICATION TIME

*Principle.* Citrated plasma is coagulated by the addition of calcium, and the interval between the addition of the calcium and the formation of a fibrin clot is recorded.

### Reagents and Apparatus
1. Stopwatch
2. M/40 calcium chloride: 2.77 g of anhydrous calcium chloride is dissolved in 1 liter of distilled water.
3. Citrated blood (see p. 4)
4. 37°C Waterbath
5. Silicon-coated tubes—10 × 75 mm
6. Siliconized syringe and needle
7. Graduated pipets—1 ml
8. Normal saline

### Method
1. Citrated plasma is centrifuged in a silicon-coated tube at 1,000 rpm for 5 minutes to obtain a platelet-rich plasma.

2. 0.1 ml of the plasma and 0.1 ml of saline are added to a prewarmed tube at 37°C; 0.1 ml of M/40 calcium chloride is added to the mixture and the stopwatch is started. The time taken for the plasma to clot is recorded.

*Normal.* 90 to 250 seconds

*Notes*

1. This test is the basis of several other coagulation procedures. Like the whole blood coagulation time, it is inherently inaccurate and difficult to standardize. The results are affected by platelet numbers; thus it is important to use siliconized glassware up to the time of recalcification.

2. Abnormal times are found in the same disorders that affect the coagulation time, as well as in thrombocytopenia.

## ONE-STAGE PROTHROMBIN TIME OF QUICK (MODIFIED)[32]

*Principle.* The plasma coagulation time in the presence of excess tissue thromboplastin and calcium is recorded and expressed as the percentage of a known normal plasma.

*Reagents and Apparatus*

1. Normal and patient's plasmas: 4.5 ml of blood is mixed with 0.5 ml of 3.8% sodium citrate. The mixture is centrifuged at 2,000 rpm for 10 minutes and the supernatant plasma removed and placed in the refrigerator until tested.

2. Commercial thromboplastin* is reconstituted according to the manufacturer's instructions.

3. M/40 Calcium chloride (see p. 240)

4. Tubes—13 × 100 mm

5. 37°C Waterbath

6. Stopwatch

7. Micropipets—0.2 ml

8. Micropipets—0.1 ml

*Method*

1. 0.1 ml of thromboplastin and 0.1 ml of M/40 calcium chloride are mixed and prewarmed at 37°C; 0.1 ml of plasma is quickly added to the mixture and a stopwatch started.

2. The mixture is left for 10 seconds and the tube removed from the waterbath. The water is wiped from its exterior and it is *gently* tilted at a rate no faster than once a second.

3. At the first appearance of a fibrin clot, the timer is stopped.

4. The procedure is repeated and the prothrombin time of the test plasma is averaged. If the repeated time falls more than ±0.5 second from the first result, other determinations are carried out until 2 within ±0.5 second are obtained. These 2 times are then averaged.

*Normal.* 11 to 15 seconds

---

* Available from numerous pharmaceutical manufacturers.

***Calculation.*** The results may be reported as the prothrombin time in seconds or as a percentage level. This level is calculated as follows, using a prothrombin activity curve.

1. Five normal oxalated plasmas are pooled and a series of dilutions prepared as shown in Table 5-9.

2. The prothrombin time of each saline dilution of plasma is determined and the times plotted against the dilution on linear graph paper.

3. A dilution curve is plotted with the pooled plasma control with no saline (tube 1) used as 100% prothrombin level.

### Notes

1. Commercial products can be obtained incorporating brain or lung thromoplastin and calcium. When such products are used, the test is modified by adding 0.2 ml of the thromboplastin-calcium mixture to 0.1 ml plasma.

2. The original one-stage prothrombin time was once throught to measure only prothrombin activity. It is now known that the test measures all the factors involved in the second and third stages of the coagulation mechanism. Dicumarol and related anticoagulants reduce the in vivo activity of Factors II, V, VII, IX and X, the tests reflecting all these plasma deficiencies with the exception of that of Factor IX.

3. The test measures the recalcification time of plasma in the presence of thromboplastin. By adding excess tissue thromboplastin, the first stage in the coagulation system is bypassed, and the test is therefore insensitive to deficiencies of Factors VIII, IX, XI and XII.

4. The final end point of fibrin clot formation is best seen against a diffuse light. Some technologists prefer to view the clot formation against a dark background. An alternate method of reading the results is to place

TABLE 5-9. Dilutions of Citrated Plasma for One-Stage
Prothrombin Test Calculation.

| Tube | Saline (ml) | Pooled Plasma (ml) | Plasma % |
|------|-------------|--------------------|----------|
| 1 | — | 1.0 | 100 |
| 2 | 0.1 | 0.9 | 90 |
| 3 | 0.2 | 0.8 | 80 |
| 4 | 0.3 | 0.7 | 70 |
| 5 | 0.4 | 0.6 | 60 |
| 6 | 0.5 | 0.5 | 50 |
| 7 | 0.6 | 0.4 | 40 |
| 8 | 0.7 | 0.3 | 30 |
| 9 | 0.8 | 0.2 | 20 |
| 10 | 0.9 | 0.1 | 10 |
| 11 | 1.0 | — | 0 |

a Nichrome wire loop in the prothrombin tube and quickly agitate it up and down at regular intervals until a fibrin clot is formed. This method has the advantage of keeping the thromboplastin-calcium-plasma mixture continually at 37°C for the entire test.

5. Fibrinogen levels below 30% of normal result in abnormal one-stage prothrombin tests.

### DETERMINATION OF THE PROTHROMBIN TIME BY THE PROTHROMBIN AND PROCONVERTIN METHOD[33]

*Principle.* This technique differs from the one-stage prothrombin time in that Factor V and fibrinogen are added to the plasma under test. This makes it possible to increase the sensitivity of the system by using dilute test plasma and also ensures that the results are affected only by changes in vitamin K dependent Factors II, VII and X.

*Reagents and Apparatus*
1. Plasma: Oxalated plasma is used, as previously described in the one-stage prothrombin time. Before use, the plasmas are diluted 1 volume to 9 in Solution B.
2. Diluents:
Solution A
   3.13% Trisodium citrate dihydrate ................. 240 ml
   Distilled water ................................. 760 ml
Veronal buffer pH 7.35
   Sodium diethyl barbiturate ........................ 5.878 g

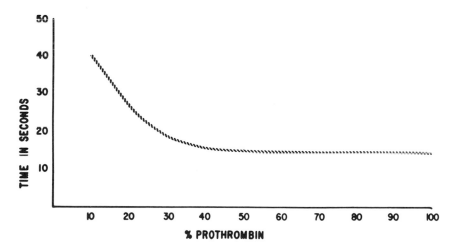

FIG. 5-13. Prothrombin dilution graph.

Sodium chloride ............................... 7.335 g
0.1 N hydrochloric acid ....................... 215.0 ml
Distilled water ............................... to 1 liter

Solution B
Veronal buffer ................................ 200 ml
0.9% Sodium chloride .......................... 600 ml
Solution A ................................... 200 ml

Solution C
3.13% Trisodium citrate dihydrate ............. 100 ml
0.9% Sodium chloride .......................... 600 ml

3. Prothrombin-free ox plasma: 50 mg of barium sulfate is added to 1 ml of oxalated ox plasma. The mixture is adsorbed for 15 minutes at 37°C and centrifuged at 2,000 rpm for 5 minutes to harvest the plasma.

4. Commercial thromboplastin*

5. M/40 Calcium chloride

6. 37°C Waterbath

7. Stopwatch

### *Method*

1. 0.1 ml of prothrombin-free ox plasma is added to 0.1 ml of diluted normal control plasma and 0.1 ml of thromboplastin. The mixture is warmed to 37°C in the bath and is recalcified by the addition of 0.1 ml M/40 calcium chloride.

2. The stopwatch is started on the addition of the calcium chloride and the clotting time of the mixture recorded, using either the "tilt" or the "wire" method previously described in the one-stage prothrombin time.

3. The procedure is repeated, using the patient's plasma in place of the normal control plasma.

### *Calculation*

1. Ten normal oxalated plasmas are pooled and dilutions set up as shown in Table 5-10.

The dilutions in the 5 tubes are rediluted by the addition of 1 volume of each of the dilutions to 9 volumes of Solution B. This gives final plasma dilutions of 1:10 to 1:160.

2. The prothrombin and proconvertin clotting times on each of these dilutions are determined and plotted against the plasma dilutions on log-log paper.

*Normal.* 30 to 40 seconds

---

* Available from Difco Laboratories, Detroit, Mich.

TABLE 5-10. Plasma Dilutions for the Prothrombin and Proconvertin
Test of Prothrombin Time.

| TUBE | NORMAL POOLED PLASMA (ML) | DILUENT SOLUTION C (ML) | PLASMA RATIO |
|------|--------------------------|------------------------|--------------|
| 1 | 1.0 | — | 1:1 |
| 2 | 1.0 | 1.0 | 1:2 |
| 3 | 1.0 from total of tube 2 | 1.0 | 1:4 |
| 4 | 1.0 from total of tube 3 | 1.0 | 1:8 |
| 5 | 1.0 from total of tube 4 | 1.0 | 1:16 |

Discard 1 ml from the final volume of tube 5.

## CONTROL OF ANTICOAGULANT THERAPY BY THE THROMBOTEST METHOD[31]

***Principle.*** The test measures the combined activities of Factors II, VII,
IX and X and was devised to be sensitive to *all* the factors depressed by
anticoagulants. The main advantage of the test appears to be its sensitivity
and its easy standardization. These claims are not universally accepted,
but the method is included to enable the student and technologist to be
familiar with its technique and theory. According to Owren's theory of

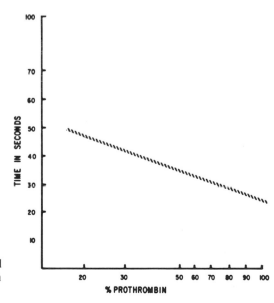

FIG. 5-14. Prothrombin and proconvertin standardization graph.

coagulation, both the intrinsic and the extrinsic pathways of thromboplastin formation are depressed by Dicumarol and related anticoagulants. The extrinsic system is altered by the depression of Factors VII and X, whereas the instrinsic pathway is altered by the reduction of Factors IX and X. Owren believes that adequate control of anticoagulated patients cannot be achieved unless the test measures all four of the depressed factors. The reagent used in the test is available commercially.* It is an active crude cephalin obtained by ether extraction of soybean and a low active thromboplastin derived from beef brain. This "total" reagent is suspended in a calcium-buffered bovine plasma (pH 7.3), which is rich in all the coagulation factors not affected by the coumarin drugs.

### Reagents and Apparatus

1. Sodium citrate: 3.13 g of sodium citrate dihydrate is dissolved in 100 ml of distilled water.
2. Thrombotest reagent dissolved in 3.2 mM calcium chloride.
3. Normal saline
4. 37°C Waterbath
5. Siliconized tubes—75 × 10 mm
6. Stopwatch
7. Micropipets—0.1 ml
8. Graduated pipets—1 ml

### Method

1. 9 volumes of venous blood is added to 1 volume of 3.13% sodium citrate and centrifuged at 2,000 rpm for 10 minutes.
2. 6 volumes of diluted plasma is further diluted with 4 volumes of normal saline.
3. 0.1 ml of the second dilution is added to 0.5 ml of prewarmed Thrombotest reagent at 37°C and the stopwatch started.

---

* Available from Baltimore Biological Laboratory, Division of B.-D. Laboratories, Inc.

TABLE 5-11. Owren's Theory of Coagulation.

| EXTRINSIC PATHWAY | | INTRINSIC PATHWAY |
|---|---|---|
| | Prothrombin | |
| Tissue Thromboplastin | | Platelets |
| Factor VII | | Factor XII |
| Factor X | | Factor VIII |
| Calcium | | Factor IX |
| Factor V | | Factor XI |
| | | Factor X |
| | | Calcium |
| | Thrombin | Factor V |

4. The clotting time of the mixture is recorded as in the one-stage pro-thrombin time.

***Calculation.*** A correlation curve is prepared by testing serial dilutions of a normal standard reference plasma in normal adsorbed plasma. This is obtained by pooling plasmas prepared from 5 male donors, each with nor-mal hematocrit, using siliconized glassware. The serial dilutions are re-diluted 3:2 with normal saline before being tested, and the coagulation time in seconds is plotted on log-log graph paper against the percentage dilution. Alternately, a standard dilution curve provided by the manu-facturers can be used.

***Normal.*** 20 to 45 seconds

## QUALITATIVE DEMONSTRATION OF FACTOR V DEFICIENCY

***Principle.*** The principle is essentially that of the one-stage prothrombin time. Normal plasma, adsorbed with barium sulfate and added to plasma having an abnormal one-stage prothrombin time, will correct the test back to normal, if the patient is deficient in Factor V. Plasma so adsorbed is rich in Factor V, but should, if correctly adsorbed, have an absence of Factors II, VII and X.

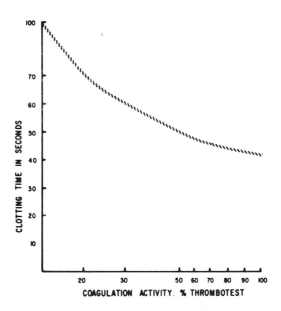

FIG. 5-15. Thrombotest standardization graph.

*Reagents and Apparatus*

1. Citrated normal and test plasmas, as described in the one-stage prothrombin time on page 241.

2. Fresh normal barium sulfate-adsorbed plasma: 100 mg of barium sulfate (Merck) is added to 1 ml of fresh normal plasma. The mixture is incubated at 37°C for 10 minutes and mixed frequently. It is then centrifuged to harvest the adsorbed plasma. If satisfactorily adsorbed, the resulting plasma will have a one-stage prothrombin time of more than 60 seconds.

3. Commercial thromboplastin
4. M/40 Calcium chloride
5. Tubes—13 × 100 mm
6. 37°C Waterbath
7. Stopwatch
8. Micropipets—0.1 ml
9. Micropipets—0.1 ml
10. Graduated pipets—1 ml

*Method*

1. The one-stage prothrombin times of the normal and test plasmas are determined as previously described.

2. 0.8 ml of normal plasma is added to 0.2 ml of barium sulfate-adsorbed plasma.

3. One-stage prothrombin times are determined in duplicate by adding 0.1 ml of the dilution made in step 2 to 0.1 of thromboplastin and 0.1 ml of M/40 calcium chloride.

4. Steps 2 and 3 are repeated, using the test plasma in place of the normal plasma.

*Results.* The one-stage prothrombin time of Factor V-deficient plasma will be shortened by the addition of 0.2 ml of the barium sulfate-adsorbed plasma. If the one-stage prothrombin time is not reduced, assays for Factors II, XII or X should be carried out.


## QUANTITATIVE DEMONSTRATION OF FACTOR V DEFICIENCY

*Principle.* Artificial Factor V-deficient plasma is made by incubating oxalated plasma for 1 to 2 weeks at 4°C. Factors I, II, VII and X are present in such a reagent in adequate amounts to determine the one-stage prothrombin time. The deficient plasma is then used as a diluent for the patient's plasma.

*Reagents and Apparatus*

1. Factor V-deficient plasma: Citrated plasma is incubated at 4°C for 1 to 2 weeks. At the end of this time, the one-stage prothrombin time should exceed 60 seconds.

2. Oxalated normal and test plasmas, as described in the one-stage prothrombin time.

3. Commercial thromboplastin

4. M/40 Calcium chloride

5. Tubes—13 × 100 mm

6. 37°C Waterbath

7. Stopwatch

8. Graduated pipets—1 ml

9. Micropipet—0.1 ml

10. Graduated micropipets—0.5 ml

### Method

1. 0.9 ml of Factor V-deficient aged plasma is added to 0.1 ml of normal plasma and a one-stage prothrombin time is determined on the mixture.

2. The procedure is repeated, using patient's plasma in place of normal plasma.

### Calculation

1. Six tubes are placed in a 37°C waterbath and dilutions set up as shown in Table 5-12.

2. 0.27 ml of aged Factor V-deficient plasma is added to each of another set of six tubes.

3. 0.03 ml of the normal diluted plasmas from Table 5-12 is added to each of the tubes prepared in 2, giving a further 1:10 dilution of these Factor V standards.

4. The one-stage prothrombin time is determined on each of these tubes and the clotting times plotted against the percentage of Factor V (in Table 5-12) on log-log graph paper.

5. The normal plasma dilution (in *Method*, part 1) should correspond to a Factor V correlation on the dilution graph. The patient's results are then read from the dilution graph and expressed as the Factor V percentage of normal.

TABLE 5-12. Plasma Dilutions for Quantitative Determination of Factor V Deficiency.

| TUBE | POOLED NORMAL PLASMA (ML) | SALINE (ML) | % FACTOR V |
|------|---------------------------|-------------|------------|
| 1 | 1.0 | — | 100 |
| 2 | 0.8 | 0.2 | 80 |
| 3 | 0.5 | 0.5 | 50 |
| 4 | 0.3 | 0.7 | 30 |
| 5 | 0.2 | 0.8 | 20 |
| 6 | 0.1 | 0.9 | 10 |

*Note.* The reagents should be prewarmed to 37°C before determining the one-stage prothrombin time.

## QUALITATIVE DEMONSTRATION OF FACTOR VII OR FACTOR X DEFICIENCY

*Principle.* Serum is aged for 3 days at 4°C. This is a rich source of Factors VII and X and, when added to a plasma which is deficient in either of these factors, it will bring the one-stage prothrombin time back to normal.

### Reagents and Apparatus
1. Aged serum: Whole blood is allowed to clot at 37°C for 1 hour. The serum is separated and left at 4°C for 3 days.
2. Commercial thromboplastin
3. M/40 Calcium chloride
4. Citrated patient and normal plasmas, as described on page 241 for the one-stage prothrombin test.
5. 37°C Waterbath
6. Stopwatch
7. Micropipets—0.1 ml
8. Micropipets—0.2 ml
9. Graduated pipets—1 ml

### Method
1. A one-stage prothrombin time is determined on the patient's plasma. If abnormal, the following procedures are carried out.
2. 0.9 ml of patient's plasma is added to 0.1 ml of aged serum.
3. A one-stage prothrombin time is determined on the plasma-serum mixture.
4. Normal plasma is substituted for patient's plasma and a one-stage prothrombin is repeated as a control.

*Results.* If there is a deficiency of either Factor VII or Factor X, the one-stage prothrombin time of the test plasma will be substantially corrected toward normal by the additon of aged serum.

## QUANTITATIVE ESTIMATION OF FACTOR VII

*Principle.* Bovine plasma, when filtered through 20% asbestos pads, contains little or no Factor VII, but does contain Factors I, II and V in adequate amounts to give a normal one-stage prothrombin time. If a test plasma contains Factor VII, it corrects the prothrombin time of this deficient substrate in proportion to the amount of Factor VII present in the test.

### Reagents and Apparatus

1. Factor VII-deficient plasma: 100 ml of oxalated bovine plasma is passed through a Seitz filter. The first 20 ml of the filtrate is discarded, because it may contain some Factor VII, the remainder being free of both Factors VII and X. A fresh Seitz asbestos pad is used for each preparation. The filtered plasma will contain Factors I, II and V and is best prepared fresh prior to use.
2. Fresh normal and test oxalated plasma
3. Normal saline
4. Commercial thromboplastin
5. M/40 Calcium chloride
6. 37°C Waterbath
7. Stopwatch
8. Micropipets—0.1 ml
9. Graduated pipets—1 ml

### Method

1. 0.1 ml of normal plasma is added to 0.9 ml of saline.
2. 0.1 ml of the diluted normal plasma is then added to 0.1 ml of the plasma deficient in Factors VII and X, and incubated for 1 minute at 37°C.
3. A one-stage prothrombin time is determined on the mixture.
4. Steps 1 to 3 are repeated, using the test plasma in place of the normal plasma.

### Preparation of Dilution Graph

1. 10 normal oxalated plasmas are pooled and serial dilutions are made as shown in Table 5-13.
2. 0.1 ml of the contents of tube 1 is added to 0.1 ml of the asbestos-filtered Factors VII and X-deficient plasma, and incubated at 37°C for 1 minute.

TABLE 5-13. Serial Plasma Dilutions for Quantitative Estimation of Factor VII.

| Tube | Normal Saline (ml) | Pooled Oxalated Plasma (ml) | % Factor VII |
|---|---|---|---|
| 1 | 1.8 | 0.2 | 100 |
| 2 | 1.0 | 1.0 from total of tube 1 | 50 |
| 3 | 1.0 | 1.0 from total of tube 2 | 25 |
| 4 | 1.0 | 1.0 from total of tube 3 | 12.5 |

Discard 1.0 ml from total of tube 4.

3. 0.1 ml M/40 calcium chloride and 0.1 ml of thromboplastin are added to the incubated mixture and the one-stage prothrombin time determined.

4. Steps 2 and 3 are repeated, using the dilutions from tubes 2, 3 and 4.

5. The prothrombin times of the dilutions are recorded and plotted on log-log paper against the percentage Factors VII and X levels.

*Calculation.* Normal plasma diluted in the test should correspond to 10% Factors VII and X correlation on the dilution graph. The patient's results are read from the graph and expressed as a percentage of the Factors VII and X complex.

*Note.* It is important to prewarm all the reagents to 37°C.


## SEPARATION OF FACTOR VII FROM FACTOR X
## (STYPVEN TIME)


*Principle.* Russell's viper venom has a thromboplastin-like activity when added to recalcified plasma. Factor VII is not needed in the reaction, the only factors involved being Factors II, V and platelets.

### Reagents and Apparatus
1. Russell's viper venom:* Dilute the venom 1:10,000 with distilled water.
2. Commercial thromboplastin
3. M/40 Calcium chloride
4. 37°C Waterbath
5. Stopwatch
6. Normal and test citrated fasting plasmas
7. Micropipets—0.1 ml

### Method
1. The one-stage prothrombin time of the patient's plasma is determined, using normal thromboplastin.

2. 0.1 ml of the patient's plasma is added to 0.1 ml of diluted venom and the mixture recalcified by the addition of 0.1 ml of M/40 calcium chloride. The clotting time of the mixture is recorded.

*Normal.* 11 to 15 seconds

### Notes
1. The Stypven time is abnormal in deficiencies of Factors II, V and X, but normal in Factor VII deficiency.

2. It is important to prewarm all the reagents to 37°C before use.

---

* Available from Sigma Chemical Co., St. Louis, Mo.

# DETECTION OF A PURE PROTHROMBIN DEFICIENCY

## Two-Stage Prothrombin Method[35]

*Principle.* Brain thromboplastin is added to citrated plasma and the mixture recalcified. Thrombin generation is assayed by adding subsamples of the mixture to a standard fibrinogen solution. The fibrinogen clotting times are converted to thrombin units, which are graphed against the subsampling times. A normal plasma is assayed and compared against the test plasma.

### Reagents and Apparatus

1. Fresh citrated normal and patient's plasmas: 1 volume of 3.8% sodium citrate is added to 9 volumes of whole blood and centrifuged at 3,000 rpm for 10 minutes.

2. 1:5 brain thromboplastin: 1 volume of thromboplastin is added to 4 volumes of normal saline.

3. M/40 Calcium chloride

4. Fibrinogen*

5. Thrombin,† 10 units per ml: 10 ml of normal saline is added to a 1,000-unit vial of thrombin. Allow to dissolve and add 1 ml of the dilution to 9 ml of saline.

6. 37°C Waterbath

7. Stopwatches—2

8. Graduated pipets—0.5 ml

9. Tubes—10 × 75 mm

10. Micropipets—0.1 ml

11. Graduated pipets—1 ml

### Method

1. 0.4 ml of fibrinogen is added to each of 10 tubes at 37°C.

2. 0.4 ml of fresh normal plasma is added to 0.4 ml of diluted thromboplastin at 37°C.

3. 0.4 ml of M/40 calcium chloride is added to the plasma-thromboplastin mixture and stopwatch 1 is started. At a time corresponding to the one-stage prothrombin time of the mixture, the plasma will clot. This hinders subsampling, and the clot should be removed as quickly as possible with an applicator stick.

4. At one-minute intervals, 0.1 ml of the thrombin generating mixture in 3 is removed and added to the fibrinogen tubes. Stopwatch 2 is started on the addition of the generating mixture to each tube.

5. The time for the fibrin clot to form is recorded and the procedure repeated for all 10 fibrinogen tubes.

---

* Available from Warner-Chilcott Co.

† Available from Parke, Davis & Co.

6. Steps 1 to 5 are repeated, using test plasma in place of normal plasma.

### Standard Thrombin-Fibrinogen Curve
1. Set up dilutions as in Table 5-14.
2. 0.1 ml of each of the 8 dilutions is withdrawn into a series of new tubes and 0.4 ml of fibrinogen is added to each in turn. Record the fibrinogen clotting time of each of the tubes.
3. The reciprocals of these times are plotted against the thrombin units on linear graph paper.

### Calculation
1. The thrombin units of both the normal and test plasma, obtained from the thrombin-fibrinogen curve, are plotted against the subsampling times.
2. The two graphs are compared by measuring the areas under the curves, and the percentage prothrombin is calculated by:

$$\frac{\text{Area under curve of test plasma} \times 100}{\text{Area under curve of normal plasma}}$$

## Owren's Method[36]

***Principle.*** Prothrombin is assayed by using deprothrombinized bovine plasma as a source of Factors II and V and aged serum as a source of Factors VII and X.

### Reagents and Apparatus
1. Oxalated normal and test plasmas
2. Commercial thromboplastin
3. M/40 Calcium chloride

TABLE 5-14. Dilutions for Standard Thrombin-Fibrogen Curve.

| TUBE | THROMBIN SOLUTION 10 UNITS/ML (ML) | NORMAL SALINE (ML) | THROMBIN UNITS |
|---|---|---|---|
| 1 | 1.0 | — | 10 |
| 2 | 0.8 | 0.2 | 8 |
| 3 | 0.5 | 0.5 | 5 |
| 4 | 0.4 | 0.6 | 4 |
| 5 | 0.3 | 0.7 | 3 |
| 6 | 0.2 | 0.8 | 2 |
| 7 | 0.1 | 0.9 | 1 |
| 8 | 0.05 | 0.95 | 0.5 |

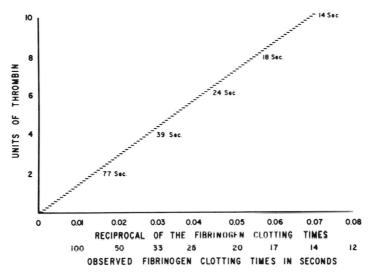

FIG. 5-16. Thrombin-fibrinogen calibration curve.

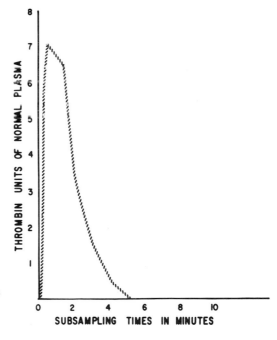

FIG. 5-17. Thrombin units of normal plasma plotted against subsampling times.

4. Deprothrombinized bovine plasma: 1 ml of oxalated bovine plasma is added to 100 mg of barium sulfate and incubated at 37°C for 10 minutes with frequent mixing. The mixture is centrifuged at 3,000 rpm for 10 minutes and the plasma harvested.

5. Aged serum: Whole blood is allowed to clot at 37°C for 1 hour. The serum is separated and left at 4°C for 3 days. 1 volume of 1.34% sodium oxalate is added to 4 volumes of serum.

6. 37°C Waterbath

7. Normal saline

8. Stopwatch

9. Graduated pipets—1 ml

10. Micropipets—0.1 ml

### Method

1. 1 ml of deprothrombinized bovine plasma is added to 1 ml of oxalated aged serum.

2. 0.1 ml of normal plasma and 0.9 ml of saline are placed in a second tube.

3. 0.1 ml of the bovine plasma-aged serum mixture from step 1 is added to 0.1 ml of the diluted normal plasma from step 2.

4. 0.1 ml of thromboplastin and 0.1 ml of M/40 calcium chloride are added to this mixture. A stopwatch is started immediately and the time required for the fibrin clot to form is recorded.

5. Repeat steps 2 to 4, using test plasma.

### Calibration Curve

1. 10 Normal oxalated plasmas are pooled together and tubes are set up as shown in Table 5-15.

2. 0.1 ml of the dilution from tube 1, 0.1 ml of bovine plasma-aged serum mixture, 0.1 ml of thromboplastin and 0.1 ml M/40 calcium chloride are added together, and the stopwatch is started on the addition of the calcium. The time for fibrin to form is recorded.

TABLE 5-15. Plasma Dilutions for the Estimation of Prothrombin by Owren's Method.

| TUBE | NORMAL SALINE (ML) | NORMAL PLASMAS (ML) | % PROTHROMBIN |
|------|------|------|------|
| 1 | 4.5 | 0.5 | 100 |
| 2 | 1.0 | 1.0 from total of tube 1 | 50 |
| 3 | 1.0 | 1.0 from total of tube 2 | 25 |
| 4 | 1.0 | 1.0 from total of tube 3 | 12.5 |

3. Step 2 is repeated for tubes 2, 3 and 4, and these clotting times are plotted against the plasma dilution.

*Calculation.* The test and normal fibrinogen clotting times are converted to per cent prothrombin from the standard calibration curve.

*Normal.* 18 to 22 seconds

*Results.* The patient's prothrombin activity is expressed both as a per cent of normal and as a time in seconds.

## PROTHROMBIN CONSUMPTION TEST
## (SERUM PROTHROMBIN)[37]

*Principle.* When normal blood clots, thrombin production continues after the clot has formed and prothrombin usage also continues. If the serum is tested at an arbitrary time after the clot has formed for the prothrombin complexes, it will be found that in normal bloods most of the factors will have been consumed in the formation of the clot. If there is a coagulation deficiency, the clot will be incompletely formed, and hence the prothrombin complex will be incompletely consumed. This will result in high levels of the prothrombin complex in the serum.

### Reagents and Apparatus

1. Patient's citrated plasma: 1 ml of 3.8% trisodium citrate is added to 9 ml of blood in a siliconized tube and centrifuged at 3,000 rpm for 10 minutes.

2. Patient's serum: Four 1-ml volumes of whole blood is allowed to clot in 8-mm diameter tubes, which are then placed in a 37°C waterbath for exactly 1 hour. At the end of that time, one-tenth of a ml of 3.8% trisodium citrate is added to the serum to inhibit the further conversion of prothrombin. The tubes are centrifuged at 1,500 rpm for 5 minutes.

3. Commercial thromboplastin

4. M/40 Calcium chloride

5. Fibrinogen—150 mg%

6. Stopwatches—2

7. 37°C Waterbath

8. Micropipets—0.1 ml

9. Micropipets—0.2 ml

10. Tubes—13 × 100 mm

### Method

1. 0.1 ml of citrated plasma is added to 0.1 ml of thromboplastin at 37°C. The reagents are allowed to warm and 0.1 ml of prewarmed M/40 calcium chloride is added. Stopwatch 1 is started on the addition of the calcium.

2. An applicator stick is placed in the tube and, at a time equivalent to

the one-stage prothrombin time, a fibrin clot forms and is removed with the stick by squeezing the clot onto the side of the tube.

3. Exactly 60 seconds after the addition of the calcium, 0.2 ml of fibrinogen is added to the tube and the second stopwatch started. The fibrinogen clotting time is recorded.

4. Steps 1 to 3 are repeated, using patient's serum. There is no fibrin clot to remove, because the conversion of prothrombin has been inhibited, thus blocking the conversion of fibrinogen.

*Calculation.* The results can be expressed two ways:

1. $$\frac{\text{Fibrinogen clotting time (plasma)}}{\text{Fibrinogen clotting time (serum)}} \times 100 = \text{Prothrombin consumption index}$$

2. Serum prothrombin time

*Normal*
Prothrombin consumption index—0 to 30%
Serum prothrombin time—greater than 30 seconds

## Modified Prothrombin Consumption Test[38]

*Reagents and Apparatus*
1. Commercial thromboplastin
2. Barium sulfate (Merck)
3. M/40 Calcium chloride
4. Pooled oxalated plasma
5. 37°C Waterbath
6. Stopwatch
7. Deprothrombinized plasma: 0.5 g of barium sulfate is added to 5 ml of pooled oxalated plasma and incubated at 37°C for 15 minutes. The mixture is inverted during the incubation to mix and ensure complete adsorption. It is then centrifuged at 2,000 rpm for 10 minutes to harvest the deficient plasma; 0.1 ml of thromboplastin, 0.1 ml of deprothrombinized plasma and 0.1 ml of M/40 calcium chloride are added together in a tube at 37°C. If no clot is formed in 5 minutes, the plasma is suitable for use. If a fibrin clot forms within that time, additional barium sulfate is added to the mixture and the adsorption repeated.
8. 5 ml of patient's blood is allowed to clot at 37°C for one hour and is centrifuged at 2,000 rpm for 5 minutes to remove the serum, which is used immediately.

*Method*
1. 0.1 ml of thromboplastin is added to 0.1 ml of deprothrombinized plasma, 0.1 ml of M/40 calcium chloride and 0.1 ml of patient's serum at 37°C. A stopwatch is started on the addition of the serum.
2. Record the time taken for the fibrin clot to form.
*Normal.* 30 to 35 seconds

*Notes*
1. Prothrombin consumption is defective in prothromboplastin factor-deficiencies, Factor V deficiency and in platelet defects.
2. In hemophilia, the serum prothrombin time is shorter than the plasma prothrombin time. The same quantitative shortening is observed when plasma is stored in glass and excess Factor V is supplied. This suggests the same basic mechanism in both and prothrombinogen is thought to be completely converted to active prothrombin. When blood lacks a primary factor such as Factor VIII, only a small amount of thromboplastin is formed and very little prothrombin consumed. At the same time, all the prothrombinogen becomes activated and, as a result, the serum prothrombin is higher than the plasma prothrombin.
3. It is important in the prothrombin consumption test to collect the blood by a standard method, using the same size syringes and needles. Deviation in technique will greatly affect the final results.

## PARTIAL THROMBOPLASTIN TIME (MODIFIED)[39]

*Principle.* Patients with abnormal partial thromboplastin times are unable to compensate for one or more factor deficiencies with the exception of Factor VII and platelet factors that involve the formation of tissue and intrinsic thromboplastin. Essentially, a one-stage prothrombin time is determined, using "partial" thromboplastin in place of the usual complete thromboplastin. The test is sensitive to Factor VIII activity to the order of 25 to 30% of normal and is comparable to the thromboplastin generation test for degree of sensitivity of the other coagulation factors.

*Reagents and Apparatus*
1. Fresh normal and test citrated plasmas
2. M/40 Calcium chloride
3. Partial thromboplastin commercially available
4. 37°C Waterbath
5. Stopwatch
6. Tubes—13 × 100 mm
7. Micropipets—0.1 ml

*Method*

1. 0.1 ml of normal plasma is added to 0.1 ml of partial thromboplastin at 37°C and is left for 30 seconds; 0.1 ml of M/40 calcium chloride is added and a stopwatch simultaneously started.

2. Gently agitate the tube and leave undisturbed for exactly 60 seconds. Observe the formation of the first sign of fibrin and record the elapsed time at that point.

3. Repeat procedures 1 and 2, using the test plasma.

*Normal.* 60 to 100 seconds

*Notes*

1. When the partial thromboplastin time of the test is within 10 seconds of the control, it can be considered normal; within 11 to 20 seconds of the control, it should be regarded as doubtful. If over 20 seconds, the test should be considered abnormal.

2. The normal range should be established for each laboratory by examining 50 to 100 normal plasmas.

3. It is extremely important to use clean glassware for this test and to add the reagents in exactly the same order.


## ACTIVATED PARTIAL THROMBOPLASTIN TIME

*Principle.* The partial thromboplastin time is a general screening test for all factors needed for thromboplastin formation, with the exception of Factor VII. To commence such a synthesis, Factor XII must be activated by a water-wettable foreign surface such as glass (in vitro) or the ruptured endothelial linings of blood vessels (in vivo).

Technically, glass presents a problem in standardizing the activation of the partial thromboplastin time. In practice, celite or kaolin is incorporated in the thromboplastin to produce this standard activation.

*Reagents and Apparatus*

1. Normal and patient's citrated plasmas: Centrifuge at 2,000 rpm for 10 minutes and store at 4°C. Use within 2 hours of collection.

2. M/40 Calcium chloride

3. Commercially available activated partial thromboplastin or ordinary partial thromboplastin can be activated by adding 1 volume of 2% kaolin or celite in 0.45% sodium chloride to 1 volume of partial thromboplastin.

4. 37°C Waterbath

5. Stopwatch

6. Tubes—10 × 75 mm

7. Micropipets—0.1 ml

*Method*

1. 0.1 ml of normal plasma is added to 0.1 ml of activated partial thromboplastin at 37°C.

2. Leave the tube for exactly 3 minutes, add 0.1 ml M/40 calcium chloride and start the stopwatch.

3. Leave the tube in the waterbath for 30 seconds, and examine for clot formation by gently tilting it back and forth at a rate no faster than *once a second*. Observe for gel formation, stopping the watch at the point of *final* gel formation. *Do not* stop the watch at the point of partial coagulation of the kaolin.

4. Repeat steps 1 to 3, using the patient's plasma.

*Normal.* 30 to 45 seconds

*Notes*

1. Deficiencies in clotting factors of all three stages of coagulation, except Factor VII, produce abnormal partial thromboplastin times.

2. The test has the advantage of being more easily controlled than the unactivated test and this is reflected in the narrow normal range.

3. The test can be easily modified to use as the basis of assaying prothromboplastin factors.


## THROMBOPLASTIN GENERATION TESTS

### Screening Technique of Hicks and Pitney[40]

*Principle.* Diluted plasma is recalcified with platelet extract and the thromboplastin generated is assayed by serial one-stage prothrombin times.

*Reagents and Apparatus*

1. Plasma: 1 volume of buffered citric acid-sodium citrate mixture (described on p. 203) is added to 9 volumes of whole blood and centrifuged at 3,000 rpm for 20 minutes to obtain platelet-poor plasma. Keep at 4°C until tested.

2. Platelet extract obtained commercially or prepared by the techniques of Bell and Alton.*

3. Substrate plasma: Citric acid-sodium citrated normal plasma is obtained by centrifuging the blood at 3,000 rpm for 10 minutes.

4. M/40 Calcium chloride

---

* Bell, W. N., and Alton, H. G.: A brain extract as a substitute for platelet suspensions in the thromboplastin generation test. Nature, *174*:880, 1954.

5. Vernonal buffer pH 7:35:
   Sodium diethyl barbiturate ..................... 5.878 g
   Sodium chloride ............................ 7.335 g
   0.1 N Hydrochloric acid .................... 215.00 ml
   Distilled water to 1 liter................... to 1.00 liter
6. 37°C Waterbath
7. Stopwatches—2
8. Tubes—13 × 100 mm
9. Micropipets—0.1 ml
10. Graduated pipets—1 ml

*Method*

1. Five tubes, each containing 0.1 ml of M/40 calcium chloride, are placed in a waterbath.

2. 1 volume of fresh normal plasma is diluted with 9 volumes of veronal buffer.

3. 0.5 ml of the diluted plasma is added to 0.5 ml of platelet substrate and allowed to warm for 1 to 2 minutes at 37°C.

4. 0.5 ml of prewarmed calcium chloride is added to the generating tube and the stopwatch started immediately.

5. At 1-minute intervals, 0.1 ml of the generating mixture and 0.1 ml of prewarmed substrate plasma are simultaneously added to the tubes set up in 1. A second stopwatch is started immediately on the addition of the substrate plasma.

6. The clotting times of the substrate are recorded and the test repeated, using diluted patient's plasma.

*Normal.* Clotting times below 14 seconds are normal at any given subsampling time.

*Notes*

1. The test is more sensitive to deficiencies of Factors XI and XII than either the partial thromboplastin time or the full thromboplastin generation test.

2. Normal results are usually found in patients receiving Dicumarol therapy but depend in part on the extent of the depression of Factors IX and X. Abnormal results are found in patients having spontaneous circulating anticoagulants.

3. Thrombocytopenic bloods produce normal generation of thromboplastin in this test, because the platelet phase is bypassed by the introduction of platelet substitutes. The test can be modified so as to detect platelet function by using patient and normal platelets in a generating tube in place of the substrate.

4. The test serves the same basic function as the partial thromboplastin time (i.e., the detection of a deficiency of one or more of the factors needed for thromboplastin formation).

### Biggs and Douglas (Modified)[41]

*Principle.* The method is essentially similar to the technique of Hicks and Pitney except that, in the latter method, 10% diluted whole plasma is used as in a generating tube, whereas here serum and adsorbed plasma are added separately. The rate of thromboplastin production is assayed by determining serial one-stage prothrombin times on the generating mixture.

#### Reagents and Apparatus

1. Patient and normal plasmas: 9 volumes of whole blood is added to 1 volume of citric acid-sodium citrate mixture (described on p. 203). The blood is centrifuged at 3,000 rpm for 10 minutes and 10 mg of barium sulfate is added for each ml of plasma. The mixture is left to adsorb for 15 minutes at 37°C and is centrifuged to separate the plasma. The adsorption should be tested by determining the one-stage prothrombin time of the plasma, which should exceed 60 seconds; 1 volume of the adsorbed plasma is added to 4 volumes of veronal buffer before use. The adsorbed plasma is the source of Factors V, VIII, XI and XII.

2. Patient and normal sera: 5 ml of whole blood is allowed to clot at 37°C and is left for 2 hours. This ensures the complete neutralization of thrombin, the maximal utilization of prothrombin and the disappearance of active thromboplastin. The serum is separated and 1 volume is diluted with 9 volumes of veronal buffer. The serum is a source of Factors IX, X, XI and XII. Veronal buffer is prepared as described on page 262.

3. Platelets (all glassware must be siliconized): 10 ml of whole blood is collected into EDTA and centrifuged at 1,000 rpm for 10 minutes to obtain platelet-rich plasma. This is removed with a Pasteur pipet, transferred to 13 × 100-mm tubes and centrifuged at 3,000 rpm for 20 minutes. The supernatant plasma is removed and retained as a source of plasma substrate. The platelet plug is washed with veronal buffer 3 times and resuspended in a volume of buffer equal to one-third of the original plasma volume.

4. Plasma substrate obtained from the platelet-poor plasma in 3.

5. M/40 Calcium chloride

6. 37°C Waterbath

7. Stopwatches—2

8. Micropipets—0.1 ml

9. Graduated pipets—0.5 ml

#### Method

1. 0.1-ml Volumes of M/40 calcium chloride are placed in 6 separate tubes at 37°C.

2. Into another tube are placed 0.4 ml of 1:10 diluted normal serum, 0.4 ml of 1:5 diluted normal adsorbed plasma, 0.4 ml of normal platelet

suspension or platelet substitute and 0.4 ml of M/40 calcium chloride. Stopwatch 1 is started on the addition of the calcium chloride. This is the generating tube.

3. At the end of the first minute, 0.1 ml of the generating mixture is added simultaneously with 0.1 ml of plasma substrate to the first tube prepared in 1. Stopwatch 2 is started immediately and the clotting time of this tube is recorded.

4. At subsequent one-minute intervals, the subsampling is repeated until 6 samples have been assayed.

5. Procedures 1 to 4 are repeated, using the following combinations of reagents in the generating tube:

    a. *Patient's adsorbed plasma*
      Normal serum
      Normal platelets
      Calcium chloride

    b. *Normal adsorbed plasma*
      Patient's serum
      Normal platelets
      Calcium chloride

*Normal.* If the clotting time for any subsample is less than 14 seconds, the specimen is considered normal.

*Results.* Typical results of the test are given in Table 5-16.

*Notes*

1. The results can be graphed by plotting the incubation times of the subsampled specimens against their individual clotting times.

TABLE 5-16. Typical Results in the Thromboplastin Generation Test

| | REAGENTS | | |
|---|---|---|---|
| FACTOR DEFICIENCY | ADSORBED PLASMA | SERUM | PLATELETS |
| V | A | N | N |
| VIII | A | N | N |
| IX | N | A | N |
| X | N | A | N |
| XI | A | A | N |
| XII | A | A | N |
| Platelets | N | N | A |

A, Abnormal; N, Normal. Thus, in a Factor VIII deficiency, the patient's adsorbed plasma produces abnormal thromboplastin generation when mixed with normal serum and platelets. The patient's serum produces normal thromboplastin generation when mixed with normal serum and platelets. The patient's serum produces normal thromboplastin generation when mixed with normal adsorbed plasma and normal platelets.

2. Alumina gel, as described by Biggs and Douglas, and commercially available aluminum hydroxide (Amphojel—obtainable in any pharmacy) can be used as alternative inorganic adsorbents.

3. All the reagents should be prewarmed to 37°C before use. When reconstituted, all reagents should be stored in crushed ice.

4. Differentiation between Factors V and VIII and between Factors IX and X can be made by the one-stage prothrombin time. Factors V and X deficiencies both produce abnormal time in this test, whereas deficiencies of Factors VIII and IX both give normal results. Differentiation between Factors XI and XII cannot be made unless plasmas deficient in these factors are available.

### Retarded Thromboplastin Generation Test of Thompson et al.[42]

*Principle.* Accelerated blood coagulation, measured by the method of Biggs and Douglas, is not easily detected. The method of Thompson, et al., differs from that of Biggs in that 1.34% sodium oxalate is used as the anticoagulant in place of citric acid-sodium citrate; barium sulfate is used as the adsorbent in place of alumina gel; and the plasma substrate is rendered incoagulable by treatment with ion exchange resin instead of sodium citrate. Further changes are that, once adsorbed, the plasma is diluted 1:50 with veronal buffer instead of the usual dilution of 1:5, and that subsamples from the generating mixture are taken for 12 minutes.

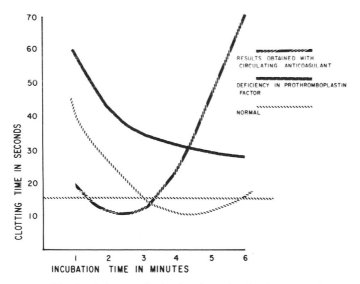

FIG. 5-18. Graph of the results in the thromboplastin generation test.

*Reagents and Apparatus.* Except for the above changes, the reagents and apparatus are as in the thromboplastin generation test described on page 261.

*Method.* As described on page 261.

*Normal.* Clotting times of 13 to 16 seconds after 11 to 16 minutes of incubation, as described on page 264.

## Cross-Correction Studies Using the Thromboplastin Generation Test

*Principle.* If a defect is found in the patient's plasma by using the thromboplastin generation test, the possible deficiency could be due to either a Factors VIII, XI or XII reduction. Similarly, if found in the serum, it could be the result of a deficiency in either Factors IX, X, XI or XII.

If dilutions of hemophilic plasma in patient's plasma are substituted for the patient's plasma in the generation test, and if this is repeated using dilutions of normal plasma in the patient's plasma, a comparison of the speed of thromboplastin generation can be obtained. If the patient has a defect in Factor VIII, the addition of a known Factor VIII-deficient plasma will not speed up thromboplastin generation. Conversely, such generation will improve if fresh normal plasma is diluted with the patient's deficient plasma. Such corrections can be carried out, using other factor-deficient plasmas.

### Reagents and Apparatus

1. As in the thromboplastin generation tests described on page 261.
2. Factor-deficient plasmas*

### Method

1. The procedure for the thromboplastin generation test is carried out as described on page 261.

2. Additional combinations of plasma and serum are assayed to compare their thromboplastin generation rates. The generating tubes are set up with the following combinations:

   a. *To detect a Factor VIII deficiency:* 1 volume patient's adsorbed plasma and 1 volume of Factor VIII-deficient adsorbed plasma; 2 volumes normal serum; 2 volumes normal platelets or platelet substitutes. Repeat, using 1 volume of normal adsorbed plasma in place of the Factor VIII-deficient adsorbed plasma.

   *Results.* If the patient's plasma is deficient in Factor VIII, the addition of normal plasma will convert the clotting time back to normal. The addition of the Factor VIII-deficient plasma will not decrease the clotting time.

---

* Available from Hyland Laboratories.

b. *To detect a Factor IX deficiency:* 2 volumes normal adsorbed plasma; 1 volume Factor IX-deficient serum and 1 volume patient's serum; 2 volumes normal platelets or platelet substitutes. Repeat, using 1 volume of normal serum in place of the Factor IX-deficient serum.

*Results.* If the patient's serum is deficient in Factor IX, the addition of normal serum will convert the clotting time back to normal. The addition of the Factor IX-deficient serum will not decrease the clotting time.

c. *To detect a Factor XI deficiency:* 1 volume of patient's adsorbed plasma and 1 volume of Factor XI-deficient adsorbed plasma; 2 volumes normal serum; 2 volumes platelets or platelet substitutes. Repeat, using 1 volume of normal adsorbed plasma in place of the Factor XI-deficient adsorbed plasma.

*Results.* If the patient's plasma is deficient in Factor XI, the addition of normal plasma will convert the clotting time back to normal. The addition of the Factor XI deficient adsorbed plasma will not decrease the clotting time.

d. *To detect a Factor XII deficiency.* 1 volume patient's adsorbed plasma and 1 volume Factor XII-deficient adsorbed plasma; 2 volumes normal serum; 2 volumes normal platelets or platelet substitutes. Repeat, using 1 volume of normal adsorbed plasma in place of the Factor XII-deficient adsorbed plasma.

*Results.* If the patient's plasma is deficient in Factor XII, the addition of normal plasma will convert the clotting time to normal. The addition of the Factor XII-deficient adsorbed plasma will not decrease the clotting time.

### Cross-Correction Studies Using the Partial Thromboplastin Time to Detect Deficiencies of Factors VIII and IX

*Principle.* If a defect is found in the patient's plasma with the partial thromboplastin time, it will be corrected to give a normal result if the patient's plasma is mixed with fresh normal plasma. Conversely, the test will not be corrected if the patient's plasma is mixed with another plasma already deficient in the same factor.

#### Reagents and Apparatus
1. As in the partial thromboplastin time described on page 260.
2. Factor-deficient plasmas*

#### Method
1. The partial thromboplastin time should be determined as described on page 260. If it is abnormal, the following tests should be carried out.

---

* Available from Hyland Laboratories.

2. 0.05 ml of patient's plasma is mixed with 0.05 ml of normal plasma and the partial thromboplastin time of the mixture is determined.

3. 0.05 ml of patient's plasma is mixed with 0.05 ml of factor-deficient plasma and the partial thromboplastin time of this mixture is also determined.

*Results.* If the patient is deficient in a specific factor, the addition of normal plasma in the mixture will correct the partial thromboplastin time to normal or near normal, whereas the mixture containing a known deficient plasma will not correct the partial thromboplastin time.

## FACTOR VIII ASSAY USING PARTIAL THROMBOPLASTIN TIME[43]

*Principle.* By extending the partial thromboplastin time method, Factor VIII assays can be determined. The assay is based upon the correcting action of the test plasma upon a prolonged partial thromboplastin time of a Factor VIII-deficient substrate. Within certain limits, the amount of correction of the substrate is proportional to the amount of Factor VIII in the plasma. The partial thromboplastin time shortening action on the test plasma is compared to that of a normal plasma and the Factor VIII content of the test is expressed as a percentage of the normal.

### Reagents and Apparatus

1. Kaolin-activated partial thromboplastin reagent as described on page 000.

2. Buffered citric acid-sodium citrate anticoagulant

3. Factor VIII-deficient plasma (less than 1%) to be used as a substrate. If the blood of a severe hemophiliac is not readily available, the reagent can be purchased commercially.*

4. M/40 Calcium chloride

5. Veronal buffer pH 7.35 (p. 243)

6. Normal control plasma: Either pool 10 normal citrated plasmas or use a 100% reference standard.*

7. Stopwatches—2

8. 37°C Waterbath

9. Test plasma: 9 volumes of blood is added to 1 volume of citric acid-sodium citrate anticoagulant and centrifuged in a refrigerated unit at 2,000 rpm for 15 minutes. Store in an ice bath.

### Method

1. The partial thromboplastin reagent is reconstituted and placed in an ice bath with the Factor VIII-deficient substrate. The calcium chloride is prewarmed to 37°C before use.

---

* Available from Hyland Laboratories.

2. Set up 4 tubes as given in Table 5-17. Add the buffer to the tubes and add the normal plasma. Place all the tubes immediately in an ice bath until used.

3. In another tube at 37°C, place 0.1 ml volumes of well-mixed kaolin partial thromboplastin reagent, Factor VIII-deficient plasma and diluted control from tube 1. Start a stopwatch immediately upon the addition of the control.

4. After exactly 3 minutes, 0.1 ml of M/40 calcium chloride is added to the mixture and stopwatch 2 is started.

5. Mix the contents of the tube quickly and leave at 37°C for exactly 30 seconds.

6. Remove the tube from the waterbath and *gently tilt* at a rate of approximately once a second. Observe for gel formation. *Do not stop* the stopwatch at the point of partial coalescence.

7. Repeat steps 3 to 8, using the dilutions in tubes 2, 3 and 4.

8. Repeat steps 2 to 6, using the patient's plasma in place of normal plasma.

*Calculation.*

1. The clotting time of each dilution is plotted against plasma concentration on semilog graph paper.

2. By interpolation, the concentrations of normal control plasma that will produce the same clotting time as 20, 10, 5 and 2.5% of test plasma are determined.

3. The resulting control plasma concentrations are multiplied by the equivalent test plasma dilutions (i.e., 2.5% concentration × 40 = 100%, 5% concentration × 20 = 100%, 10% concentration × 10 = 100%, and 20% concentration × 5 = 100%).

4. The 4 assays are averaged to give the overall Factor VIII concentration.
*Normal.* 70 to 145%

*Notes*

1. It is essential that, after the reagents are made up, they be kept in a bath of crushed ice.

TABLE 5-17. Plasma Dilutions for Partial Thromboplastin Time to Assay Factor VIII.

| TUBE | VERONAL BUFFER (ML) | NORMAL CONTROL PLASMA (ML) | PLASMA CONCENTRATION % |
|------|------|------|------|
| 1 | 0.4 | 0.1 | 20 |
| 2 | 0.9 | 0.1 | 10 |
| 3 | 1.9 | 0.1 | 5 |
| 4 | 3.9 | 0.1 | 2.5 |

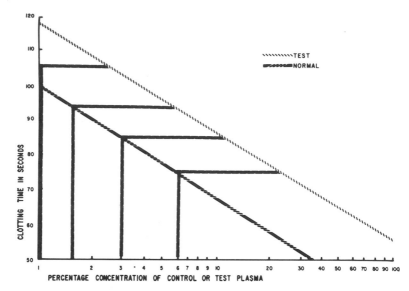

FIG. 5-19. Calculation of Factor VIII, using the partial thromboplastin time.

2. The method suffers from the fact that a severely deficient plasma must be used as a substrate in the test. If this plasma has a Factor VIII concentration of more than 1%, it is unsuitable for use as a substrate.

3. Factor VIII assays are difficult methods to master. The main difficulty lies in the preparation and stability of the reagents and in the choice of a normal control plasma. It has been demonstrated that Factor VIII levels vary with age and sex, being higher in males than in females. The availability of a normal assayed control plasma helps greatly in the standardization of the test.

TABLE 5-18. Example of the Calculation of Factor VIII Using the Partial Thromboplastin Time.

| PLASMA CONCENTRA-TION % | CLOTTING TIME OF | | EQUIVALENT CONTROL PLASMA CONCENTRATION | MULTIPLICA-TION OF CONTROL PLASMA BY DILUTION FACTOR | FACTOR VIII ACTIVITY OF TEST PLASMA |
|---|---|---|---|---|---|
| | NORMAL CONTROL | TEST PLASMA | | | |
| 20 | 58 | 75 | 6 | 6　× 5 | 30 |
| 10 | 68 | 85 | 3 | 3　× 10 | 30 |
| 5 | 77 | 95 | 1.5 | 1.5 × 20 | 30 |
| 2.5 | 87 | 104 | 1 | 1　× 40 | 40 |
| | | | | | Average 32% |

## FACTOR VIII ASSAY BY THE THROMBOPLASTIN
## GENERATION TEST

***Principle.*** Thromboplastin generation tests are carried out using substrates deficient in Factor VIII but containing all the other coagulation factors needed to produce thromboplastin. Patient's plasma is added to the substrate in a thromboplastin generation test, and the clotting times are compared with those obtained by adding dilutions of standard normal plasma to the test.

### Reagents and Apparatus

1. Substrate hemophilic plasma: 1 volume of 3.8% sodium citrate is added to 9 volumes of severely affected hemophilic blood having a Factor VIII assay of less than 1%. Centrifuge at 3,000 rpm for 15 minutes and store the plasma in small aliquots in the freezer. Prior to use, 0.1 g of barium sulfate is added to 1 ml of the thawed plasma, and the mixture is incubated at 37°C for 5 minutes and centrifuged. The barium sulfate adsorbs Factors II, VII, IX and X, leaving Factors V and VIII. A one-stage prothrombin time is carried out on the plasma to ensure adequate adsorption. The time should be in excess of 60 seconds. The adsorbed plasma is diluted 1:5 with veronal buffer before use.

2. Normal serum: 5 ml of whole blood is allowed to clot and is incubated for 4 hours at 37°C. It is reincubated at 4°C overnight, diluted 1:10 with veronal buffer pH 7.35 and once more left for 4 hours at 4°C. The diluted serum can be frozen at −20°C and kept for a maximum of 2 weeks.

3. Platelets: Normal platelets are prepared as described on page 275, or commercially obtainable platelet substitutes can be used.

4. Fresh normal plasma: 5 ml of fresh citrated normal plasma is mixed

TABLE 5-19. Plasma Dilutions for Factor VIII Assay by the
Thromboplastin Generation Test.

| Tube | Fresh Normal Citrated Plasma (ml) | Veronal Buffer (ml) | Final Dilution | % Factor VIII |
|------|-----------------------------------|---------------------|----------------|---------------|
| 1 | 0.1 | 1.9 | 1:20 | 100 |
| 2 | 1.0 from total of tube 1 | 1.0 | 1:40 | 50 |
| 3 | 1.0 from total of tube 2 | 1.0 | 1:80 | 25 |
| 4 | 1.0 from total of tube 3 | 1.0 | 1:160 | 12.5 |
| 5 | 1.0 from total of tube 4 | 1.0 | 1:320 | 6.25 |

with 0.5 g of barium sulfate and incubated at 37°C for 5 minutes. The plasma is centrifuged and dilutions set up as in Table 5-19, using veronal buffer and the diluent.

5. Fresh patient's plasma: This is obtained and treated in the same way as the normal plasma in 4.

6. M/40 Calcium chloride
7. Stopwatches—2
8. 37°C Waterbath
9. Substrate plasma. Normal citrated plasma is used.
10. Micropipets—0.1 ml
11. Graduated pipets—1 ml

### Method

1. 0.1-ml volumes of calcium chloride are added to 8 tubes.

2. 0.1-ml volumes of 1:20 normal diluted plasma in tube 1, 1:10 normal serum, platelet suspension and prewarmed calcium chloride are added to the generating tube. Stopwatch 1 is started on the addition of the calcium chloride.

3. After 8 minutes of incubation, 0.1 ml of the generating mixture from 2 is added simultaneously with 0.1 ml of plasma substrate to one of the calcium tubes in 1. Stopwatch 2 is started on the addition of the last reagent.

4. The procedure is repeated, using the dilutions set up in tubes 2, 3, 4 and 5, and Factor VIII concentrations are plotted against the clotting times of the samples.

5. Steps 1 and 2 are repeated, using the same dilutions of patient's plasma and the results are graphically recorded.

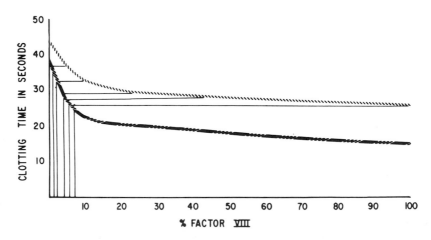

FIG. 5-20. Calculation of Factor VIII, using the thromboplastin generation test.

*Calculation.* The dilution of normal plasma producing the same clotting time as the patient's is found from the graph and allowance is made for the initial dilution of the plasma.

As an example, taking the 1:20 dilution as 100% Factor VIII, if a 1:80 dilution of the patient's plasma corresponds to a clotting time of 5% Factor VIII of 1:20 dilution, the level of Factor VIII in the patient is:

$$5\% \times (80/20) = 5\% \times 4 = 20\%$$

TABLE 5-20. Example of the Calculation of Factor VIII Using the Thromboplastin Generation Test.

| PLASMA CONCENTRA- TION % | CLOTTING TIME OF | | EQUIVALENT CONTROL PLASMA CONCENTRATION | MULTIPLICA- TION OF CONTROL PLASMA BY DILUTION FACTOR | FACTOR VIII ACTIVITY OF TEST PLASMA |
|---|---|---|---|---|---|
| | NORMAL CONTROL | TEST PLASMA | | | |
| 1:20 (100) | 15 | 26 | 8 | 8 × 1 | 8 |
| 1:40 (50) | 17 | 27 | 7 | 7 × 2 | 14 |
| 1:80 (25) | 19 | 29 | 5 | 5 × 4 | 20 |
| 1:160 (12.5) | 21 | 34 | 3 | 3 × 8 | 24 |
| 1:320 (5.25) | 29 | 38 | 1 | 1 × 16 | 16 |
| | | | | | Average 14.4% |

*Notes*

1. The main disadvantage of both Factor VIII Assay methods described is that Factor VIII-deficient plasma is essential to the test.

2. Bergna's method[44] can be used as an alternative procedure and is based upon the use of bovine serum in place of hemophilic plasma. Such serum contains all the clotting factors necessary for the generation of thromboplastin, with the exception of Factor VIII.

3. An alternate technique includes the use of an artificially prepared hemophilic plasma. The preparation involves aging normal plasma until the one-stage prothrombin time is in excess of 60 seconds. This aging produces a plasma deficient in Factors V and VIII. If commercial Factor V is added back to the aged plasma, the sole deficient substance is Factor VIII. This plasma is used as a substrate for either of the two assays described.

4. A third method of assaying without the use of hemophilic plasma is to use thrombocytopenic serum derived from platelet-poor plasma. The high level of Factor V and the absence of Factor VIII in this reagent make it an alternative to hemophilic plasma.

5. Factor VIII assays can be used as an aid in the diagnosis of mild cases of hemophilia, in controlling therapy in such cases and in controlling necessary surgical procedures. Knowledge of the level of Factor VIII is also useful in the diagnosis of von Willebrand's disease.

## FACTOR IX ASSAY

Fresh or fresh-frozen Factor IX-deficient citrated plasma is used as substrate. If Factors V and VIII have deteriorated, they can be replaced by adding an equal volume of fresh barium-sulfate absorbed normal plasma or of absorbed prothrombin-free rabbit plasma to the substrate plasma. The remainder of the procedure is the same as described under Factor VIII assay.

## FACTORS XI AND XII ASSAY

The assay of these coagulation factors presents many technical problems. Unlike the assay of Factor VIII, no substitutes are readily available to use as factor-deficient substrates. If a severely deficient plasma is available, the assays can be carried out by procedures similar to those previously described for Factor VIII assays. The main difference in the method used to assay Factors XI and XII is that siliconized glassware must be used throughout the test.

## DETECTION OF INHIBITORS OF FACTORS VIII AND IX

*Principle.* If inhibitors of either Factor VIII or IX are present in the patient's plasma they will neutralize the corresponding factor in normal plasma.

### Reagents and Apparatus
1. Normal and patient's citrated plasma.
2. Reagents as listed under Factor VIII or IX assay (p. 268).

### Method
1. The following dilutions are made and kept on ice until assayed.

TABLE 5-21. Dilutions Used in the Detection of Inhibitors.

| TUBE | 1 | 2 | 3 |
|---|---|---|---|
| Patient's plasma (ml) | 0.5 | — | 0.1 |
| Normal plasma (ml) | — | 0.5 | 0.5 |
| Veronal buffer (ml) | 0.1 | 0.1 | — |

2. Each tube is incubated at 37°C for 1 hour and activated partial thromboplastin times are determined (p. 260).

3. Alternatively the amount of factor inhibited can be measured by assaying the respective factor in each of the dilutions.

*Interpretation.* If an inhibitor is present in the patient's plasma, the addition of this plasma to the normal plasma will, after incubation, disproportionately reduce the factor assay (increase the partial thromboplastin time) in tube 3 lower than in tube 2.

*Note.* By setting up a series of dilutions, a semiquantitative estimation can be made as to the strength of the inhibitor.

## PLATELET FACTOR 3 ASSAY[45]

*Principle.* Thromboplastin generation depends upon adequate plasma factors, calcium ions, and upon functional activity and quantity of the platelets. If the adsorbed plasma and serum are from a normal source in the thromboplastin generation test and it the platelets are abnormal, an estimate of thromboplastin platelet activity can be made. Controls of pooled platelets are prepared and dilutions of the pool in buffer are assayed to give a standard reference curve.

### Reagents and Apparatus

1. Normal platelets: 9 ml of whole blood is collected in a siliconized syringe from 10 normal subjects and added to 1 ml of 3.8% sodium citrate. Each blood is centrifuged at 2,000 rpm for 3 minutes to obtain platelet-rich plasma. The plasmas are transferred with a siliconized pipet to 2 siliconized tubes and centrifuged at 3,000 rpm for 30 minutes to obtain a platelet button. The platelet harvest is washed at least 3 times with clean saline and the platelets pooled into 1 tube; 0.1 ml of the pool is added to 9.9 ml of clean saline in a volumetric flask, and 0.1 ml of this 1% platelet suspension is added to 2.9 ml of saline to obtain a 0.033% suspension.

2. Patient's platelets: 1% and 0.033% saline suspensions of patient's platelets are prepared in a manner similar to the normal platelet preparation in step 1.

3. Substrate plasma as previously described in the thromboplastin generation test on page 263.

4. Adsorbed plasma as previously described in the thromboplastin generation test on page 263.

5. Serum as previously described in the thromboplastin generation test on page 263.

6. 37°C Waterbath

7. Stopwatches—2

8. M/40 Calcium chloride

9. Siliconized tubes

10. Micropipets—0.1 ml
11. Graduated pipets—0.5 ml
12. Tubes—13 × 100 mm

### Method

1. 0.1 ml of the substrate plasma is added to each of 8 tubes at 37°C.

2. 0.4-ml Volumes of 1:10 buffered serum diution, 1:5 buffered adsorbed plasma, 1% normal platelets and M/40 calcium chloride are added together in a generating tube. Stopwatch 1 is started on the addition of the calcium chloride.

3. After exactly 60 seconds, 0.1 ml of the generating mixture is added simultaneously with 0.1 ml of M/40 calcium chloride to one of the plasma substrate tubes prepared in step 1. Stopwatch 2 is started and the time needed for fibrin formation is recorded.

4. At 1-minute intervals for a maximum of 8 minutes, the subsampling described in 3 is repeated.

5. Steps 1 to 4 are repeated, using the 0.033% normal platelet suspension.

6. Steps 1 to 4 are repeated, using the patient 1% and 0.033% platelet suspension.

*Normal.* Normal 1% platelet suspension produces clotting times of 9 to 16 seconds in the 4 minutes of incubation.

Normal 0.033% platelet suspension produces clotting times of 14 to 19 seconds in 5 minutes of incubation.

### Calculation

Preparation of platelet Factor 3 dilution curve:

1. Set up 4 tubes as given in Table 5-22.

2. To a generating tube, add 0.2-ml volumes of platelet dilution from tube 1, 1:5 diluted adsorbed plasma, 1:10 serum and M/40 calcium chloride. Start the stopwatch on the addition of the calcium and incubate for exactly 5 minutes.

TABLE 5-22. Plasma Dilutions for Platelet Factor 3 Dilution Curve.

| TUBE | 0.033% PLATELET SUSPENSION (ML) | SALINE (ML) | % PLATELET CONCENTRATION |
|------|------|------|------|
| 1 | 1.0 | — | 100 |
| 2 | 1.0 | 1.0 | 50 |
| 3 | 1.0 from total of tube 2 | 1.0 | 25 |
| 4 | 1.0 from total of tube 3 | 1.0 | 12.5 |

Discard 1.0 ml from tube 4.

3. Subsample 0.1-ml volumes of the mixture to 0.1 ml of plasma substrate and to 0.1 ml of M/40 calcium chloride. Start stopwatch 2 on the addition of the calcium and record the clotting time of the mixture.

4. Steps 2 and 3 are repeated, using the platelet dilutions from tubes 2, 3 and 4.

5. The clotting times of these tubes are plotted against the platelet concentrations on log-log graph paper.

6. The platelet activity is calculated by comparing the shortest patient-clotting time against the pooled normal and expressing the result as a percentage of platelet activity.

### Notes

1. Platelet functional tests are time consuming and suffer from the difficulty of obtaining a standardized platelet suspension. If a sufficiently weak dilution of platelets is used, the test can demonstrate abnormalities when compared against the normal.

2. An alternate technique is to use a two-stage partial thromboplastin time in which a brain residue, normal serum and standard platelet suspension is recalcified. At regular intervals, thromboplastin activity is assayed by adding the suspension to additional calcium and to normal plasma.

## REPTILASE TEST[46]

*Principle.* Reptilase is a thrombin-like enzyme isolated from the venom of *Bothrops atrox*, capable of clotting fibrinogen. The fibrin monomers formed by thrombin polymerize side to side, whereas the monomers found by Reptilase are only capable of polymerizing end to end.

Thrombin inhibitors such as heparin, heparinoids, and hirudin do not inhibit the activity of this enzyme and it is unabsorbed by fibrin. The enzyme does not activate plasminogen and is uninhibited by antifibrinolytics such as EACA.

Inhibition of this material can be accomplished by specific antibodies contained in antibothrops-serum.

### Reagents and Apparatus
1. Reptilase.* 1.0 ml of distilled water is added to a vial of the enzyme.
2. Citrated plasma
3. 37°C Waterbath
4. Stopwatch

### Method
1. 0.1 of Reptilase is added to 0.3 ml of citrated plasma and a stopwatch started.

---

* Available from Abbott Scientific Products Division, North Chicago, Ill.

2. The tube is mixed and at the first appearance of a fibrin clot, the timer is stopped.

3. The test is repeated using a normal citrated plasma as a control.

*Normal.* 18 to 22 seconds.

*Notes*

1. Unlike the inhibition of thrombin-formed fibrin monomers by FDP, the polymerization of monomers obtained by Reptilase is slightly or not at all influenced by fibrinogen or fibrin split products.

2. The test is basically used as a substitute for the thrombin time when the patient is heparinized.

## DEMONSTRATION OF CIRCULATING ANTICOAGULANTS

### Method Using Whole Blood Coagulation Time

*Principle.* If a volume of blood containing a circulating anticoagulant is added to normal blood, the whole blood coagulation time of the normal is prolonged.

*Reagents and Apparatus*
1. Normal and patient's compatible whole blood
2. Siliconized syringes
3. Unsiliconized tubes—8 × 75 mm
4. 37°C Waterbath
5. Stopwatch
6. Graduated pipets—1 ml

*Method*

1. Patient's and normal blood is obtained by venipuncture, using siliconized syringes. A stopwatch is started as soon as the blood appears in the syringe.

2. Five unsiliconized tubes are placed in a waterbath and set up as in Table 5-23.

TABLE 5-23. Dilutions for Measurement of Circulating Anticoagulants by Whole Blood Coagulation Times.

| TUBE | PATIENT'S WHOLE BLOOD (ML) | NORMAL WHOLE BLOOD (ML) |
|------|-----------------------------|--------------------------|
| 1 | 1.0 | — |
| 2 | 0.9 | 0.1 |
| 3 | 0.5 | 0.5 |
| 4 | 0.1 | 0.9 |
| 5 | — | 1.0 |

3. The tubes are mixed by inversion and the coagulation time of each tube is measured.

**Results.** In the presence of a circulating anticoagulant, tubes 1 to 4 will all show prolonged coagulation time.

## Method Using Recalcification Times

*Principle.* This is similar to the whole blood method, except that platelet-rich plasma is used in place of the whole blood and the plasma is re-calcified.

### Reagents and Apparatus
1. Patient's and normal citrated plasmas: Citrated plasma is centrifuged at 1,000 rpm for 5 minutes.
2. M/40 Calcium chloride
3. 37°C Waterbath
4. Stopwatch
5. Tubes—8 × 75 mm
6. Graduated pipets—1 ml

### Method
1. Five tubes are placed in a waterbath and set up as in Table 5-24.
2. At the addition of the calcium chloride, a stopwatch is started and the recalcification time of each tube recorded.

**Results.** In the presence of a circulating anticoagulant, the recalcification times of tubes 1 to 4 will be prolonged. Tube 5 will be normal.

## Method Using the Thromboplastin Generation Test

*Principle.* A circulating anticoagulant can sometimes be detected by using the thromboplastin generation test. If the anticoagulant is present, the adsorbed patient's plasma and the serum will show prolonged coagulation after the initial subsampling. Differentiation between this and Factors XI- and XII-deficient states can be made by showing that the addition

TABLE 5-24. Plasma Dilutions for Measuring Circulating Anticoagulants by Recalcification Times.

| TUBE | PATIENT'S PLASMA (ML) | NORMAL PLASMA (ML) | CALCIUM CHLORIDE (ML) |
|------|------|------|------|
| 1 | 1.0 | — | 1.0 |
| 2 | 0.9 | 0.1 | 1.0 |
| 3 | 0.1 | 0.5 | 1.0 |
| 4 | 0.1 | 0.9 | 1.0 |
| 5 | — | 1.0 | 1.0 |

of 1 volume of patient's plasma to 9 volumes of normal plasma will not correct the time.

### Detection of Antitissue Thromboplastin[47]

*Principle.* The presence of an antitissue thromboplastin will produce prolonged one-stage prothrombin times. These are compared with the normal test.

#### Reagents and Apparatus
1. Brain thromboplastin—commercially available
2. Normal and patient's oxalated plasmas
3. M/40 Calcium chloride
4. 37°C Waterbath
5. Stopwatch
6. Tubes—13 × 100 mm
7. Micropipets—0.1 ml
8. Graduated pipets—1 ml
9. Graduated pipets—10 ml
10. Volumetric flask—50 ml
11. Volumetric flask—100 ml

#### Method
1. Dilute tissue thromboplastin with sodium chloride as in Table 5-25.
2. 0.1 ml of each thromboplastin dilution is added to a prewarmed tube.
3. The one-stage prothrombin time is determined on both the normal and patient's plasmas, using the 6 different dilutions of thromboplastin made in 1.

*Results.* If an anticoagulant is present against tissue thromboplastin, it will produce increasing one-stage prothrombin times as the thromboplastin becomes more dilute.

TABLE 5-25. Thromboplastin Dilutions for Detection of
Antitissue Thromboplastin.

| TUBE | SALINE (ML) | TISSUE THROMBO-PLASTIN (ML) | FINAL DILUTION |
|------|-------------|------------------------------|----------------|
| 1 | — | 0.5 | 1:1 |
| 2 | 0.4 | 0.1 | 1:1 |
| 3 | 0.9 | 0.1 | 1:10 |
| 4 | 9.9 | 0.1 | 1:100 |
| 5 | 49.9 | 0.1 | 1:500 |
| 6 | 99.9 | 0.1 | 1:1,000 |

TABLE 5-26. Typical Results in the Detection of
Antitissue Thromboplastin.

| Thromboplastin Dilution | 0 | 1:5 | 1:10 | 1:100 | 1:500 | 1:1,000 |
|---|---|---|---|---|---|---|
| 1-Stage Prothrombin Time on Normal Blood | 12 | 16 | 65 | 90 | 65 | 90 |
| 1-Stage Prothrombin Time on Patient's Blood | 13 | 25 | 40 | 100 | 150 | 200 |

*Note.* Do not use commercial thromboplastin which contains added calcium. If serial dilutions of this are made, the calcium is also diluted in proportion to the thromboplastin.

## DETECTION OF PLASMA ANTITHROMBIN

*Principle.* The presence of heparin-like substances in plasma can be detected by showing that the thrombin clotting time is delayed and that this inhibition can be neutralized by the addition of protamine sulfate to the plasma.

### Reagents and Apparatus

1. Stock thrombin 1,000 units per vial (Parke, Davis): 10 ml of normal saline is added to a vial of thrombin; 1 ml of this dilution is added to 9 ml of saline. This produces a concentration of *10 units per ml.*
2. Normal and patient's oxalated plasmas
3. 37°C Waterbath
4. Stopwatch
5. Tubes—13 × 100 mm
6. 0.25% Aqueous protamine sulfate
7. Graduated pipets—1 ml
8. Micropipets—0.1 ml

### Method

1. Thrombin dilutions are added to 6 tubes at 37°C, as designated in Table 5-27.
2. 0.1 ml of normal plasma and normal saline are added to tube 1 and the stopwatch is started. The time for the fibrin clot to form is recorded.
3. Step 2 is repeated, using tubes 2 to 6.
4. Steps 2 and 3 are repeated, using patient's plasma in place of normal plasma.
5. If the thrombin times of the patient's plasma are longer than those of

TABLE 5-27. Thrombin Dilutions for Detection of
Plasma Antithrombin.

| TUBE | THROMBIN (ML) | SALINE (ML) | FINAL DILUTION |
|------|---------------|-------------|----------------|
| 1 | 0.5 | — | 1:1 |
| 2 | 0.5 | 0.5 | 1:2 |
| 3 | 0.5 from total of tube 2 | 0.5 | 1:4 |
| 4 | 0.5 from total of tube 3 | 0.5 | 1:8 |
| 5 | 0.5 from total of tube 4 | 0.5 | 1:16 |
| 6 | 0.5 from total of tube 5 | 0.5 | 1:32 |

Discard 0.5 ml from total volume of tube 6.

the normal, 0.1 ml of 0.25% protamine sulfate is added to the patient's plasma in place of normal saline and the test is repeated.

*Results.* If the thrombin time of the patient is corrected to normal by the addition of protamine sulfate (a heparin inhibitor), the presence of a heparin-like anticoagulant is confirmed.

## HEPARIN ASSAY

*Principle.* The amount of protamine required for the neutralization of heparin in a test plasma is titrated by using a system based on the thrombin time.

### *Reagents and Apparatus*
1. Tubes—10 × 75 mm
2. Waterbath
3. Pipets—0.2 ml
4. Timer
5. Stock protamine sulfate—10 mg/ml. (Available from hospital pharmacy.)
6. Veronal buffer, pH 7.35 (p. 243)
7. Thrombin reagent. A 1,000 U/ml vial of thrombin is diluted with veronal buffer pH 7.35, until it produces a clotting time greater than 20 seconds with normal citrated plasma.
8. Citrated plasma

*Method*

1. The stock protamine sulfate solution is diluted as follows:

TABLE 5-28.

| TUBE | PROTAMINE SULFATE (ML) | BUFFER (ML) | FINAL CONCENTRATION OF PROTAMIN SULFATE ($\mu$G/ML) |
|------|------------------------|-------------|------------------------------------------------------|
| 1 | 1.0 stock | 99.0 | 100.0 |
| 2 | 0.5 from total of tube 1 | 4.5 | 10.0 |
| 3 | 2.0 from total of tube 2 | 2.0 | 5.0 |
| 4 | 2.0 from total of tube 3 | 2.0 | 2.5 |
| 5 | 2.0 from total of tube 4 | 2.0 | 1.25 |

2. 0.1 ml of citrated plasma is pipeted into each of 5 tubes, and 0.1 ml of each of the protamine dilutions added to each tube.

3. 0.1 ml of diluted thrombin is added to each tube and the timer started. Record the time of clot formation.

*Results*

1. The lowest concentration of protamine which completely corrects the thrombin time is the point at which the heparin has been completely neutralized by the protamine.

2. 85 units of heparin are neutralized by 1 mg of protamine sulfate.

## DETECTION OF FIBRINOLYSINS

*Principle.* Serial dilutions of patient's plasma are made in pooled normal plasma and 10 units of thrombin are added per ml of plasma. The fibrin clots are incubated at 37°C overnight and examined for zones of lysis.

*Reagents and Apparatus*

1. Thrombin (Parke, Davis): 10 ml of saline is added to a 1,000-unit vial of thrombin, giving a concentration of 100 units per ml.

2. Normal and patient's oxalated plasmas

3. 37°C Waterbath

4. Tubes—13 × 100 mm

*Method*

1. Five tubes are set up at 37°C with the plasma combinations given in Table 5-29.

2. 0.1 ml of 100 units per ml thrombin is added to each tube.

3. The tubes are mixed by inversion and incubated at 37°C. They are inspected for zones of lysis of the clot at hourly intervals for 3 hours and left to incubate overnight.

*Results.* In the presence of a fibrinolysin, tubes 2 to 5 will show marked lysis of the fibrin clot in proportion to the amount of patient's plasma. Tube 1 will show less lytic effect. In severe fibrinolytic states, lysis will frequently begin within 5 minutes of incubation, and often will be complete within 30 minutes.

*Notes*

1. When preparing the reagents for the test, it is important to use fresh plasma and to pool at least 5 normal plasmas to use as the normal control.

2. Fibrinolysins can be increased in moderate exercise, under stress conditions including fear, and after the injection of epinephrine, nicotinic acid or acetylcholine.

## THE DETECTION OF FIBRINOGEN-
## FIBRIN DEGRADATION PRODUCTS[48] (Modified)[49]

### *Staphylococcal Clumping Test*

*Principle.* Suspensions of certain staphylococcal cells will clump in the presence of fibrinogen, some fibrinogen degradation products, some fibrin degradation products, and insoluble fibrin monometer or polymer complexes. While only "early" fibrinogen-fibrin degradation products (FDP) are detected by this test, it has been shown that "late" products form nonclottable soluble fibrin monomers or polymer complexes which are also detectable by the test.

TABLE 5-29. Combinations of Normal and Patient's Plasmas for Detection of Fibrinolysins.

| Tube | Normal Plasma (ml) | Patient's Plasma (ml) |
|---|---|---|
| 1 | 1.0 | 0 |
| 2 | 0.9 | 0.1 |
| 3 | 0.7 | 0.3 |
| 4 | 0.5 | 0.5 |
| 5 | — | 1.0 |

To detect such degradation products, blood is collected in the presence of excess thrombin to ensure complete conversion of fibrinogen to fibrin and its subsequent removal in the clot. In addition, epsilon-aminocaproic acid (EACA) is added to inhibit conversion of plasminogen to plasmin. When excess preformed plasmin is expected (in patients undergoing streptokinase therapy), trypsin inhibitor is added instead of the EACA. The blood is incubated at 37°C to allow for completion of coagulation, clot retraction, and inactivation of excess thrombin. The blood is centrifuged, and the separated serum diluted in a saline buffer and mixed with the staphylococcal cell suspensions.

An estimate of the degradation products present (in $\mu$g fibrinogen equivalents/ml) is provided by a comparison of the amount of clumping of cells produced by the test serum with the clumping produced by known levels of fibrinogen.

### Reagents and Apparatus

1. Glass plates (20 × 20 cm) marked off into approximately 2 cm squares
2. Microdiluters—0.5 ml
3. Calibrated pipet droppers—0.05 ml
4. 37°C Waterbath
5. Imidazole-buffered saline

Base: 680 mg of Imidazole (0.2m) is dissolved in distilled water and diluted to 50 ml

Buffer: 2.5 Volumes of base are added to 1.86 volumes of 0.1N hydrochloric acid and 5.64 volumes of distilled water to give a concentration of 0.05M. The pH is adjusted to 7.3. To each 100 ml of buffer made, 0.585 g of sodium chloride is added.

Imidazole-buffered saline: 1 volume of the buffer (above) to 2 volumes of 0.85% sodium chloride

6. Phosphate-citrate-albumin buffer

3.2 g disodium hydrogen phosphate, 7.2 g potassium dehydrogen phosphate, 14.7 g of trisodium citrate, 4.0 g bovine albumin, and 10 ml of 0.1% sodium azide are dissolved in 800 ml of warm distilled water. The volume is made up to 1 liter with distilled water.

7. 1% Soybean trypsin inhibitor*. Store at −20°C.
8. Thrombin—1000 units/ml*
9. Lyophilized preparations of *Staphylococcus aureus* (Newman D$_2$C strain)

140 mg of lyophilized bacteria are added to 45 ml of Imidazole-buffered saline, and the resulting clumps gently broken up by stirring. The suspension is filtered through a fine mesh nylon filter, aliquoted

---

* Available from Parke, Davis & Co., Detroit, Mich.

in 3 ml volumes and stored at 4°C. The preparation can also be commercially obtained. This cell suspension should not be thawed until all sample dilutions are made and must be used within 30 minutes of preparation.

10. Working fibrinogen standards. The fibrinogen level of normal plasma is determined (p. 295) and the plasma diluted with phosphate-citrate-albumin buffer to produce a final concentration of 10 μg/ml. This stock standard is aliquoted in 2.5 ml volumes and stored frozen at −20°C.

The working standard is made up by thawing one of the frozen vials of stock and diluting as follows (Table 5-30):

TABLE 5-30. The Preparation of Working Fibrinogen Standards.

| STOCK (ML) | PHOSPHATE-CITRATE-ALBUMIN BUFFER (ML) | FINAL CONCENTRATION (μG/ML) |
|---|---|---|
| 0.6 | 0 | 10.0 |
| 0.6 | 0.2 | 7.5 |
| 0.6 | 0.4 | 6.0 |
| 0.6 | 0.6 | 5.0 |
| 0.6 | 2.4 | 2.5 |
| 0.3 | 2.7 | 1.0 |
| 0.5 from 1.0 μg/ml tube | 0.5 | 0.5 |
| 0.5 from 0.5 μg/ml tube | 0.5 | 0.25 |

11. Preparation of test serum:

5 ml of blood are added to a tube containing 1 drop of 36% EDTA and 1 drop of 1% trypsin inhibitor. The blood is mixed by inversion and allowed to clot. It is incubated at 37°C for 2 hours, the clot loosened, and centrifuged at 2000 rpm for 10 minutes (the serum sample can be stored frozen for 2 to 3 months).

Serial dilutions of the test serum are carried out as follows (Table 5-31):

TABLE 5-31. Preparation of Test Serum in FDP Detection.

| TUBE | SERUM (ML) | IMIDAZOLE BUFFERED SALINE (ML) | DILUTION |
|------|------------|-------------------------------|----------|
| 1 | 0.1 | 0.1 | 1:2 |
| 2 | 0.1 from total of tube 1 | 0.1 | 1:4 |
| 3 | 0.1 from total of tube 2 | 0.1 | 1:8 |
| 4 | 0.1 from total of tube 3 | 0.1 | 1:16 |
| 5 | 0.1 from total of tube 4 | 0.1 | 1:32 |
| 6 | 0.1 from total of tube 5 | 0.1 | 1:64 |
| 7 | 0.1 from total of tube 6 | 0.1 | 1.128 |

Discard 0.1 ml from total of tube 7

### Method

1. 0.05 ml of each serum dilution is pipeted onto glass slides or a glass tile.

2. 0.5 ml of each fibrinogen dilution is pipeted onto the glass slides or tile.

3. A blank control, composing of 0.05 ml of imidazole-buffered saline is separately pipeted onto the tile.

4. To each dilution and to the blank, 0.05 ml of a freshly prepared, well-mixed staphylococcal suspension is added.

5. Each suspension is mixed and spread about 2 cm in diameter with fresh applicator sticks. The slides or tile are gently rocked over a black nonreflective background having indirect lighting from below.

6. The fibrinogen control most closely matching the *clumping intensity* of the end point of the test is noted.

7. The fibrinogen equivalents of the serum are obtained by multiplying the reciprocal of the dilution of the serum end point by the micrograms of fibrinogen in the closest matching control. For example, the serum end point 1:64 and the matching control contains 5.0 $\mu$g/ml fibrinogen. Serum equivalent is $64 \times 5 = 320$ $\mu$g/ml.

*Normal.* 0 to 4 $\mu$g fibrinogen equivalents/ml

### Notes

1. The results are interpreted as fibrinogen equivalents/ml. While the test measures fibrin-fibrinogen degradation products remaining after

fibrinogen removal, the results are based on activities equivalent to known amounts of fibrinogen.

2. Serum FDP levels are increased in primary and secondary fibrinolytic states. Primary states may arise from increased levels of circulating plasminogen producing plasmin with resulting lysis of fibrinogen. Secondary fibrinolytic states are characterized by intravascular coagulation and fibrinolysis (disseminated intravascular coagulation).

3. Some conditions showing increases in serum FDP include: alcoholic cirrhosis, following cesarean section, preeclamptic toxemia, and abruptio placentae or intrauterine deaths. Moderate-to-marked increases are often present in postoperative pulmonary embolism or venous thrombosis. Peripheral vascular occlusions treated with streptokinase show marked increases in serum FDP.

4. Additional thrombin may be required to ensure complete clotting in blood from patients undergoing heparin or streptokinase therapy. While heparin does not interfere with the clumping reaction, increased levels may inhibit coagulation, producing falsely elevated results due to the presence of unconverted fibrinogen. When possible, blood should be collected prior to the initiation of therapy.

5. Unless reagents are brought to room temperature, false-normal results can be obtained.

6. Active or recent staphylococcal infections occasionally stimulate the production of circulating anti-staphylococcal antibodies which will cause false elevations of serum FDP levels.

Anti-staphylococcal antibodies may be demonstrated by heating the serum at 60°C for 10 minutes. Staphylococcal clumping of the serum is destroyed, while the antibodies are unaffected.

**Fibrin Degradation Products** (Thrombo-Wellcotest Kit*)

*Principle.* A suspension of latex particles in buffer is sensitized with specific antibodies to purified fibrinogen degradation products. The sensitivity of the reagent is adjusted to that, in the presence of fibrinogen concentrations of 2 $\mu$g/ml or greater; the latex particles clump together giving macroscopic agglutination. By testing two unknown samples at different dilutions, the approximate concentration of FDP can be determined.

The agglutination pattern can be seen most clearly when the slide is viewed against a distant dark background, with bright diffused daylight as illumination.

*Reagents.* Thrombo-Wellcome Test Kit

---

* Burroughs Wellcome & Co., Research Triangle Park, North Carolina 27709

### Method
1. 2 ml of blood is added to a tube (provided in the kit) containing thrombin and an enzyme inhibitor.
2. Mix well by inverting the tube and allow the blood to clot and retract at 37°C for 30 minutes.
3. Centrifuge the clotted sample and remove the serum.
4. Prepare 1:5 and 1:20 dilutions of the patient's serum in glycine buffer.
5. Transfer 1 drop of each serum dilution to the test slide (provided in the kit).
6. Mix the latex suspension by vigorously shaking the tube, and add 1 drop of the suspension to each serum dilution on the slide.
7. Using a disposable mixing rod, stir each of the serum latex mixtures in turn, spreading each pool of liquid to fill its respective circle.
8. Rock the slide gently for a maximum of 2 minutes.

*Results* Agglutination in each of the two dilutions indicates the presence of FDP at a final concentration greater than 2 μg/ml. Agglutination of the 1:20 dilution indicates a level greater than 40 μg/ml.

### Note
1. If blood is collected from patients on heparin therapy, the thrombin of the sample collection tube may be inhibited to such an extent that the blood will fail to clot. In such cases, the whole blood should be treated with Reptilase,* which is a "thrombin-like" enzyme which will clot fibrinogen in the presence of heparin and other antithrombins.
2. The contents of one bottle of Reptilase are reconstituted in 1 ml of distilled water; 0.1 ml of this solution should be sufficient to clot 1 ml of heparinized blood at 37°C.

## Serum Fi Test† (Screening)

*Principle.* This test utilizes latex particles coated with antifibrinogen antisera. It can be used for the detection of those complexes which do not clot with thrombin but which react with antifibrinogen antisera.

### Reagents and Apparatus
1. Fi Test Kit‡
2. Thrombin†—1,000 units/ml
3. Citrated plasma
4. 0.01 ml of thrombin is added to 0.2 ml of patient's citrated plasma. The mixture is incubated at 37°C for 5 minutes and the resulting clot re-

---

* Available from Abbott Scientific Products Division, North Chicago, Ill.
† Available from Hyland Laboratories, Costa Mesa, Calif.
‡ Available from Parke, Davis & Co., Detroit, Mich.

moved with an applicator stick. The procedure is repeated twice and the defibrinated plasma centrifuged at 2,000 rpm for 5 minutes.

*Method.* One drop of defibrinated plasma and 2 drops of the Fi reagent are mixed together on a slide and examined within 2 minutes.

*Results.* A positive reaction is shown by latex agglutination, which can be quantitated by serially diluting the patient's defibrinated plasma with saline.

*Notes*
1. A normal blood should always be defibrinated in parallel with the test plasma.
2. The laboratory normal range should be determined from the testing of known normal individuals.


## TANNED RED CELL HEMAGGLUTINATION INHIBITION TEST[50]

*Principle.* Formalin-treated sheep cells are sensitized to human fibrinogen. Aliquots of an antifibrinogen serum are added to serial dilution of the sample to be assayed. If fibrinogen is present it will combine with the antifibrinogen serum, and the sensitized red cells subsequently added will fail to agglutinate. The amount of fibrinogen or antigentically reacting split products can be calculated by comparison with a known fibrinogen standard.

*Reagents and Apparatus*
1. Microtiter Kit* consisting of a plate 13 × 8.3 cm having 8 rows of 12 "V" bottom wells; calibrated 0.025 ml dropper and microdiluters holding 0.025 ml.
2. Fibrinogen coated red cells:
    9 volumes of Group O human red cells are mixed with 1 volume of 0.1M sodium oxalate, centrifuged at 2,000 rpm for 5 minutes, and washed 4 times with 0.85% formol saline.
3. 3% Formol-saline pH 7.2-74. 3 ml of concentrated formaldehyde is added to 97 ml of normal saline and the pH adjusted with sodium hydroxide.
4. Phosphate-citrate-buffer:
    3.2 g of disodium hydrogen phosphate, 7.2 g of potassium dihydrogen phosphate, and 14.7 g trisodium citrate are dissolved in 800 ml of warm distilled water; 10 ml of 1% sodium azide is added and the volume made up to 1 liter.
5. One volume of 3% formol-saline is added to 1 volume of an 8% saline suspension of washed red cells. The cells are kept suspended with a mag-

---

* Available from Flow Laboratories, Inc., Rockville, Md.

netic stirrer at a slow speed for 24 hours at 37°C and are washed 3 times with saline. They are stored as a 20% suspension at 4°C in phosphate-citrate-buffer. These cells are stable for 2 to 3 months.

6. Tanning:

The 20% suspension of formolized red cells are diluted 1:10 with the phosphate-citrate-buffer. Equal volumes of the resulting 2%-cell suspension and a 1:40,000 freshly prepared tannic acid solution in the same buffer are incubated for 1 hour at 56°C with gentle mixing every 20 minutes. After this incubation, the cells are washed 3 times with the phosphate-citrate-buffer.

7. Fibrinogen coated red cells:

A 4% suspension of the formolized tanned red cells in buffer is added to an equal volume of fresh oxalated normal human plasma previously diluted 1:250 with the same buffer. The mixture is incubated for 1 hour at 37°C and washed 3 times in the buffer, before suspending to make a 10% concentration in phosphate-citrate-albumin buffer (0.4% bovine serum albumin* added to the phosphate-citrate-buffer).

When stored at 4°C this stock suspension is stable for 2 to 3 months.

8. Test serum:

The patient's freshly drawn blood is mixed with soybean trypsin inhibitor† in the ratio of 2 mg/2 ml of blood to prevent fibrinolysis after collection. The mixture is inverted 3 times and allowed to clot at room temperature until clot retraction becomes evident. The serum is removed and stored at −20°C. At this temperature it is stable indefinitely.

9. Antifibrinogen rabbit serum:‡

One volume of human Group O red cells is added to 4 volumes of the serum and incubated at 4°C overnight. The serum is first serially diluted to determine the highest dilution which will strongly agglutinate fibrinogen-coated cells. Antiserum is substituted for the patient's serum and the coated cells are added.

*Method*

1. The test serum is serially diluted using a 0.025 ml dropper, 1 drop of phosphate-citrate-buffer is added to the microtiter plate wells.

2. 0.025 ml of the test serum is added to the first well of each row with microdiluters.

3. The serum and buffer are mixed by swirling the microdiluters 20 times and the microdiluters transferred to the next wells of the rows with 0.025 ml of the mixture.

4. These doubling dilutions are carried out to the end of the rows and the residual 0.025 ml volumes discarded.

---

* Available from Cohn Fraction V, Nutritional Biochemical Corp., Cleveland, Ohio
† Available from Type I-S, Sigma Chemical Co., St. Louis, Missouri
‡ Available from Hyland Laboratories, Costa Mesa, California

5. 0.025 ml of the antifibrinogen serum (diluted to 1 tube less than the titration on 9 above) is added with a pipet dropper.

6. The microtiter plate is vibrated for 1 minute using a Model JIA* oscillator and incubated at room temperature for 10 minutes.

7. 0.025 ml of a 1:1250 suspension of formalized tanned fibrinogen-coated red cells in phosphate-citrate-albumin buffer is added to each well.

8. The microtiter plate is reincubated at room temperature for 10 minutes and the plate centrifuged at 1,500 rpm for 30 seconds (GLC-1 Sorvall centrifuge).

9. The plate is placed almost vertically against a white light source and the button of cells in each well observed for 5 to 15 minutes for the developing pattern. Each well is graded 0 to 4+.

10. A negative pattern (inhibition of agglutination) is represented by early migration of the cell button into a narrow line or tail. 4+ agglutination is represented by an absence of tailing and the persistance of the agglutinated cell button in its original rounded form.

Grades 1+, 2+, and 3+ represent intermediate stages between prominent tailing with a small residual button and only little tailing with a prominent button.

The titer of the inhibition is the highest dilution of the test serum yielding less than a 3+ pattern.

11. Fibrinogen control. Normal plasma is diluted in phosphate-citrate-buffer so that the fibrinogen concentration is 1 mg/dl (usually the dilution approximates 1:300). The diluted plasma is titrated simultaneously as the tests on every plate.

### Calculations

If 1 mg/dl solution of fibrinogen reaches an agglutination-inhibition end point at a dilution of 1:8, the concentration of fibrinogen in the plasma in the final well is 0.125 mg/dl or 1.25 $\mu$g/ml.

Any serum is believed to have fibrinogen split products equivalent to 1.25 $\mu$g/ml of fibrinogen/ml at its own end point.

The concentration of split products is thus the reciprocal dilution of the serum multiplied by 1.25 expressed as $\mu$g/ml.

$$\text{FDP } (\mu g/ml) = \frac{\text{Fibrinogen in Control plasma} \times \text{Inhibition titer of control plasma}}{\text{Inhibition titer of test serum}}$$

***Normal.*** 1 to 6 $\mu$g/ml.

---

* Syntron Jagger, Homer City, Pa.

*Notes*

1. Mild intravascular coagulation-fibrinolysis syndromes produce FDP levels between 10 and 40 $\mu$g/ml. Severe cases of intravascular coagulation often show levels up to 200 $\mu$g/ml.

2. This method utilizes human red cells, eliminating the problem of human anti-sheep red cell antibodies.

## ETHANOL-GEL SOLUBILITY TEST[51]

*Principle.* The addition of ethanol to the soluble fibrin present in the plasma of patients with intravascular coagulation causes a gel to form.

### *Reagents and Apparatus*

1. Platelet-poor plasma:
   5 ml of blood obtained using a plastic syringe are added to 0.5 ml of buffered sodium citrate (p. 4). The blood is centrifuged at 1,500 rpm for 15 minutes using a GLC-1 centrifuge (Sorvall).

2. 50% Ethyl alcohol

### *Method*

1. 0.15 ml volumes of 50% ethyl alcohol is added to 0.5 ml of platelet-poor test plasma and to 0.5 ml of normal platelet-poor plasma.

2. The tubes are inverted to mix and inspected at 5-minute intervals at room temperature.

### *Results*

Visible gel formation is seen within 5 minutes in patients having FDP. The formation of a granular precipitate is read as a negative test.

### *Notes*

1. Ethanol in a final concentration of 10 to 15% causes soluble fibrin to gel promptly at room temperature. The reaction is independent of the fibrinogen level and it is unaltered by the presence of fibrinolytic activity, heparin, or red cell contamination.

2. Gel formation after the first 5 minutes should be tested by adding 1 drop of 0.1N sodium hydroxide and gently shaking the tube. Nonspecific precipitates will promptly return to solution while the fibrin gel will remain.

## EUGLOBULIN LYSIS TIME[52]

*Principle.* Euglobulin is separated from the plasma by adjusting the pH with acetic acid at 4°C. A buffer composed of sodium chloride and sodium borate is added and the mixture recalcified. The resulting clot is examined for lysis at hourly intervals.

### Reagents and Apparatus

1. Citrated blood. 9 volumes of whole blood is added to 1 volume of 3.8% sodium citrate.
2. M/40 Calcium chloride. 2.77 g of anhydrous calcium chloride is dissolved in 1 liter of distilled water.
3. 1% Acetic acid
4. Borate solution. 9 g of sodium chloride and 1 g of sodium borate are dissolved in 1 liter of distilled water. This produces a reagent having a pH of 9.
5. Distilled water
6. Graduated pipets—10 ml
7. Oswald-Folin pipets—0.5 ml
8. Graduated pipets—0.1 ml
9. 37°C Waterbath
10. Refrigerator
11. Timer

### Method

1. The citrated blood is centrifuged at 3,000 rpm for 10 minutes to separate the plasma.
2. 0.5 ml of plasma is added to 9 ml of distilled water.
3. 0.1 ml of 1% acetic acid is added to the plasma dilution.
4. The mixture made in step 3 is placed in a refrigerator at 4°C for 30 minutes, to allow the euglobulin fraction to precipitate out.
5. The euglobulin precipitate is separated by centrifuging at 3,000 rpm for 5 minutes.
6. Decant the supernatant and drain the tube by inverting onto filter paper.
7. 0.5 ml of borate solution is added to the precipitate. Place in a 37°C waterbath, and stir *gently*, using a glass rod, for 5 to 10 minutes.
8. 0.5 ml of M/40 calcium chloride is added and the timer started.
9. The clot is inspected at hourly intervals for signs of lysis.

*Normal.* Normal clots require more than 2 hours for complete lysis to take place.

### Notes

1. After collection the blood should be kept on ice. The test should be set up as rapidly as possible, preferably within 30 minutes of collection.
2. Lysis time is the time at which the clot is no longer visible and only shreds of fibrin remain.
3. A normal control should always be set up with the test for comparison.
4. Pathological fibrinolysis can produce lysis times as short as 5 to 10 minutes.

5. The euglobulin fraction contains fibrinogen, plasmin, and plasminogen activator. Thus the euglobulin lysis time is considered a measure of activator and plasmin activity. Some antiplasmins remain in the discarded supernatant, accelerating the time needed for lysis and an end point.

6. The euglobulin time can be moderately shortened by leaving the tourniquet on for a prolonged period, by rubbing the vein vigorously, or by pumping the fist excessively. These activities apparently release plasminogen activator from the endothelial cells.

7. Platelets prolong the euglobulin lysis time by their antiplasmins and antiplasminogen activator activities.

8. The lower the pH of the plasma-acid mixture, the longer the lysis time. Maximal lysis is obtained by precipitation of the globulins at pH 6.2 with increasing prolongation of the time as the pH approaches 5.3.

9. If the sample is not drained and the inside of the tube not wiped clean, antiplasmins will drain back into the sediment causing prolongation of the lysis time.

## QUANTITATIVE ESTIMATION OF FIBRINOGEN

### Method 1[53]

*Principle.* Thrombin times are determined on serial dilutions of plasma. The titer of the plasma producing a fibrin clot is proportional to the fibrinogen concentration.

### Reagents and Apparatus
1. Veronal buffer pH 7.35 (p. 262)
2. Thrombin 100 units/ml
3. Tubes—12 × 75 mm
4. Patient's citrated plasma

### Method
1. The following dilutions are made in ten tubes and set up as in Table 5-32.
2. 0.2 ml of thrombin is added to each tube and all of the tubes are left at room temperature for 30 minutes.
3. The highest dilution of plasma which forms a visible fibrin clot is recorded.

*Normal.* >1:160.

*Notes.* The test can be modified by making plasma dilutions in (a) buffer containing EACA, to prevent fibrinolysis, (b) buffer containing protamine sulfate to overcome the inhibitory effect of fibrin.

TABLE 5-32. Quantitative Estimation of Fibrinogen.

| Tube | Patient's Plasma (ML) | Veronal Buffer (ML) | Plasma Dilution |
|:---:|:---:|:---:|:---:|
| 1 | 1.0 | — | 1:1 |
| 2 | 0.2 | 1.8 | 1:10 |
| 3 | 1.0 from total of tube 2 | 1.0 | 1:20 |
| 4 | 1.0 from total of tube 3 | 1.0 | 1:40 |
| 5 | 1.0 from total of tube 4 | 1.0 | 1:80 |
| 6 | 1.0 from total of tube 5 | 1.0 | 1:160 |
| 7 | 1.0 from total of tube 6 | 1.0 | 1:320 |
| 8 | 1.0 from total of tube 7 | 1.0 | 1:640 |
| 9 | 1.0 from total of tube 8 | 1.0 | 1:1280 |
| 10 | 1.0 from total of tube 9 | 1.0 | 1:2560 |

Discard 1.0 ml from tube 10

## Method 2[54]

*Principle.* Fibrinogen is salted out of the plasma, using 17.33% ammonium sulfate.

### Reagents and Apparatus
1. 0.85% Sodium chloride
2. 17.33% Aqueous ammonium sulfate. This reagent is stable for 2 weeks at 4°C.
3. Spectrophometer
4. Stopwatch
5. EDTA anticoagulated patient's and control plasma
6. Fibrinogen standard*

---

* Available from Warner-Chilcott, Morris Plains, N.J.

*Method*

1. 1 ml of control plasma is added to each of 2 spectrophometer cuvets.

2. 3.0 ml of 0.85% sodium chloride is added to one cuvet, and the spectrophometer adjusted with this blank to 100% transmission at 510 nm.

3. 3.0 ml of ammonium sulfate reagent is added to the second cuvet and the stopwatch started.

4. The cuvet is gently inverted to mix and remixed after approximately 2 minutes.

5. The percentage transmission is read exactly after 3 minutes have elapsed from the addition of the ammonium sulfate and is converted to fibrinogen in mg% from the standard graph.

6. The procedure is repeated using the patient's plasma.

*Standard Graph*

1. The standard graph is constructed by reconstituting lyophilized fibrinogen standard*

   a. 300 mg%: Two vials of standard are prepared by adding 2.0 ml of distilled water to each vial.

   b. 225 mg%: Two vials of standard are prepared by adding 2.0 ml of distilled water and 1.0 ml of saline to each vial.

   c. 150 mg%: One vial of standard is prepared by adding 2.0 ml of distilled water and 2.0 ml of saline.

2. The 3 standard dilutions are tested in duplicate as described above (1-5) and the percentage transmission plotted against the standard values as semilogarithmic graph paper.

*Normal.* 200 to 400 mg%.

*Notes*

1. The control plasma is made by pooling normal plasma. A good control should read approximately 300 mg% and should always be used to check the validity of the standard curve. Once prepared it can be aliquoted and stored at 4°C for up to 1 month.

2. The timing (after the addition of the ammonium sulfate) is critical, since the salt will continue to precipitate out other proteins.

3. The test is nonspecific for fibrinogen. It will measure large molecules of fibrin-split products (clottable split products) and other large molecular weight abnormal proteins.


## QUALITATIVE ESTIMATION OF FIBRINOGEN (THROMBIN TIME)

*Principle.* A rapid thrombin titer is determined. The fibrin clot formed is proportional to the amount of fibrinogen present.

---

* Available from Warner-Chilcott, Morris Plains, N.J.

***Reagents and Apparatus***

1. Thrombin 1,000 units per ml (Parke, Davis): 1 ml of saline is added to a vial containing 1,000 units thrombin per ml.
2. Normal and patient's citrated plasmas
3. Tubes—13 × 100 mm
4. Graduated pipets—1 ml
5. Micropipets—0.1 ml

***Method.*** 1 ml of fresh plasma is added to 0.1 ml of thrombin and the tube is mixed by inversion.

***Results.*** In the absence of fibrinogen, no fibrin clot will form, but if a small amount of fibrinogen is present, a small clot that ultimately shrinks will be seen. Normal fibrinogen levels of 150 to 400 mg% will produce a fibrin clot which remains rigid for at least 20 minutes.

***Note***

1. The test is also sensitive to the presence of fibrinolysins.
2. Low fibrinogen levels may be either inherited or acquired. Inherited hypofibrinogenemia is rare. Acquired hypofibrinogenemia is often caused by obstetrical accidents such as abruptio placentae or amnioniotic fluid embolism, causing intravascular clotting which will result in a depletion of fibrinogen. In these cases, the fibrinogen will be rapidly removed from the circulation as micro clots which may in turn be lysed by secondary fibrinolysis.

## CONTACT ACTIVATION TEST[55]

***Principle.*** Normal plasma, previously exposed to kaolin or celite, will shorten the clotting time of uncontacted normal plasma in a siliconized tube. The degree of shortening indicates the amount of activity developed in the test plasma by standard exposure to contact. This activation is defective when the test plasma is deficient in either Factor XI or XII.

***Reagents and Apparatus***

1. Siliconized syringe and needle
2. Siliconized tubes
3. Citrated platelet-poor test and normal plasmas: 9.8 ml of blood is anticoagulated with 0.2 ml of 20% sodium citrate and centrifuged at 3,000 rpm for 20 minutes.
4. Kaolin or celite
5. Soybean phospholipid, Inosithin*: 1 g of Inosithin is added to 20 ml

---

\* Available from Associated Concentrates, Inc., Woodside, N.Y.

of diethyl ether in a flask. The soybean is dissolved by constant shaking and 100 ml of saline is added to the mixture. The ether is allowed to evaporate at room temperature and the stock reagent is stored frozen. For use, 1 ml of the stock is diluted with 9 ml of saline to give a 0.1% suspension.

6. Phospholipid-calcium mixture: Equal volumes of M/40 calcium chloride and Inosithin are combined.

7. Unsiliconized tubes—10 × 75 mm
8. Siliconized tubes—10 × 75 mm
9. Stopwatch
10. 37°C Waterbath
11. Graduated pipets—1 ml
12. Micropipets—0.1 ml

*Method*

1. 0.4 ml of test plasma is added to 1 mg of celite in an unsiliconized 10 × 75-mm tube and mixed at 37°C for 3 minutes.

2. The tube is centrifuged at 3,000 rpm for 5 minutes to deposit the celite.

3. 0.4 ml of uncontacted normal plasma is pipeted into a siliconized tube, and 0.2 ml of the supernatant plasma from 2 is immediately added to produce a 1:3 dilution (i.e., 0.2 ml in a total volume of 0.6 ml).

4. 0.4 ml of uncontacted plasma and 0.2 ml of the 1:3 dilution from 3 are added to a second siliconized tube. This produces a 1:9 dilution.

5. Repeat this threefold dilution, using the 1:9 dilution obtained in 4 to give a 1:27 final dilution.

6. The 3 dilutions (1:3, 1:9, 1:27) are placed in a 37°C waterbath with a fourth tube containing 0.4 ml of uncontacted normal plasma.

7. 0.1 ml of the phospholipid-calcium mixture is added to each of the 4 tubes and the clotting time of each is recorded.

*Results.* Typical results are shown in Table 5-33.

TABLE 5-33. Typical Results in the Contact Activation Test.

| CONTACTED PLASMA | DILUTIONS OF TEST PLASMA IN INTACT NORMAL PLASMA | | | INTACT NORMAL PLASMA |
|---|---|---|---|---|
| | 1:3 | 1:9 | 1:27 | |
| Normal | 240 | 340 | 420 | 610 |
| Factor XI deficiency | 470 | 560 | 620 | 590 |
| Factor XII deficiency | 540 | 620 | 650 | 605 |

## CELITE-6 TEST FOR FACTOR XI DEFICIENCY[56]

*Principle.* Factor XI can be removed from normal plasma by contact with celite followed by incubation at 37°C. This Factor XI-deficient plasma, which contains Factor XII, is used in the contact activation test.

### Reagents and Apparatus
1. With the exception of the following, all reagents and apparatus are as described for the contact test on page 298.
2. Celite-6-treated plasma: 1 ml of normal uncontacted plasma is incubated with 6 mg of celite in a siliconized tube at 37°C for 10 minutes. The tube is mixed frequently and centrifuged at 3,000 rpm for 5 minutes to deposit the celite. The supernatant plasma is transferred to a new siliconized tube and incubated at 37°C for 18 to 24 hours. This plasma is found to contain Factor XII but very little Factor XI.

### Method
1. 0.3 ml of celite-6-treated normal plasma and 0.1 ml of test plasma are mixed and incubated for 5 minutes with 1 mg of celite at 37°C.
2. Steps 2 to 6 are performed as in the contact activation test.

*Results.* Typical results are shown in Table 5-34.

TABLE 5-34. Typical Results in the Celite-6 Test.

| PLASMA | DILUTIONS OF TEST PLASMA IN INTACT NORMAL PLASMA | | | INTACT NORMAL PLASMA |
|---|---|---|---|---|
| | 1:3 | 1:9 | 1:27 | |
| Normal | 320 | 430 | 470 | 605 |
| Factor XI deficiency | 502 | 620 | 630 | 620 |
| Factor XII deficiency | 355 | 430 | 485 | 630 |

## QUANTITATIVE TEST FOR FACTOR XIII DEFICIENCY[57]
## (FIBRIN STABILIZING FACTOR)

*Principle.* Normal plasma clots are insoluble in 5 M urea, whereas clots formed in the absence of Factor XIII are soluble.

### Reagents and Apparatus
1. 5 M Aqueous urea: 30.0 g of urea is dissolved in 100 ml of distilled water.
2. M/40 Calcium chloride
3. Citrated normal and test plasmas

*Method*

1. 0.5 ml of normal plasma is added to tube 1 and 0.5 ml of test plasma is added to tube 2.

2. 0.5 ml of normal plasma is added to 9.5 ml of test plasma, and 0.5 ml of this dilution is added to tube 3.

3. Add 0.5 ml of M/40 calcium chloride to each of the 3 tubes. Mix by inversion and incubate for 30 minutes at 37°C.

4. Pipet a 5-ml volume of 5 M urea into each of 3 tubes. Transfer the loosened clots from 3 to the urea tubes and leave at room temperature.

*Results.* In the absence of Factor XIII, the clot will dissolve within 2 to 3 hours, whereas the normal clot and that obtained from the plasma mixture will remain intact for at least 24 hours.

If the mixed clot also dissolves, it suggests that dissolution of the test clot may *not* have been due to Factor XIII deficiency but to fibrinolytic activity.

*Notes*

1. 1% Factor XIII is sufficient to render a clot insoluble in 5 M urea.

2. If, when determining clot retraction, it is found that the clot is unusually fragile, Factor XIII-deficiency test should be carried out.

## CLINICAL CONSIDERATIONS

### Hemorrhagic Defects

*Hemophilia (Antihemophilic Globulin Deficiency; Factor VIII Deficiency).* This is an inherited disease, manifested in childhood and remaining as a lifelong affliction. Hemorrhages can occur both externally and internally, the commonest sites being the nose, mouth, eyes, gastrointestinal tract, urinary tract, joints, and sometimes superficial abrasions. The hemorrhages resulting from this condition frequently form large hematomas, which often cause secondary conditions. A clinical feature sometimes found in hemophilia is the presence of hemarthrosis, usually in the elbow and knee.

This disease is found to affect the Germanic races more than the Eastern peoples. One of the true characteristics of hemophilia is its mode of transmission, a peculiarity also found in PTC deficiency (Factor IX deficiency). Hemophilia is inherited as a sex-linked recessive character, the gene being carried by the X chromosome. The condition is thus passed on to affected males by the mother, who appears normal but carries a gene for the disease. Such a person is phenotypically normal, but genotypically affected. This implies that she appears outwardly normal but has an abnormal genetic makeup.

***Mode of Inheritance.*** A mating of a normal female and normal male is shown in Figure 5-21. Normal female genes are shown as XX and normal male genes as XY.

The resulting siblings will be 50% normal females (XX); 50% normal males (XY).

A mating of a female carrier and a normal male is shown in Figure 5-22. The gene responsible for carrying hemophilia is designated as $X$.

The resulting siblings will be: 25% hemophilic males ($X$Y); 25% normal males (XY); 25% normal females (XX); 25% hemophilic female carriers ($XX$).

A mating of a female carrier and a hemophilic male is shown in Figure 5-23.

The resulting siblings will be: 25% hemophilic male ($X$Y); 25% normal male (XY); 25% hemophilic female carriers ($X$X); 25% hemophilic females ($XX$).

Homozygote female hemophilics who exhibit the characteristics of classical hemophilia have been reported but such individuals are extremely rare.

A mating of a hemophilic male with a normal female is shown in Figure 5-24.

The resulting siblings will be: 50% hemophilic female carriers ($XX$); 50% normal males (XY).

A mating of a true homozygote hemophilic female and a normal male is shown in Figure 5-25.

The resulting siblings will be: 50% hemophilic female carriers ($XX$); 50% hemophilic males ($X$Y).

In severe hemophilia, the laboratory findings are clear-cut, but when the disease is present in a mild form, care is needed to establish a correct diagnosis.

The platelet count, tourniquet test, bleeding time, clot retraction, one-stage prothrombin time, and two-stage test are all normal. The prothrombin consumption is abnormal only when the Factor VIII level falls to 10% of normal. The most sensitive tests are the partial thromboplastin time and the thromboplastin generation test. Using either of these in conjunction with cross-correction studies, deficiencies of Factor VIII, producing assay values of 30 to 40% of normal, will be detected. Both of these tests can also be used as the basis of Factor VIII assays. The corresponding sensitivity of the Lee and White coagulation time is such that only patients with Factor VIII values of 1% or less will normally be detected.

***PTC Deficiency (Factor IX Deficiency).*** Clinically, PTC deficiency has a mode of inheritance and symptoms resembling hemophilia, although it is often found in a milder form.

Normal Female

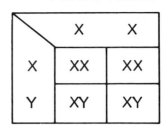

FIG. 5-21. Mating of a normal male and a normal female.

The results of the tests used in the diagnosis of hemophilia are very similar in this disease. The exception is the thromboplastin generation test, which locates the abnormality as being in the patient's seru, whereas that of hemophilia is in the plasma. The partial thromboplastin time is also a sensitive method of detecting the abnormality; cross-correction studies have the same diagnostic use. A minor difference is sometimes noticed in the coagulation time, tests exceeding 30 minutes being rare and results over this figure usually being indicative of hemophilia.

*PTA Deficiency (Factor XI Deficiency).* The clinical findings in PTA are normally milder than those in either hemophilia or PTC deficiency. Less than half of the patients show hemarthrosis, but a large proportion have gum bleeds and epistaxis. The condition is not sex-linked and therefore affects both males and females in a similar manner.

The coagulation time, platelet count, bleeding time, prothrombin time and tourniquet test are all normal. The diagnostic test is again the thromboplastin generation test, in which the inherent defect is found in both the serum or barium sulfate-adsorbed plasma, whereas hemophilia is found in the plasma alone, and PTC deficiency in the serum. Abnormalities are also found in the prothrombin consumption test and the activated partial thromboplastin time.

*Von Willebrand's Disease:* This disease occurs early in life and takes the form of generalized hemorrhages from the nose, gums and gastric

Female Carrier

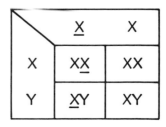

FIG. 5-22. Mating of a normal male with a female carrier.

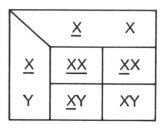

FIG. 5-23. Mating of a hemophilic male with a female carrier.

tract. It is thought to be due to a capillary defect that is inherited as a simple mendelian dominant. The disease shows a prolonged bleeding time, and platelet adhesiveness, but normal platelet count, coagulation time and clot retraction. Variable results are found in the tourniquet test, prothrombin consumption test, thromboplastin generation test and partial thromboplastin time, 50% of the patients having reduced Factor VIII levels.

***Functional Platelet Deficiency.*** The main feature of this disease is marked purpura, usually with an abnormal bleeding time, prothrombin consumption test, platelet adhesiveness, platelet Factor III assay and clot retraction. Platelet aggregation is usually abnormal in the presence of ADP. Clinically, the condition resembles thrombocytopenia, although the platelets do not show any reduction in numbers. Inheritance is by simple mendelian dominance, the disease first being noticed in infancy.

***Idiopathic Thrombocytopenia.*** Clinically, this disease shows purpuric hemorrhages. The patient has a variable degree of anemia and a low platelet count; the clot retraction is reduced, but the coagulation time is normal. The diagnostic laboratory test is the bleeding time, which is often increased to over 40 minutes. The bone marrow may occasionally show changes in the distribution and morphology of the megakaryocytes, although the appearance is often normal. Platelet antibodies can be detected in approximately 50% of all patients.

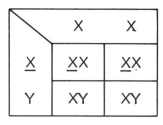

FIG. 5-24. Mating of a hemophilic male and a normal female.

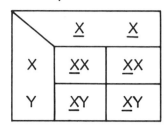

FIG. 5-25. Mating of a normal male with a homozygote hemophilic female.

*Symptomatic Thrombocytopenia.* Clinically, the symptoms are the same as those found in essential thrombocytopenia. The disease is divided into two groups, one caused by splenic dysfunction, the other by a marrow dyscrasia. The former shows hyperactivity of the spleen, resulting in the overdestruction of the platelets, whereas the latter is a maturation defect of the marrow, usually caused by drugs or by toxemia.

*Capillary Purpura.* Investigation of this disease shows a normal platelet count, bleeding time and clotting time. The diagnostic test is found to be the tourniquet test. The disease is thought to be due to an abnormality of the endothelial lining of the capillaries, and can be caused by pyrexia, poisons, allergies or vitamin deficiencies.

*Vitamin K Deficiency.* This usually manifests itself as an aprothrombinemia. When this occurs, the one-stage and two-stage prothrombin times, the bleeding time, and often the coagulation time are abnormal.

*Idiopathic Hypoprothrombinemia.* This is a congenital disease, laboratory findings being identical with those of the vitamin K deficiency.

*Fibrinogenopenia.* Clinically, there is severe bleeding following minor abrasions. The bleeding time is prolonged and a variable platelet count is also found. The major laboratory finding is the absence of clot formation by any of the usual tests. The absence or low value of fibrinogen is confirmed by the failure of citrated plasma to clot on the addition of thrombin.

*Factor V Deficiency.* The symptoms are similar to those of hemophilia. The laboratory findings show an abnormal one-stage prothrombin time and thromboplastin generation test. The bleeding time, tourniquet test and platelet counts are all normal. Differentiation can be made by the shortening of the one-stage prothrombin time by the addition of 10% normal adsorbed plasma, rich in Factor V.

*Factor VII Deficiency.* This disease resembles Factor V deficiency and related conditions in both symptoms and laboratory findings. These results are similar to those of Factor V deficiency, with the exception that the one-stage prothrombin test is not shortened by the addition of adsorbed plasma, but is shortened by 10% normal serum, rich in Factor VII.

## CIRCULATING ANTICOAGULANTS

Circulating anticoagulants are found in several clinical situations. They may complicate laboratory investigations of most of the congenital coagulation factor deficiencies, due to the presence of antibodies to Factors VIII and IX and occasionally to Factors V and VII. Antifibrinogens (fibrinolysins-plasmin) are probably the commonest anticoagulants found in the laboratory.

The laboratory findings in the presence of anticoagulants against Factors VIII or IX reveal low factor assays. They can be differentiated by assaying mixture of patient's plasma and normal plasma, patient's plasma and buffer, and normal plasma and buffer. Anticoagulant effect is demonstrated by the patient's plasma reducing the normal plasma assay proportionally to the strength of the antibody.

Other abnormal tests are the coagulation time, recalcification time, partial thromboplastin time, etc. In general, any test involved in that specific factor will be abnormal and will usually be indistinguishable from a true factor assay.

The presence of fibrinolysins (increased plasmin) can be detected by clot lysis tests, and the euglobulin lysis time.

In addition to the hemorrhagic conditions already mentioned, there are other rare disorders having characteristic clinical symptoms. These include Factor X deficiency, David's disease, Ehlers-Danlos syndrome, Henoch-Schönlein purpura, hereditary telangiectasia, and the presence of platelet antibodies.

One rare condition, which is not truly a hemorrhagic state, is Hageman factor deficiency (Factor XII). Patients with such an abnormality are characteristic in that, clinically, they do not hemorrhage; the diagnostic laboratory test is the thromboplastin generation test or the partial thromboplastin time. Separation in the laboratory between this deficiency and a Factor XII deficiency rests mainly on suitable cross-correction of either the thromboplastin generation test or the partial thromboplastin time with Factors XI- and XII-deficient plasma.

## REFERENCES

1. A Manual of Methods for the Coagulation Laboratory. Baltimore, Baltimore Biological Laboratory Division, B-D Laboratories, Inc., 1965.
2. Reference Manual of Coagulation Procedures. ed. 2, p. 6. Los Angeles, Hyland Laboratories, 1964.
3. Ivy, A. C., Shapiro, P. R., and Melnick, P.: The bleeding tendency in jaundice. Surg. Gynec. Obstet., *60*: 781, 1935.
4. Duke, W. W.: The relation of blood platelets to hemorrhagic disease. JAMA, *55*: 1185, 1910.

5. Borchgrevink, C. F., and Waaler, B. A.: The secondary bleeding time. Acta. Med. Scand., *162*: 361, 1958.
6. Mielke, C. H., Kaneshiro, M. M., Maher, I. A., Weiner, J. M., and Rappaport, S. I.: The standardized normal ivy bleeding time and its prolongation by aspirin. Blood, *34*: 204, 1969.
7. Quick, A. J.: Aspirin Tolerance Test. Hemorrhagic Diseases and Thrombosis. ed. 3, p. 386. Philadelphia, Lea & Febiger, 1966.
8. Tocantins, L. M.: Measurement of the rate and extent of clot retraction. *In* Tocantins, L. M., and Kazal, L. A. (eds.): Blood Coagulation, Hemorrhage and Thrombosis. ed. 2, p. 41. New York, Grune & Stratton, 1964.
9. Brecher, G., and Cronkite, E. P.: Morphology and enumeration of human blood platelets. J. Appl. Physiol., *3*: 365, 1950.
10. Dacie, J. V., and Lewis, S. M.: Practical Hematology. ed. 4, p. 70. New York, Grune & Stratton, 1968.
11. Tocantins, L. M.: Technical methods for the study of blood platelets. Arch. Pathol., *23*: 850, 1937.
12. Lempert, H.: Modified technique for enumeration of blood platelets. Lancet, *1*: 151, 1935.
13. Oettle, A. G., and Spriggs, A. I.: Recent Advances in Clinical Pathology. ed. 2, p. 406. London, J. & A. Churchill, 1951.
14. Cramer, W., and Bannerman, R. G. (As quoted by Britton, C. J. C.): Disorders of the Blood. ed. 9, p. 759. New York, Grune & Stratton, 1963.
15. Dameshek, W.: Method for simultaneous enumeration of blood platelets and reticulocytes with consideration of normal platelet counts in man and woman. Arch. Int. Med., *50*: 579, 1932.
16. Coulter Platelet Method. Bulletin L103-66C. Evanston, Scientific Products, 1966.
17. Technical Manual: Autocounter. Tarrytown, N.Y., Technicon Instruments Corp., 1970.
18. Technical Manual: Thrombocounter. Hialeah, Fla., Coulter Electronics, 1973.
19. Hellem, A. J.: The adhesiveness of human blood platelets "in vitro." Norwegian monographs on medical science. Oslo, University of Oslo Press, 1960.
20. Salzman, E.: Measurement of platelet adhesiveness. J. Lab. Clin. Med., *62*: 724, 1963.
21. Borchgrevink, C. F.: A method of measuring platelet adhesiveness in vivo. Acta. Med. Scand., *168*: 157, 1960.
22. Blakely, J. A.: Basic Techniques of Platelet Aggregation. Instructor's Manual. Buffalo, N.Y., Payton Aggregometer, 1970.
23. Van de Wiel, T. W. M., van de Weil-Dorfmeyer, H., and Van Loghem, J. J.: Studies on platelet antibodies in man. Vox Sang., *6*: 641, 1961.
24. Harrington, W. J., Minnich, V., and Arimura, G.: The auto-immune thrombocytopenia. *In* Tocantins, L. M. (ed.): Progress in Hematology. vol. 1, p. 177. New York, Grune & Stratton, 1956.
25. Dausset, J., Colombari, J., and Colombari, I.: Study of leukopenias and thrombocytopenias by the direct antiglobulin consumption test on leukocytes and/or platelets. Blood, *18*: 672, 1961.
26. Aster, R. H., Cooper, H. E., and Singer, D. L.: Simplified complement fixation test for the detection of platelet antibodies in human serum. J. Lab. Clin. Med., *63*: 161, 1964.

27. Kabat, E., and Mayer: Experimental Immunochemistry. Springfield, Ill., Charles C Thomas, 1961.
28. Aster, R. H.: Detection of antiplatelet antibodies: Inhibition of clot retraction. *In* Williams, W. J., *et al.* (eds.) p. 1417. Hematology. New York, McGraw-Hill, 1972.
29. Lee, R. I., and White, P. D.: A clinical study of the coagulation time of blood. Am. J. Med. Sci., *145*: 495, 1913.
30. Margulies, H., and Barker, N. W.: The coagulation time of blood in silicon tubes. Am. J. Med. Sci., *218*: 42, 1949.
31. Dale, H. H., and Laidlaw, P. P.: A simple coagulometer. J. Pathol., *16*: 351, 1911.
32. Quick, A. J.: The prothrombin in hemophilia an in obstructive jaundice. J. Biol. Chem., *109*: 73, 1935.
33. Owren, P. A., and Aas, K.: The control of dicumarol therapy and the quantitative determination of prothrombin and proconvertin. Scand. J. Clin. Lab. Invest., *3*: 201, 1951.
34. Owren, P. A.: Thrombotest. A new method for controlling anticoagulant therapy. Lancet, *11*: 1115, 1960.
35. Biggs, R., and MacFarlane, R. G.: Human Blood Coagulation. ed. 3, p. 389. Philadelphia, F. A. Davis, 1962.
36. Owren, P. A.: A quantitative one-stage method for the assay of prothrombin. Scan. J. Clin. Lab. Invest., *1*: 81, 1949.
37. Dacie, J. V., and Lewis, S. M.: Practical Hematology. ed. 4, p. 275. New York, Grune & Stratton, 1968.
38. Darmady, E. M., and Davenport, S. G. T.: Hematological Technique. ed. 3, p. 180. New York, Grune & Stratton, 1963.
39. Rodman, N. F., Jr., Barrow, E. M., and Graham, J. B.: Diagnosis and control of the hemophiloid states with the partial thromboplastin test. Am. J. Clin. Pathol., *29*: 525, 1958.
40. Hicks, N. D., and Pitney, W. R.: A rapid screening test for disorders of thromboplastin generation. Br. J. Haemat., *3*: 227, 1957.
41. Biggs, R., and Douglas, A. S.: The thromboplastin generation test. J. Clin. Pathol., *6*: 23, 1953.
42. Thompson, J. H., Jr., Owen, C. A., Jr., Spittel, J. A., Jr., and Pascuzzi, C. A.: The "retarded" thromboplastin generation test: Its use in the study of accelerated blood coagulation. Am. J. Clin. Pathol., *37*: 63, 1962.
43. Reference Manual of Coagulation Procedures. ed. 2, p. 19. Los Angeles, Hyland Laboratories, 1964.
44. Bergina, L. J. A.: A simple method for the assay of Factor VIII. Blood, *15*: 637, 1960.
45. Weiss, H. J., and Eichelberger, J. W., Jr.: The detection of platelet defects in patients with mild bleeding disorders. Am. J. Med., *32*: 872, 1962.
46. Blomback, B., Blomback, M., and Nilsson, I. M.: Coagulation studies on "Reptilase", an extract of the venom from Bothrops Jararaca. Thromb et Diath Haem., *1*: 1, 1957.
47. Margolius, A., Jr., Jackson, D. P., and Ratnoff, O. D.: Circulating anticoagulants. A study of 40 cases and a review of the literature. Medicine, *40*: 145, 1961.
48. Hawiger, J., Niewlarowski, S., Gurewich, V., and Thomas D. P. Measurement of fibrinogen and fibrin degradation products in serum by Staphylococcal clumping test. J. Lab. Clin. Med., *75*: 93, 1970.

49. Leavelle, D. E., Mertens, B. F., Bowie, E. J. W., and Owen, C. A., Jr.: Staphylococcal clumping on microtiter plates: A rapid, simple method for measuring fibrinogen split products. Am. J. Clin. Pathol., *75*: 452, 1971.
50. Mertens, B. F., McDuffie, F. C., Bowie, E. J. W., and Owen, C. A., Jr.: Rapid sensitive method for measuring fibrinogen split-products in human serum. Mayo Clin. Proc., *441*: 1141, 1969.
51. Breen, F. A., and Tullis, J. L.: Ethanol gelation: A rapid screening test for intravascular coagulation. Ann. Int. Med., *69*: 1197, 1968.
52. Bucknell, M.: The effect of citrate on euglobulin methods of estimating fibrinolyte activity. J. Clin. Pathol., *11*: 403, 1958.
53. Schneider, C. L.: Rapid estimation of plasma fibrinogen concentration and its use as a guide to therapy of intravascular defibrination. Am. J. Obstet. Gynecol., *64*: 141, 1952.
54. Fowell, A. H.: Turbidometric method of fibrinogen assay results with a Coleman Jr. Spectrophometer. Am. J. Clin. Pathol. *25*: 340, 1955.
55. Margolis, J.: Initiation of blood coagulation by glass and related surfaces. J. Physiol., *137*: 95, 1957.
56. Nossel, H. L.: As described in Hardisty, R. M., and Ingram, G. I. C.: Bleeding Disorders, Investigation and Management. p. 314. London, Blackwell Scientific Publications, 1965.
57. Josso, F., Prov-Wartelle, O., and Alagille, D., and Soulier, J. P.: Le deficit congenital en facteur stabilisant de la fibrine (facteur XIII). Etude de deux cas Nouv. Rev. Franc. Hemat., *4*: 267, 1964.

# 6

# *Staining Techniques*

## RED CELLS

### *Staining of Siderocytes (Prussian Blue Technique)*

*Principle.* Siderocytes are red cells containing nonhemoglobin iron-containing granules, which stain with a potassium ferrocyanide-hydrochloric acid mixture.

### *Reagents and Apparatus*
1. Absolute methyl alcohol
2. 2% Potassium ferrocyanide
3. 0.2 N Hydrochloric acid
4. 0.1% Aqueous eosin
5. 56°C Waterbath

### *Method*
1. Blood or bone marrow smears are air dried and fixed in absolute methyl alcohol for 15 minutes at room temperature. The smears are allowed to dry free of alcohol.

2. Equal volumes of 2% potassium ferrocyanide and 0.2 N hydrochloric acid are mixed, giving a 1% solution of potassium ferrocyanide in 0.1 N acid.

3. The dried smears are placed in a Coplin jar filled with the acidified ferrocyanide solution for 10 minutes at 56°C.

4. The slides are washed in running tap water for 20 to 30 minutes, rinsed in distilled water and counterstained for 5 to 10 seconds in 0.1% aqueous eosin.

*Normal.* Normal blood contains 0.4 to 0.6% siderocytes. The findings in some diseases are as follows:

|  | % |
| --- | --- |
| Microcytic hypochromic anemia | 1-3 |
| Infections | 6-10 |
| Severe burns | 3-10 |
| Pernicious anemia | 8-14 |
| Lead poisoning | 10-30 |

*Notes*

1. Siderocytes are occasionally seen as basophilic granules in Romanowsky stained smears. These are then known as Pappenheim bodies.

2. Siderocytes can be found in normoblasts of bone marrow and in reticulocytes. When this occurs in a normal marrow, it is thought to represent iron taken into the cell in excess of that required for immediate incorporation into heme.

3. The Prussian blue technique can be applied to old blood smears previously stained by Romanowsky dyes.

4. Sideroblasts are normoblasts with siderocytic granules in the cytoplasm.

## *Staining of Thick Smears for Malarial Parasites*[1]

*Principle.* The smears are not fixed. Aqueous methylene blue and aqueous eosin are added to the smear; this lyses the red cells and stains the parasites.

*Reagents and Apparatus*

1. Stain A

   Methylene blue . . . . . . . . . . . . . . . . . . . . . . . . . . . . . . . . . 1.3 g
   Disodium hydrogen phosphate . . . . . . . . . . . . . . . . . . . 12.6 g
   Potassium dihydrogen phosphate . . . . . . . . . . . . . . . . . 6.25 g
   Distilled water . . . . . . . . . . . . . . . . . . . . . . . . . . . . . to 500 ml

The methylene blue and disodium hydrogen phosphate are dissolved in 50 ml of distilled water. The solution is boiled and evaporated in a waterbath to near dryness; 500 ml of freshly boiled distilled water and the potassium dihydrogen phosphate are added and the stain mixed until dissolved. The solution is left for 24 hours and filtered.

   Stain B

   Eosin . . . . . . . . . . . . . . . . . . . . . . . . . . . . . . . . . . . . . . . . 1.3 g
   Disodium hydrogen phosphate . . . . . . . . . . . . . . . . . . 12.6 g
   Potassium dihydrogen phosphate . . . . . . . . . . . . . . . . 6.25 g
   Distilled water . . . . . . . . . . . . . . . . . . . . . . . . . . . . . to 500 ml

2. Buffered distilled water (pH 7.2)
3. Coplin jars

*Method*

1. The unfixed smears are dipped into Stain A for 2 to 3 seconds and rinsed in buffered distilled water (pH 7.2) until the stain ceases to flow from the smear.

2. They are dipped into Stain B for 1 to 2 seconds and rinsed rapidly in buffered distilled water.

3. The slide is set upright to dry without blotting.

## WHITE CELLS

### *Feulgen's Stain for Desoxyribonucleic Acid*[2]

*Principle.* The reaction is based on the capacity of fuchsin sulfurous acid to develop a red color with the aldehyde group produced by acid hydrolysis of desoxyribonucleic acid (DNA).

### *Reagents and Apparatus*

1. Stain: 1 g of basic fuchsin is dissolved in 200 ml of boiling distilled water, filtered and cooled to room temperature; 20 ml of N hydrochloric acid and 1 g of anhydrous sodium bisulfite are added. The solution is kept in the dark and not used for at least 24 hours.

2. Susa's fixative:

| | |
|---|---|
| Mercuric chloride | 4.5 g |
| Sodium chloride | 0.5 g |
| Trichloracetic acid | 2.0 g |
| Glacial acetic acid | 4.0 g |
| Formalin | 20 ml |
| Distilled water | 80 ml |

3. 1% Aqueous light green
4. 1% Sodium thiosulfate
5. Lugol's iodine:

| | |
|---|---|
| Iodine | 1 g |
| Potassium iodide | 2 g |
| Distilled water | 100 ml |

6. N hydrochloric acid
7. 56°C Waterbath
8. Bisulfate acid mixture:

| | |
|---|---|
| 10% Aqueous anhydrous sodium bisulfate | 10 ml |
| N Hydrochloric acid | 10 ml |
| Distilled water | to 200 ml |

### *Method*

1. The blood smears are placed in Susa's fixative for 1 hour.

2. The mercury deposits are removed from the smear by immersing in Lugol's iodine for 5 minutes. The iodine is removed by immersing in 1% sodium thiosulfate for 5 minutes.

3. The smears are rinsed in running tap water and are hydrolzyed in N hydrochloric acid at 56%C for 5 minutes. They are dipped in acid at room temperature and thoroughly rinsed in distilled water.

4. Immerse in Feulgen's stain for 2 hours and wash in the bisulfate acid mixture for 20 minutes. Rewash 3 more times, rinse in running tap water for 10 minutes and counterstain with 1% aqueous light green for 2 to 3 seconds.

*Results.* Leukocytes and nucleated red cells take up the stain according to the concentration of DNA in the nucleus. Cytoplasm and mature red cells do not stain. The nuclei of the mature cells stain pale pink and the nucleoli show up as definite spaces in the cytoplasm.

*Note.* The stain has value in that it distinguishes between mature and immature cells and is especially useful in the differentiation between lymphocytes and micromyeloblasts. The nucleoli are clearly defined by this technique, enabling them to be more easily counted. The cellular reaction to the stain is shown in Table 6-1.

### Identification of DNA by the Digestion Technique

*Principle.* DNA stains well with the basophilic dyes of the Romanowsky stains. When DNA is digested with desoxyribonuclease and restained with Wright's or Giemsa stain, the area digested loses its affinity for the stain.

#### Reagents and Apparatus

1. Deosxyribonuclease solution: 1.4 g of sodium acetate is dissolved in 10 ml of dissolved water; 2.46 g of magnesium sulfate is disolved in 10 ml of distilled water and the 2 solutions added together with 80 ml of distilled water; 8 mg of desoxyribonuclease* is added to the solution.

2. Giemsa stain 1:10.1 ml Giemsa stain is added to 9 ml distilled water.

3. Coplin jar

#### Method

1. Two thin blood smears, both from the same source, are made as described under differential white counts (pp. 99-100).

---

* Available from Sigma Chemical Co., St. Louis, Mo.

TABLE 6-1. Cellular Reaction to Feulgen's Stain.

| Feulgen Positive | Feulgen Negative |
|---|---|
| L. E. Cells | Lymphoblasts |
| Lymphocytes | Monocytes |
| Segmented granulocytes | Myelocytes |
| Bands | Early megaloblasts |
| Metamyelocytes | |
| Rubricytes | |

2. One slide is placed in the desoxyribonuclease solution for 1 hour at 37°C, washed well in distilled water and allowed to air dry.

3. Both the treated and untreated slides are stained in dilute Giemsa stain or by any conventional Romanowsky procedure for 30 minutes and air dried.

*Results.* DNA containing chromatin is stained basophilic on the control slide but is colorless on the test slide.

### Unna-Pappenheim Stain for Ribonucleic Acid (Modified)[3]

*Principle.* The stain is a combination of pyronin and methyl green. The pyronin stains the cell components containing the ribonucleic acid and the methyl green stains the chromatin.

#### Reagents and Apparatus
1. Susa's fixative as described on page 312.
2. Unna-Pappenheim stain:

Pyronin . . . . . . . . . . . . . . . . . . . . . . . . . . . . . . . . . . . . . . . . . . . . 0.3 g
Methyl green . . . . . . . . . . . . . . . . . . . . . . . . . . . . . . . . . . . . . 0.7 g
Glycerin . . . . . . . . . . . . . . . . . . . . . . . . . . . . . . . . . . . . . . . . . . . 20 ml
Absolute ethyl alcohol . . . . . . . . . . . . . . . . . . . . . . . . . 2.5 ml
0.5% Aqueous phenol . . . . . . . . . . . . . . . . . . . . . . . to 100 ml

The stains are ground with the glycerin and ethyl alcohol, and the phenol solution is added. The resulting stain is boiled for 2 minutes and filtered.

3. Lugol's iodine as described on page 312.
4. Tertiary butyl alcohol
5. 5% Aqueous sodium thiosulfate

#### Method
1. The blood smears are immersed in Susa's fixative for 1 hour.

2. The mercury deposits are removed from the smear by the same technique previously described in the Feulgen's stain (p. 312).

3. The smears are washed in running tap water for 10 minutes and stained in Unna-Pappenheim stain for 1 hour. They are rinsed in distilled water for 2 minutes, dehydrated in tertiary butyl alcohol for 1 minute, cleared by rinsing in xylol and mounted in a neutral media.

*Results.* RNA is stained bright red, and chromatin, green-black.

*Notes.* RNA is found mainly in the cytoplasm of mature plasma cells but is also present in the nucleoli of the immature cells.

### Identification of RNA by the Digestion Technique

*Principle.* The basic principle is similar to that of the DNA digestion method. Ribonuclease derived from ox pancreas is used as the digesting enzyme. It is available from the same companies that produce the desoxyribonuclease.

### Reagents and Apparatus

1. Ribonuclease solution: 1.4 g of sodium acetate is dissolved in 10 ml of distilled water; 2.46 g of magnesium sulfate is also dissolved in 10 ml of distilled water, and the sodium acetate and magnesium sulfate solutions mixed together with 80 ml of distilled water; 8 mg of ribonuclease* is dissolved in the above solution.

2. Giemsa stain 1:10.1 ml Giemsa stain is added to 9 ml distilled water.

3. Coplin jar

### Method

1. Two thin blood smears, both from the same source, are made as described under differential white counts (p. 99).

2. One slide is placed in the ribonuclease solution for 1 hour at 37°C, washed well in distilled water and allowed to air dry.

3. Both the treated and untreated slides are stained with dilute Giemsa stain or by any conventional Romanowsky procedure for 30 minutes and air dried.

**Results.** RNA-containing areas are stained with the basic component on the control slide but are colorless on the test slide.

### Identification of Glycogen by the Periodic Acid Schiff Reaction[4]

**Principle.** The reaction depends on the liberation of carbohydrate radicals from combination with protein and their oxidation to aldehydes by Schiff's reagent, producing a magenta color.

### Reagents and Apparatus

1. Solution 1: 1 g of periodic acid is added to 100 ml of distilled water.

2. Solution 2: *Schiff's leukobasic fuchsin*—1 g of basic fuchsin is added to 400 ml of boiling distilled water. The solution is cooled to 50°C and filtered; 1 ml of thionyl chloride is added and the mixture allowed to stand in the dark for 12 hours; 2 g of activated charcoal is added and the stain shaken for 1 minute, stored in a dark bottle at 4°C and filtered before use.

3. 40% Formalin

---

* Available from Sigma Chemical Co., St. Louis, Mo.

4. Sulfur dioxide water: Bubble sulfur dioxide through distilled water until a saturated solution is obtained or make up the following solution:

10% Sodium metabisulfite ........................ 6 ml
N hydrochloric acid ............................ 5 ml
Distilled water ................................ 100 ml

5. 5.2% Aqueous Ehrilich's hematoxylin ............ 100 ml

### Method

1. Blood or bone marrow smears are air dried and fixed by exposing to formalin vapor for 5 minutes.

2. The smears are washed in running tap water for 15 minutes and treated with 1% periodic acid solution for 10 minutes.

3. They are immersed in Schiff's leukobasic fuchsin for 20 minutes and rinsed in two changes of saturated sulfur dioxide water for 3 minutes each time.

4. The smears are washed in distilled water for 5 minutes, counterstained with 2% aqueous hematoxylin for 1 minute and allowed to "blue" in tap water for 5 minutes.

5. Control smears are exposed to salivary digestion for 30 minutes at stage 2.

*Results.* A magenta staining reaction indicates the presence of glycogen.

### Notes

1. Developing granulocytes react at all stages of maturation. Mature neutrophil polymorphonuclear cells react most strongly, the cytoplasm containing large amounts of glycogen, especially in the granules. Earlier cells in the same series show decreasing glycogen content but still stain weakly with a PAS reaction.

2. Lymphocytes and monocytes stain weakly for glycogen, but occasionally a few fine granules are demonstrated.

3. Red cell precursors are normally glycogen-negative.

4. In pathological states, the PAS stain is positive in many cells in which glycogen is absent or present only in small amounts.

Lymphocytes in chronic lymphatic leukemia, lymphosarcoma, or Hodgkin's disease sometimes show glycogen reactions. Erythroblasts in DiGuglielmo's disease and in thalassemia have been reported to produce positive PAS reactions.

5. Evidence exists to show that the glycogen content of hemopoietic cells parallels alkaline phosphatase activity.

### *Identification of Leukocyte Alkaline Phosphatase by the Modified Azo Dye Method[5]*

*Principle.* The enzyme is present in the cytoplasm of granulocytes. The method depends upon the hydrolysis of alpha-naphthyl phosphate, which liberates free naphthol. This, in turn, unites with a diazotized amine to form an insoluble color precipitate, which is proportional to the concentration of the enzyme present.

### Reagents and Apparatus

1. Fixative: 10 ml of 40% formalin is added to 90 ml of absolute ethyl alcohol. This fixative is stored *in the freezer* and prepared fresh at least *once a week*.

2. Stock propanediol buffer 0.2 M: 10.5 g of 2-amino-2-methyl propane-1,3-diol is added to 500 ml of distilled water.

3. Working buffer 0.05 M (pH 9.75): 25 ml of stock buffer, 5 ml of 0.1 N hydrochloric acid and 70 ml of distilled water are added together.

4. Azo dye:

Sodium alpha-naphthyl phosphate .............. 35 mg
Brentamine fast garnet ........................35 mg
Working buffer................................ 35 ml

The brentamine fast garnet is unstable in solution and the azo dye should be made immediately prior to use. The dye and naphthyl substrate do not always dissolve easily, and the dye should be filtered directly onto the slide.

5. 2% Mayer's aqueous hematoxylin
6. Kaiser's glycerine jelly kept at 60°C
7. Freshly taken blood or bone marrow smears
8. Coplin jar

### Method

1. The blood smears are fixed in fixative at 4°C for 2 minutes. Once fixed, the smears can be stored overnight before staining.

2. The smears are rinsed in tap water and stained in a Coplin jar with the azo dye for 10 minutes at room temperature. They are rinsed in distilled water and counterstained for 10 minutes with Mayer's hematoxylin.

*Calculation.* The slides should be examined within a few hours of preparation, because the stain fades quickly. Enzyme activity is indicated by a brown pigment in the cytoplasm, the amount varying from a faint diffuse coloration to a dense aggregation of red-brown granules. This variation can be used to roughly measure the amount of enzyme present in the cell.

100 Segmented neutrophils are individually scored in a range from 0 to 4+. The individual scores are totaled and compared with the normal.

0—negative
1+—barely visible diffuse staining
2+—diffuse staining with moderate granule formation
3+—strong positive with numerous granules
4+—very strong positive with very numerous coarse granules.

### Normal

```
Low range ..........................................0-8
Normal ...........................................8-100
High .............................................100+
```

### Notes

1. EDTA blood should not be used to make the smears, because it has an inhibitory effect on the staining reaction. For best results the blood smears should be made directly from capillary blood and fixed and stained within 30 minutes of preparation.

2. High alkaline phosphatase activity is found in infections, non-leukemic myeloproliferative diseases, pregnancy and Hodgkin's disease. Low scores are often found in chronic and acute granulocytic leukemia, paroxysmal nocturnal hemoglobinuria, infectious mononucleosis and acute monocytic leukemia. Normal values are present in chronic lymphatic leukemia, lymphosarcoma, multiple myeloma and Naegli monocytic leukemia.

## Identification of Lipids by Sudan Black B

### Technique 1[6]

*Principle.* The inert diazo dye, Sudan black B, stains neutral fat droplets and phospholipids. The exact nature of the staining reaction is not fully understood.

### Reagents and Apparatus

1. Sudan black B stock solution: 0.3 g of the stain is dissolved in 100 ml of absolute ethyl alcohol.

2. Buffer diluent: 16 g of crystalline phenol is dissolved in 30 ml of absolute ethyl alcohol and added to 100 ml of distilled water, in which has been dissolved 0.3 g of hydrated disodium hydrogen phosphate.

3. Sudan black B working solution: 40 ml of the buffer is added to 60 ml of the stock solution. The stain is filtered by suction. It keeps well at room temperature for 3 months.

4. 40% Formalin

5. 70% Ethyl alcohol

6. Fresh capillary blood smears

7. Coplin jar

### Method

1. Fix air-dried blood smears by exposing them to formalin vapor for 10 minutes. Wash them in running tap water for 10 minutes and immerse in a Coplin jar containing working stain for 1 hour.

2. Wash the smears in 70% ethyl alcohol for 3 minutes to differentiate

the stain, wash in tap water for 2 minutes and counterstain with any Romanowsky stain.

### Technique 2[7]

#### Reagents and Apparatus

1. Stain: Saturated Sudan black B in 70% ethyl alcohol. Allow the stain to stand for 24 hours before using.
2. Fixative: 9 volumes of 95% ethyl alcohol is added to one volume of 40% formalin.
3. 0.1% Aqueous safranin
4. Coplin jar

#### Method

1. Air-dried blood or bone marrow smears are fixed in formal alcohol for 5 seconds. The smears are air dried and stained for 1 hour in saturated alcoholic Sudan black B in a Coplin jar at 37°C.
2. The stain is drained away, the smears quickly rinsed in distilled water, and counterstained by dipping for 1 to 2 seconds in 0.1% aqueous safranin.

#### Notes

1. There is a close correlation between sudanophilia and positive peroxidase stain.
2. Cells of the granulocytic series show increasing distribution of lipids as they mature. Eosinophils of all stages of maturity show a strong reaction at the periphery of the specific granules, which retain an unstained central core. Basophils show a variable reaction, whereas lymphocytes are usually negative. Monocytes and megakaryocytes show scattered lipid deposits, whereas the red cell series are normally negative.

### Peroxidase Reaction

*Principle.* The cytoplasm of mature granulocytes, monoblasts, myeloblasts and promyelocytes possesses granules that contain a peroxidase enzyme. Bone marrow or blood smears are fixed in alcohol and treated with benzidine hydrogen peroxide and sodium nitroprusside, which form a blue compound in the presence of the enzyme.

### Technique 1[7]

#### Reagents and Apparatus

1. Absolute ethyl alcohol
2. 40% Neutral formaldehyde

3. Saturated aqueous sodium nitroprusside

4. Saturated aqueous benzidine

5. 2 Drops of 10% (v/v) hydrogen peroxide is added to 10 ml of distilled water.

6. 0.1% Aqueous eosin: Before use, 1 volume of saturated sodium nitroprusside is added to 99 volumes of saturated benzidine.

*Method*

1. Blood smears are fixed in a fluid containing 90 ml of absolute ethyl alcohol and 10 ml of 40% neutral formaldehyde and left for 1 minute at room temperature.

2. The smears are rinsed in running tap water, and 1 volume of peroxide solution is added to 2 volumes of nitroprusside-benzidine solution. The smears are flooded with this mixture and left for 1 minute.

3. Wash in distilled water for 2 to 3 minutes and counterstain with 0.1% aqueous eosin for 5 to 10 seconds.

*Results.* The peroxidase-containing granules appear as blue-black dots.

### Sato's and Sekiya's Method[8]

*Reagents and Apparatus*

1. 0.5% Copper sulfate

2. Saturated aqueous benzidine: The solution is filtered and 2 drops of 3% hydrogen peroxide added to 100 ml.

3. 0.1% Aqueous safranin

4. Fresh blood or bone marrow smears

*Method*

1. The copper sulfate solution is applied to the smears and left for 60 seconds. They are drained free of the copper sulfate, and the benzidine-peroxide reagent is added for 2 minutes.

2. The smears are rinsed well in running tap water, air dried, and counterstained with 0.1% safranin for 2 to 5 seconds.

*Results.* Peroxidase granules stain blue-green.

### Goodpasture's Method[9]

*Reagents and Apparatus*

1. 0.05 g of sodium nitroprusside is dissolved in 2 ml of distilled water, and 98 ml of absolute ethyl alcohol is added; 0.05 g of benzidine and 0.05 g of basic fuchsin are added to the solution. This stain will keep for 3 to 6 months at room temperature.

2. 1 ml of 10% (v/v) hydrogen peroxide is diluted to 200 ml with distilled water. Prepared fresh before use.

3. Fresh blood or bone marrow smears

*Method*

1. A freshly prepared smear is flooded with 1 volume of the nitroprusside reagent and left for 1 minute.

2. An equal volume of hydrogen peroxide is added to the smear and the mixture is allowed to stain for 4 minutes.

3. The smears are washed well in running tap water for 2 to 3 minutes and air dried.

*Results.* Peroxidase-containing granules stain a deep blue, whereas cell nuclei appear red and the cytoplasm pink. Red cells stain a buff color.

## Jacoby's Method[10]

*Reagents and Apparatus*

1. 40% Formalin
2. Absolute ethyl alcohol
3. 0.05% Aqueous 2,6-dichlorophenol-indophenol: This solution should be stored at 48°C or lower.
4. Hydrogen peroxide—4 volumes
5. Aqueous safranin—0.1%
6. Fresh blood or bone marrow smears

*Method*

1. Freshly prepared air-dried smears are fixed in a mixture of 1 volume of formalin and 9 volumes of absolute alcohol for 3 minutes.

2. The smears are washed well in running tap water, stained for 5 minutes with a mixture composed of 5 ml of dichlorophenol-indophenol and 4 drops of hydrogen peroxide, and washed in running tap water for 3 minutes.

3. The smears are counterstained with 0.1% aqueous safranin.

*Results.* Peroxidase-containing granules stain deep purple.

*Notes*

1. Peroxidases are hemoprotein enzymes consisting of a protein moiety attached to a prosthetic iron-porphyrin complex. In the presence of hydrogen peroxide, they catalyze the oxidation of many substances, including phenols, some amino acids and some aromatic acids.

2. The cytochemical demonstration of peroxidases depends on the use of an oxidizable substrate having brightly colored oxidation products. The most commonly used substrate is benzidine, which yields blue and brown compounds on oxidation.

3. The distribution of peroxidases in hemic cells is well established. Most of the cells of the granulocytic series show some peroxidase staining reactions, the intensity of which progress as the cells become more mature.

4. In practice, the stain is of limited value, inasmuch as it yields equivocal results in the blast and procyte stages of cellular development.

## Supravital Staining

*Principle*. This is the process of staining living material with nontoxic dyes so that the dye penetrates without killing the cell. The two commonest stains used are Janus green and neutral red. The former stains the mitochondria blue-green; the latter stains the specific granules and the vacuoles. Granules in the neutrophils are stained yellow; in the eosinophil, orange; and in the basophil, scarlet.

### Reagents and Apparatus
1. Saturated alcoholic neutral red
2. Saturated alcoholic Janus green
3. Neutral red-Janus green mixture: 5 ml of absolute ethyl alcohol is added to 0.2 ml of saturated alcoholic neutral red; 1.5 ml of this solution is delivered into each of 2 tubes. Into one tube is added 0.02 ml of saturated alcoholic Janus green and into the other tube 0.05 ml of the Janus green.
4. Grease-free slides
5. 37°C Incubator

### Method
1. Stains from the 2 tubes are spread on clean grease-free slides and dried by placing in an incubator at 37°C.
2. One drop of fresh blood is added to the slide, mounted with a coverslip and ringed with wax to keep airtight.
3. The preparation is placed in a 37°C incubator for 15 minutes and examined on a warm stage of a microscope.

### Results
Eosinophils   —actively ameboid
Basophils    —slightly ameboid
Neutrophils  —ameboid
Monocytes    —slightly ameboid
Lymphocytes—variable

### Notes
1. For successful supravital staining, it is necessary to have clean glassware and to avoid the use of concentrated dyes that will kill the cells. A warm microscope stage is also useful in obtaining good preparations.
2. Death of a cell is indicated by staining of the nucleus. In a good preparation, the Janus green stains the mitochrondria a brilliant blue-green, whereas the neutral red stains the specific granules and the vacuoles in varying shades, depending on their pH.
3. This method of staining is useful in distinguishing between myeloblasts and lymphoblasts. In the former, the mitochondria are fine and

scattered throughout the cytoplasm; in the latter, they are larger, oval and frequently grouped around the nucleus.

### Nitroblue-Tetrazolium Reduction Test (Modified)[11]

*Principle.* Neutrophils in fatal granulomatous disease ingest bacteria naturally but have a diminished capacity to kill the organisms. They also fail to reduce nitroblue-tetrazolium dye at a normal rate during in vitro phagocytosis of latex particles.

#### Reagents and Apparatus
1. Pooled normal human serum in frozen aliquots.
2. Nitroblue-tetrazolium (NBT)
0.28 g of NBT are dissolved in sterile isotomic saline and sterilized by filtering through a sintered glass filter. The dye is stored frozen in small aliquots, and thawed immediately before use.
3. Latex particles 0.81 µ (Bacto-Latex. Difco).
4. Safranin O:
1.0 g of safranin is dissolved in 100 ml of distilled water, and 40 ml glycerine added.
5. Incubation medium. Add into 2 small tubes:
   a. 0.5 ml Pooled human serum
      0.3 ml Sterile isotonic saline
      0.6 ml NBT
This is a control tube not containing phagocytosable material
   b. 0.5 ml Pooled human serum
      0.2 ml Sterile istonic saline
      0.6 NBT
      0.1 ml Latex particles
6. Capillary blood (fresh)
7. Absolute methyl alcohol
8. Alcohol clean coverglasses and slides
9. Petri dish
10. 1% Aqueous safranin

#### Method
1. One drop of capillary blood, obtained from a fingerstick, is placed on each of 2 clean coverglasses.
2. The coverglasses are placed on stoppers resting on damp sponges in a small deep tray with a cover. The tray is incubated at 37°C for 25 minutes.
3. One coverglass is removed and the red cell clot is gently washed away with sterile saline, leaving the granulocytes adhering to the coverglass.

4. The coverglass is drained of excess saline and is immediately inverted over a drop of incubation medium (a) on a clean glass slide.

5. Excess incubation media is removed from the underside of the coverglass with filter paper and the slide is placed in a moist covered chamber (Petri dish with damp wool).

6. Procedures 3 through 5 are repeated using incubation medium (b).

7. The moist chambers containing the coverglasses and slides are incubated at 37°C for 20 minutes; the coverglasses are removed, air dried, and fixed in absolute methyl alcohol for 1 minute.

8. The coverglasses are gently washed with running tap water for 10 seconds allowed to air dry and stained with 1% aqueous safranin for 2 to 5 minutes.

9. Differentiate by gently washing in running tap water for 10 seconds. Carefully blot to dry and counterstain using any Romanowsky stain.

10. The coverglass preparations are examined under the oil immersion lens and 100 neutrophils counted. The percentage of cells having large black deposits are classified as NBT-positive and recorded.

*Normals.* 3 to 10%

*Notes*

1. A second control consisting of test granulocytes incubated in saline can be used.

2. The formazan cytoplasmic deposits (reduced NBT) are seen in mature granulocytes and in juvenile forms. Occasionally, similar deposits are present in monocytes and in platelet clumps.

3. Normal results are found in patients with rheumatoid arthritis, systemic lupus erythematosus, measles, chickenpox, mumps, and primary tuberculosis.

4. Increases in NBT-positive neutrophils are seen in bacterial meningitis. *Candida albicans* septicemia and in other acute bacterial infections.

5. Decreases in NBT-positive neutrophils are seen in granulomatous disease of children.

### REFERENCES

1. Field, J.W.: Further note on a method of staining malarial parasites in thick blood films. Trns. Roy. Soc. Trop. Med. Hyg., *35*: 35, 1941.
2. Feulgen, R., and Rossenbeck, H.: Mikroskopisch-chemischer Nachweis einer Nucleinsaüre von Typens der Thyronucleinsaüre und die darant behrunde Elective Farbung von Zellkernen in mikroskopischen Pröparaten. Z. Phys. Chem., *135*: 203, 1924.
3. Perry, S., and Reynolds, J.: Methyl green pyronin as a differential nucleic acid stain for peripheral blood smears. Blood, *11*: 1132, 1956.
4. McManus, J. F. A.: Lipid morphology of tubercle. Nature, *157*: 772, 1946.

5. Kaplow, L. S.: A histochemical procedure for localizing and evaluating leucocyte alkaline phophatase activity in smears of blood and marrow. Blood, *10*: 1023, 1955.
6. Sheehan, H. L., and Storey, G. W.: Improved method of staining leucocyte granules with Sudan black B. J. Pathol. Bact., *59*: 336, 1947.
7. Dacie, J. V., and Lewis, S. M.: Practical Hematology. ed. 4, p. 95. New York, Grune & Stratton, Inc., 1968.
8. Sato, A., and Sekiya, N.: As quoted by Bover, G. F.: Atlas of Blood Cytology. p. 46. New York, Grune & Stratton, 1964.
9. Goodpasture, E. W.: A peroxidase reaction with sodium nitroprusside and benzidine in blood smears and tissues. J. Lab. Clin. Med., *4*: 442, 1919.
10. Jacoby, F.: As quoted by Darmady, E. M., and Davenport, S. G. T.: Haematological Technique. ed. 3, p. 127. New York, Grune & Stratton, 1963.
11. Park, B H., Holmes, B., Rodey, G., and Grood, R.: Nitroblue-tetrazolium test in children with fatal granulomatous disease and newborn infants. Lancet, *1*: 157, 1969.

# 7

# *Miscellaneous Tests*

## SEDIMENTATION RATES

If an anticoagulant is added to blood and the mixture set up in a vertical tube, the red cells gradually fall, and the plasma is displaced upward. The rate of this action is constant in health and is known as the sedimentation rate. The cells settle because their density is greater than that of the plasma. The cause of this phenomenon is not clear but it is thought to be associated with the albumin, globulin and fibrinogen fractions of the plasma.

The sedimentation of the red cells takes place in three stages:

1. The red cells begin to cling together, starting rouleaux formation during the first 5 minutes.

2. When the size of the red cell aggregate is at a maximum, the falling rate remains constant.

3. The sedimentation slows down for a period, due to the packing of the cells at the bottom of the tube.

### Factors Influencing the Sedimentation Rate

1. Room temperature: If the room temperature is raised, the sedimentation rate is likewise raised.

2. Vertical tube: If the tube is inclined, the cells sink to its lower edges and gradually slide down the tube. The result is an increased rate of sedimentation.

3. Tube bore: The internal bore of the tube is standardized at 2.5 mm; a smaller diameter retards the sedimentation rate.

4. The apparatus must be clean.

5. The blood used for the test must be set up within 2 hours of its collection.

6. Hemolyzed blood is unsuitable for the test.

7. Blood containing any trace of coagulation is also unsuitable.

8. The effects of anemia: The sedimentation rate is raised in most anemias, with the exception of sickle cell anemia, in which the sedimentation rate is normal. This is due to the low oxygen tension which

induces sickling. By bubbling oxygen through the blood prior to setting up the test, this effect can be eliminated.

Blood is collected in an anticoagulant that produces little alteration in cell size. The sedimentation tube is filled and allowed to stand in a vertical position. There are two main methods of recording sedimentation rates: (a) by the time taken for the cells to settle to a certain arbitrary distance, or (b) by the degree of sedimentation taking place in a given time. The latter method is generally used. The rate of fall depends on the method employed.

### Wintrobe's Method[1]

#### Reagents and Apparatus
1. Wintrobe tube: This is a thick-walled tube, 120 mm long, having an internal diameter of 2.5 mm. The tube is graduated from 0 to 100 millimeters.
2. Anticoagulated blood: Either balanced oxalates of EDTA can be used (see p. 2).
3. Long-stemmed Pasteur pipet
4. Sedimentation rack

#### Method
1. The venous anticoagulated blood is mixed well and the Wintrobe tube is filled to the zero mark, using the Pasteur pipet.
2. The tube is allowed to stand in a vertical position for exactly 1 hour at room temperature.
3. The distance the red cell meniscus has fallen in 1 hour is recorded as the sedimentation rate.

#### Normal Values
Male—4 to 7-mm fall in 1 hour
Female—5 to 10-mm fall in 1 hour

#### Notes
1. Care should be taken to avoid air bubbles in the sedimentation tube. The Pasteur pipet should be placed at the bottom of the tube and pressure gradually reduced on the bulb of the pipet. It is slowly raised and the pressure adjusted so that the tube is filled without bubbles or frothing.
2. The main advantage of Wintrobe's method is that a macrohematocrit determination can be carried out by centrifuging the blood for 30 minutes at 3,000 rpm.
3. Wintrobe and Landsberg originally observed that the sedimentation rate can be corrected for anemia, and a correction chart was devised. The main disadvantage of using such a chart is that the results are often overcorrected; such corrections are now seldom used.

4. The test is nonspecific, the sedimentation rate being increased in all conditions in which tissue destruction and inflammation are present. This makes the test a useful guide in assessing the progress and the value of treatment of a disease, and is especially useful in following the conditions or rheumatoids and of tuberculosis patients.

5. The sedimentation rate remains constant for up to 2 hours at room temperature. All determinations should be started within this time after drawing the blood.

## Westergren's Method[2]

### Reagents and Apparatus

1. Westergren pipet. This is a thick-walled pipet, 300 mm long, having an internal diameter of 2.5 mm. It is graduated from 0 to 200 in millimeters.

2. Anticoagulated blood: 1 volume of 3.8% sodium citrate is added to 9 volumes of venous blood.

3. Westergren stand

### Method

1. A Westergren pipet is filled by pipeting anticoagulated blood by mouth to the zero mark.

2. The tube is clamped in a vertical stand and left for exactly 1 hour at room temperature.

3. The distance the red cell meniscus falls in that time is recorded as the sedimentation rate.

### Normal Values

> Male   —0 to 9-mm fall in one hour
> Female—0 to 20-mm fall in one hour

*Note.* The normal sedimentation rate is less in this method than in the Wintrobe technique, despite the longer tube used.

## Landau Micro Method[3]

### Reagents and Apparatus

1. Landau-Adams Tube: This tube resembles a red cell Thoma pipet, having a capillary stem 50 mm in length, which is graduated in millimeters. A small rubber bulb is fitted onto the end of the pipet, allowing capillary blood to be drawn into the stem.

2. 5% Sodium citrate

3. Capillary blood

4. Landau-Adams stand

**Method**

1. 5% Sodium citrate is slowly drawn into the stem of the pipet to the first line marked, using the rubber bulb.

2. Capillary blood is drawn into the pipet in the same manner until the fluid reaches the upper mark.

3. The external surface of the pipet is wiped clean of blood and the anticoagulant and blood mixture is slowly drawn up into the bulb of the pipet.

4. The contents of the pipet are mixed in the bulb and transferred back into its stem, adjusting the upper level of the diluted blood so that it coincides with the zero graduation.

5. The end of the pipet is closed with the thumb, the rubber suction bulb is removed, and the pipet is placed in a vertical position in the Landau-Adams stand.

6. It is left for 1 hour at room temperature and the distance the red cell meniscus falls in that time is recorded.

**Normal Values**

Males —0 to 5-mm fall in one hour

Female—0 to 20-mm fall in one hour

**Notes**

1. Care should be taken to avoid the introduction of air bubbles into the stem of the pipet.

2. This micro method is of particular value in children and arthritic patients in whom difficulty may be met in obtaining venous blood.

**Zetafuge**

*Principle.* The Zetafuge is a device which implements a new approach to sedimentation rate analysis. When the apparatus is in operation, a low centrifugal force is applied to a tube containing a blood sample. This force causes the red cells to migrate across the diameter of the tube toward the outer wall where rouleaux formation is accelerated.

After the centrifugal force has been applied for 45 seconds, the Zetafuge stops, the sample tube is rotated 180° and the apparatus restarts. During the second cycle, centrifugal force removes the red cell rouleaux from what is now the inner wall of the capillary tube. The rouleaux are partially dispersed, move across the diameter of the tube and reform on the opposite wall. Each time the rouleaux traverses the tube diameter, they sediment gently toward the bottom of the tube as a result of the downward force of gravity. After four 45-second cycles, the Zetafuge stops. The Zeta sedimentation ratio is expressed as a percentage, and is determined by a comparison of the zetacrit per cent to the hematocrit per cent.

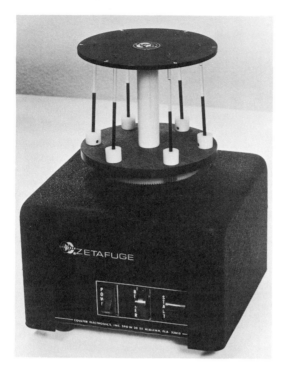

FIG. 7-1. The Zetafuge. (Courtesy of Coulter Electronics, Inc., Hialeah, Fla.)

### Reagents and Apparatus

1. Capillary tube*—75 mm (internal diameter 2.0 mm, external diameter 2.3 mm).
2. Zetafuge
3. EDTA anticoagulated blood

### Method

1. Fill the capillary tube approximately 3/4 full with anticoagulated blood. (A mark on each tube designates the amount of blood to be used.)
2. Plug one end of each tube with clay to a depth of approximately 5 mm.
3. Place the tubes immediately into the spin plate. If less than 6 samples are to be processed, place the sample tubes into the unit so that a balanced condition exists (tubes should be placed 180° apart).
4. Push the power switch up to turn the Zetafuge on. The switch will light to indicate that power is applied.
5. Start the unit by depressing the Start switch. As the plate spins, the

---

* Available from Coulter Diagnostics, Inc.

speed indicator will move to a horizontal position, indicating that the motor is turning at full speed.

6. The buzzer setting is at the option of the operator. It is set by pushing the buzzer switch up. The switch will light to indicate that the buzzer is set. When the complete cycle has finished, the unit will stop and the buzzer will sound. The buzzer will remain set for the next cycle, however, unless the switch is returned to the Down position.

7. Read or mark the tubes immediately.

*Calculation*

1. For the Zeta Sedimentation Ratio (ZSR) to be calculated, the hematocrit of the sample must be determined.

2. The ZSR can be most easily determined using conventional hematocrit readers. After obtaining a packed cell volume (hematocrit) the ZSR is calculated from the formula:

$$\frac{\text{True hematocrit \%} \times 100}{\text{Zetacrit \%}} = \text{ZSR\%}$$

*Normal.* 40 to 51% (for both sexes)

Values between 51 to 54% are considered doubtful; 55 to 59% mildly elevated; 60 to 64% moderately elevated; and over 65% markedly elevated.

## DETECTION OF HETEROPHIL ANTIBODIES

### Presumptive Test[4]

*Principle.* The serum of patients with infectious mononucleosis agglutinates sheep cells in high titers. Antibodies against sheep cells are normally present at titers of up to 1:56, but in cases of severe infectious mononucleosis, the titer can rise to 1:2,000.

*Reagents and Apparatus*

1. 2% Suspension of washed sheep cells—1 to 7 days old.

2. Normal saline

3. Patient's inactivated serum. The serum is incubated at 56°C for 30 minutes to destroy complement.

4. Tubes—13 x 100 mm

5. Graduated pipet—1 ml

*Method*

1. Twelve tubes are set up as in Table 7-1.

2. Each tube is shaken, incubated at 37°C for 2 hours, and *gently* reshaken to resuspend the sheep cells. The highest dilution of serum showing agglutination is recorded as the titer.

*Normal.* 1:7 to 1:56

TABLE 7-1. Serum Dilutions for Detection of Heterophil Antibodies
by the Presumptive Test.

| TUBE | SALINE (ML) | PATIENT'S SERUM | SHEEP CELLS (ML) | SERUM DILUTION |
|------|-------------|-----------------|------------------|----------------|
| 1 | 0.8 | 0.2 | 0.2 | 1:7 |
| 2 | 0.5 | 0.5 from total of tube 1 | 0.2 | 1:14 |
| 3 | 0.5 | 0.5 from total of tube 2 | 0.2 | 1:28 |
| 4 | 0.5 | 0.5 from total of tube 3 | 0.2 | 1:56 |
| 5 | 0.5 | 0.5 from total of tube 4 | 0.2 | 1:112 |
| 6 | 0.5 | 0.5 from total of tube 5 | 0.2 | 1:224 |
| 7 | 0.5 | 0.5 from total of tube 6 | 0.2 | 1:448 |
| 8 | 0.5 | 0.5 from total of tube 7 | 0.2 | 1:896 |
| 9 | 0.5 | 0.5 from total of tube 8 | 0.2 | 1:1,792 |
| 10 | 0.5 | 0.5 from total of tube 9 | 0.2 | 1:3,584 |
| 11 | 0.5 | 0.5 from total of tube 10 | 0.2 | 1:7,168 |
| 12 | 0.5 | 0 | 0.2 | Control |

Discard 0.5 ml from total of tube 11 before adding the sheep cells.

### Notes

1. The presumptive test for heterophil antibodies is nonspecific.

2. Centrifugation of the tubes after the incubation period produces false-positive results, due to mechanical adhesion of the red cells.

3. In the presence of clinical and hematological findings suggestive of infectious mononucleosis, a titer of 1:224 or higher can be interpreted as confirming the diagnosis. In this disease, positive heterophils almost always appear during the first two weeks of illness.

### Differential Absorption Test[5]

*Principle.* The Forssman antibody present in the serum of normal persons is completely absorbed by tissues containing the Forssman antigen. Examples of such tissues are guinea pig kidney and horse kidney. The antibody is only partially absorbed by ox cells. The antibody commonly found in infectious mononucleosis is not absorbed to the same extent by the Forssman antigen but is taken up by the ox cells. Heterophil antibodies in high titer are also found in serum sickness, but can be differentiated from those of infectious mononucleosis and from the Forssman antibody by the fact that they are absorbed by both Forssman antigens and ox cells.

### Reagents and Apparatus
1. Sheep cells as in the presumptive test
2. Guinea pig kidney antigen: 20% guinea pig kidney antigen is obtained commercially or prepared by the following technique:

The capsules and fat are stripped from 2 pairs of kidneys and washed in running water. The tissue is placed in a sieve partly immersed in normal saline and ground through the mesh with a pestle. The mashed tissue is autoclaved at 15 lb pressure for 20 minutes, resieved twice and centrifuged; 1 volume of packed tissue is suspended in 4 volumes of 0.5% phenol.

3. 20% ox cell antigen: Commercially obtained or prepared by the following technique:

Ox cells are washed 3 times in saline and a 30% suspension is autoclaved at 15 lb pressure for 20 minutes. The cells are allowed to cool to room temperature, filtered through gauze, and the hematocrit adjusted to 20% with normal saline. An equal volume of 1% phenol in saline is added to give a final 10% suspension.

4. Patient's inactivated serum: The serum is incubated at 56°C for 30 minutes to destroy complement.

5. Normal saline
6. Tubes—13 × 100 mm
7. Graduated pipets—1 ml

### Method
1. 0.2 ml-Volumes of inactivated patient's serum are added to 2 tubes containing 0.8 ml of guinea pig kidney and 0.8 ml of ox cells, respectively.

2. The contents of the tubes are mixed well and allowed to stand at room temperature for 3 minutes, centrifuged at 1,500 rpm for 3 minutes. The supernatant fluids are transferred to 2 clean tubes labeled "absorbed guinea pig kidney" and "absorbed ox cells."

3. Two rows of 10 tubes each are placed in a rack and doubling dilutions, 1 set for each absorption, are set up as in Table 7-2.

4. The tubes are shaken to mix, allowed to stand for 2 hours at 37°C and *gently* reshaken to resuspend the sheep cells. The highest dilution of absorbed serum showing agglutination is recorded as the titer.

### Results
1. The antibody in normal serum is completely absorbed by exposure to guinea pig kidney and only partially absorbed by exposure to ox cells.

2. In serum sickness, treatment with guinea pig kidney and ox cells completely absorbs the antibody.

TABLE 7-2. Serum Dilutions for Detection of Heterophil Antibodies
by the Differential Absorption Test.

| TUBE | SALINE (ML) | ABSORBED SERUM (ML) | SHEEP CELLS (ML) | SERUM DILUTION |
|------|-------------|---------------------|------------------|----------------|
| 1 | — | 0.25 | 0.1 | 1:7 |
| 2 | 0.25 | 0.25 | 0.1 | 1:14 |
| 3 | 0.25 | 0.25 from total of tube 2 | 0.1 | 1:28 |
| 4 | 0.25 | 0.25 from total of tube 3 | 0.1 | 1:56 |
| 5 | 0.25 | 0.25 from total of tube 4 | 0.1 | 1:112 |
| 6 | 0.25 | 0.25 from total of tube 5 | 0.1 | 1:224 |
| 7 | 0.25 | 0.25 from total of tube 6 | 0.1 | 1:448 |
| 8 | 0.25 | 0.25 from total of tube 7 | 0.1 | 1:896 |
| 9 | 0.25 | 0.25 from total of tube 8 | 0.1 | 1:1,792 |
| 10 | 0.25 | 0.25 from total of tube 9 | 0.1 | 1:3,584 |

Discard 0.25 ml from total volume of tube 10 before adding the sheep cells.

3. In infectious mononucleosis, the antibody is completely absorbed by ox cells and will show a minimum 3 tube drop in titer when compared to the unabsorbed serum.

*Notes*

1. The sheep cells used should be 1 to 7 days old.

2. The test is between 80 to 90% accurate and will detect antibodies by the twenty-first day of the disease. These antibodies will persist in the patient's serum for as long as 4 to 5 months.

3. When investigating a suspected case of infectious mononucleosis, the technologist should remember that atypical mononuclear cells are frequently seen in the peripheral blood before the heterophil titer becomes abnormal, and that the cells disappear from the blood before the titer reverts to the normal range.

4. The Forssman antibody present reacts against a common antigen in animal tissues. These antibodies can be stimulated by injecting a guinea pig kidney emulsion into rabbits, the resulting antibody reacting with tissues from horses, dogs, cats and mice, but not with human red cells or with those from oxen or rats.

5. The results obtained by differentially absorbing the antibody are sometimes manifested as hemolysins instead of agglutinins, if complement is present.

6. The heterophil antibody is of the warm type, better agglutination being observed when the test is incubated at 37°C instead of at the frequently suggested temperature of 20°C.

7. The varying degree of sensitivity of the sheep cells used causes fluctuation in the day-to-day reproducibility of the test.

8. The serum dilutions of the tubes in the differential absorption should be explained. In tube 1, 0.25 ml of absorbed serum and 0.1 ml of sheep cells are added together. The initial dilution of the serum was 0.2 ml in a total volume of 1 ml (0.8 + 0.2); there is 0.05 ml of serum in 0.25 ml of diluted serum, and 0.05 ml of serum in a total volume of 0.35 (0.25 ml of dilution + 0.1 ml of sheep cells). Thus the total serum dilution is 0.05 ml in 0.35 ml or 1:7.

## Slide Test for Heterophil Antibodies

(Monospot)*

*Principle.* The test is based on agglutination of horse red cells by the heterophil antibody of infectious mononucleosis. Since horse red cells conain both Forssman and infectious mononucleosis antigens, a differential absorption of the patient's serum is necessary to distinguish the specific heterophil antibody of infectious mononucleosis from those of the Forssman type. This is accomplished by absorbing the serum or plasma with both guinea pig kidney and beef erythrocyte stroma.

Guinea pig kidney contains only the Forssman antigen while beef red cells contain only the antigen associated with infectious mononucleosis. Therefore, guinea pig kidney will absorb only heterophil antibodies of the Forssman type while beef red cells will absorb only the heterophil antibody of infectious mononucleosis. Agglutination of horse red cells by the absorbed patient specimen is indicative of a positive reaction.

### Reagents and Apparatus

1. 11% Suspension of guinea pig kidney antigen (Reagent I) preserved with sodium azide.

2. 11% Suspension of beef red cell stroma antigen (Reagent II) preserved with sodium azide.

3. 20% Suspension of stabilized horse red cells preserved with chloromycetin and neomycin sulfate.

4. Patient's serum or plasma—EDTA, citrate, heparin, oxalate

5. Glass Monospot slides—ruled into 2 squares, I and II

6. Microcapillary pipets—10

7. Wooden applicators for mixing

8. Stopwatch.

---

* Ortho Pharmaceuticals, Raritan, N.J.

**Method**

1. Shake all of the reagent cell suspension to mix.
2. Place the Monospot slide on a flat surface under a direct light.
3. Invert the indicator horse cells several times to uniformly suspend the cells, and deliver 10 λ of cells to one corner of both squares on the slide.
4. Place 1 drop of the guinea pig kidney antigen (Reagent I) in the center of Square I.
5. Place 1 drop of the beef red cell suspension (Reagent II) in the center of Square II.
6. Using a disposable plastic pipet, add 1 drop of the serum or plasma being tested to the center of each square on the slide.
7. Mix the patient's serum or plasma with the guinea pig kidney and beef cells on each square.
8. Using no more than 10 stirring motions, blend in the horse cells to each mixture.
9. Start a stopwatch upon completion of the final mixing.
10. Observe for agglutination for no longer than 1 minute after final mixing.

(**Note:** Do not pick up or move the slide during the reaction period.)

**Results**

1. Stronger agglutination in Square I (patient's plasma or serum, guinea pig kidney antigen, horse cells) indicates a positive result.
2. Stronger agglutination in Square II (patient's plasma or serum, beef red cells, horse cells) indicates a negative result.
3. If no agglutination appears on either side of the slide (Square I or Square II) or if agglutination is equal on both squares, the test is negative.

**Notes**

1. Because of a delayed heterophil antibody response, it is possible that clinical and hematologic symptoms of infectious mononucleosis may appear before serologic confirmation is possible.
2. False-positive results with Monospot test have been reported in patients with pancreatic carcinoma,[6] rubella,[7] and rheumatoid arthritis.[8]

## ESTIMATION OF BLOOD VOLUMES

### Radioactive Method

*Principle.* A small volume of patient's red cells is tagged with radioactive chromium and injected back into the circulation. After allowing time for the cells to become thoroughly mixed, a sample is withdrawn and the decrease in radioactivity is measured.

### Reagents and Apparatus

1. Hexavalent sodium chromate ($Cr^{51}$) as described in the Ashby Cell Survival on page 174.
2. Scintillation counter
3. Sterile ACD solution
4. Sterile graduated pipet—5 ml
5. Sterile volumetric flask—50 ml
6. Sterile graduated centrifuge tubes
7. Sterile syringes—20 ml
8. Microhematocrit centrifuge
9. Hematocrit capillary tubes
10. Volumetric flask—100 ml
11. Saponin

### Method

1. 15 ml of patient's whole blood is added to 5 ml of sterile ACD solution.
2. 50 ml of hexavalent sodium chromate is added to the blood and the solution is mixed by inversion and allowed to stand at room temperature for 30 minutes. The cells are washed 3 times in sterile saline to remove the unattached $Cr^{51}$.
3. Sufficient saline is added to the red cell button to make the volume up to 25 ml, 20 ml of which is injected intravenously into the patient's arm.
4. The labeled red cells are allowed to equilibrate throughout the circulation for 20 to 30 minutes, and 5 to 10 ml of blood is collected from the vein in the other arm. The blood is anticoagulated with EDTA.
5. The hematocrit of the postinjected blood is determined by the method described on page 73.
6. 1 ml of the noninjected red cell residue from 3 is diluted to 100 ml with distilled water.
7. 1 ml of the postinjection blood sample from 4 is hemolyzed by the addition of saponin (the amount on a knife point), and the radioactivity of both the noninjected and the postinjection blood is measured with the scintillation counter.

### Calculation

1. The red cell volume is calculated from the following:

$$\frac{\text{Hematocrit} \times \text{radioactivity of standard in counts/min/ml} \times \text{dilution of standard} \times \text{volume in ml injected}}{100 \times \text{radioactivity of postinjected sample}}$$

2. The total blood volume is calculated from the following:

$$\frac{\text{Red cell volume} \times 100}{\text{Hematocrit}}$$

3. The total plasma volume is calculated from the following: Total blood volume − red cell volume = plasma volume.

### Evans Blue Dye Method[9]

*Principle.* Evans blue dye (T-184a) is bound up with serum albumin after injection and is quantitatively estimated by a colorimetric method.

#### Reagents and Apparatus

1. Evans blue dye: 75 mg of Evans blue dye is dissolved in 100 ml of saline, and 4 ampules, each containing 25 ml of the dilution, are autoclaved at 15 lb pressure for 15 minutes.
2. Spectrophotometer
3. Centrifuge
4. Sterile syringes—20 ml
5. Micropipets—0.05 ml
6. Graduated pipets—10 ml

#### Method

1. 20 ml of patient's blood is heparinized and centrifuged at 2,000 rpm for 10 minutes.
2. 20 ml of a sterile saline dilution of Evans blue is injected intravenously into the patient's arm.
3. 10 ml of patient's blood is taken into a heparinized syringe 15 minutes later from a vein in the other arm.
4. A second sample of blood is collected 30 minutes after the original injection and both blood samples are centrifuged at 2,000 rpm for 10 minutes immediately after collection.
5. A standard dye solution is prepared by adding 0.05 ml of Evans blue to a 7.45-ml sample of patient's preinjected plasma.
6. The dye concentrations are read spectrophotometrically at a wavelength of 620 nm, using the preinjected plasma in 1 as a blank.

#### Calculation

1. Dye concentration of sample 1 is calculated from the following:

$$\frac{\text{Optical density of plasma at 15 min} \times 100}{97.5}$$

2. Dye concentration of sample 2 is calculated from the following:

$$\frac{\text{Optical density of plasma at 30 min} \times 100}{95}$$

3. The concentrations of 1 and 2 are averaged.
4. The plasma volume in milliliters is determined by the following:

$$\frac{\text{Vol of dye injected} \times \text{optical density of stnd. dye} \times \text{dilution of stnd.}}{\text{Average concentration of dye postinjection (3 above)}}$$

*Notes*
1. The above technique is difficult to carry out accurately. One of the practical difficulties is the deep blue color of the dye, which makes it hard to achieve accurate measurement in the syringe.
2. Dye measurements are best determined on fasting patients, because a control on the opacity of the plasma is made possible.
3 In most cases, there is a close correlation between peripheral blood volumes and red cell volumes, but there are occasionally discrepancies if the plasma volume is reduced or increased disproportionately.
4. The measurement of red cell volume is useful in the diagnosis of polycythemia, in which an increase in the cell mass is of diagnostic value, in the investigation of obscure anemic conditions, and in investigating the effects of large blood losses on the circulation.

## CEREBROSPINAL FLUID CELL COUNTS

*Reagents and Apparatus*
1. Diluting fluid:
      Methyl violet crystals........................ 0.2
      Glacial acetic acid ........................ 10 ml
      Distilled water ........................... 90 ml
The fluid is filtered before use.
2. White cell Thoma pipet
3. Improved Neubauer hemocytometer or Fuchs-Rosenthal hemocytometer

*Method*
1. Diluting fluid is pipeted to the 1 mark on the Thoma pipet.
2. Spinal fluid is drawn up to the 11 mark on the pipet and the pipet is shaken well to mix the dilution. The first few drops of fluid are expelled by vigorously shaking the pipet.

3. The hemocytometer is filled in the way described on page 50, and the cells are allowed to settle for 5 minutes at room temperature in a moist chamber.

4. All the cells seen in the entire counting chamber are counted.

*Note.* It is desirable to use a magnification of about 200× to determine the count.

### Calculation

1. Using improved Neubauer hemocytometer:

The dimensions of the ruled area are 3 × 3 mm = 9 sq mm.

The depth of the chamber is 0.1 mm. Thus the total volume of fluid within the ruled area is 3 × 3 × 0.1 mm = 0.9 cu mm.

If 22 cells are counted in the total volume of 0.9 cu mm, the total number of cells in 1 cu mm of diluted fluid is 22/9. But because there is a 1.1 dilution of spinal fluid in the pipet, there are 22/0.9 (1.1) cells in 1 cu mm of undiluted fluid (i.e., 27 cells per cu mm). Multiply the number of cells counted in the entire ruled area by 1.22 to calculate the number of cells per cubic millimeter of fluid.

2. Using the Fuchs-Rosenthal hemocytometer:

The dimensions of the ruled area are 4 × 4 mm = 16 sq mm.

The depth of the chamber is 0.2 mm. Thus the total volume of fluid within the ruled area is 4 × 4 mm × 0.2 mm = 3.2 cu mm. If 42 cells are counted in the total volume of 3.2 cu mm, the total number of cells in 1 cu mm of diluted fluid is 42/3.2. But because there is a 1.1 dilution of spinal fluid in the pipet, there are 42/3.2 × 1.1 cells in 1 cu mm of undiluted fluid (i.e., 14 cells per cu mm). Multiply the number of cells counted in the entire ruled area by 0.34 to calculate the number of cells per cubic millimeter of fluid.

## Alternative Method (on Purulent Fluids When the White Count Is Greatly Increased)

### Reagents and Apparatus

1. 0.1N Hydrochloric acid at 2% acetic acid
2. White cell Thoma pipet
3. Improved Neubauer hemocytometer

### Method

1. A 1:10 or a 1:20 dilution of spinal fluid is made with 0.1N hydrochloric acid.

2. The 4 corner squares (1 × 1 mm) are scanned and the cells counted in this area.

3. A differential count is carried out by first centrifuging the spinal fluid and making thin smears of the sediment.

4. Proceed to stain and count the cells as in a routine white cell differential count.

### Calculation

Report differential in percentage based on the total number of cells counted. For example, 15 cells counted in 9 cu mm, of which 8 were neutrophils and 7 lymphocytes

$$\frac{8 \times 100}{15} = \quad \begin{array}{l} 53\% \text{ neutrophils} \\ 47\% \text{ lymphocytes} \end{array}$$

## INVESTIGATION OF $B_{12}$ ABSORPTION[10]

*Principle.* Vitamin $B_{12}$ is tagged with radioactive $Co^{57}$ and given orally to the patient. Urine and fecal $B_{12}$ extraction is estimated and the proportion of $B_{12}$ absorbed can be calculated.

### Reagents and Apparatus
1. Well-type scintillation counter
2. $Co^{57}$ $B_{12}$

### Method
1. 1 $\mu$g of $Co^{57}$ $B_{12}$ is given orally to a fasting patient.
2. A sample of this cobalt is kept as a standard.
3. All feces passed subsequent to the administration of the $B_{12}$ are collected and their radioactivity measured in a scintillation counter. Collection is carried out for 4 days or until less than 2% of the radioactive dose appears in a 24-hour sample.
4. The percentage of the dose absorbed is calculated from the following:

$$\% \text{ absorbed} = \frac{\text{counts/minute standard} - \text{counts/minute feces} \times 100}{\text{counts/minute standard}}$$

*Normal.* Greater than 0.45 $\mu$g

### Notes
1. Patients with pernicious anemia or intestinal malabsorption absorb less than 0.2 to 0.3 $\mu$g. These two conditions can be separated by adding to the radioactive tagged $B_{12}$ 100 mg of concentrated hog's stomach as a source of intrinsic factor. Under these conditions, patients having pernicious anemia absorb normal quantities of $B_{12}$.

2. A urinary excretion technique can be used in place of the fecal extraction. The method is similar, except that 1,000 $\mu$g of intramuscular nonradioactive $B_{12}$ is given in addition to the radioactive dose. Urine is collected over one 24-hour period only. The percentage of radioactive $B_{12}$ excreted in the urine is calculated from the following:

$$\frac{\text{Total counts/minute in 24-hour urine sample} \times 100}{\text{counts/minute in standard}}$$

4. Normal excretion of $B_{12}$ is more than 15% of the test dose. In pernicious anemia, the excretion is less than 5%.

## SEPARATION OF LEUKOCYTES FOR CHEMICAL ANALYSIS[11]

*Principle.* Citrated blood is mixed with fibrinogen and allowed to sediment under gravity. The red cells settle out first, leaving a concentration of white cells and platelets.

### Reagents and Apparatus
1. Bovine fibrinogen commercially obtained
2. Citrated blood
3. Tube—13 × 100 mm
4. Centrifuge

### Method
1. 20 ml of fresh citrated blood is added to a saline solution of fibrinogen so that the hematocrit is between 30 and 35% and the fibrinogen level approximates 7 mg per ml.
2. The head of foam is carefully removed from the blood-fibrinogen mixture and is allowed to stand for 30 minutes at room temperature.
3. The supernatant plasma, which is rich in platelets and white cells, is pipeted off and centrifuged at 1,000 rpm for 3 minutes.
4. The supernatant plasma is removed and the leukocytes resuspended in normal saline.
5. All tests should be carried out in duplicate and negative and positive controls should be included with each test. The latter may consist of immune rabbit serum if positive human serum is unavailable.

As a further control, the serum under test should be added to a red cell suspension from the leukocyte donor to exclude antigens common to red cells and leukocytes.

## DEMONSTRATION OF LEUKOAGGLUTININS

### Method 1

*Principle*. Defibrinated whole blood and PVP are mixed and allowed to stand, to separate the red cells from the white cells and the platelets. The white cell suspension is added to the inactivated test serum, and later examined for the presence of white cell agglutination.

#### Reagents and Apparatus
1. Defibrinated blood
2. Polyvinylpyrrolidone (PVP)
3. Patient's serum inactivated at 56°C for 30 minutes
4. 1% Acetic acid
5. 37°C and 56°C Waterbaths
6. Glass beads
7. Erlenmeyer flask—100 ml
8. Graduated pipet  5 ml
9. Micropipet—0.1 ml
10. Tube—10 × 75 mm

#### Method
1. 30 ml of normal whole blood is defibrinated with glass beads by gently swirling in an Erlenmeyer flask for 5 to 10 minutes.
2. 4 ml of PVP is added to 20 ml of the defibrinated blood and is mixed and allowed to stand at 37°C in a stoppered tube.
3. 0.1 ml of inactivated serum is added to 0.05 ml of the supernatant leukocyte suspension harvested from 2 in a tube (10 × 75 mm). The mixture is incubated at 37°C for 2 hours.
4. 0.1 ml of 1% acetic acid is added to the tube and the leukocytes are examined under the 10× objective as a thick drop.

*Results*. The presence of antibodies is confirmed by the presence of agglutinates of three or more white cells.

### Method 2[13]

#### Reagents and Apparatus
1. Siliconized tubes (16 mm OD) containing 1 ml 5% disodium EDTA
2. Plasmagel*
3. 37°C Waterbath
4. Siliconized Pasteur pipets
5. Centrifuge (GLC-1 Sorvall)
6. EDTA buffer
2.6 g of disodium hydrogen phosphate, 3.0 g of disodium EDTA, and

---

* Available from Laboratoire Roger Bellon, Seine, France

8.5 g sodium chloride are dissolved in distilled water and the volume made up to 1 liter.

7. Siliconized tubes—6 × 50 mm, 13 × 100 mm, 7 × 100 mm
8. Patient's serum
9. Clean glass slides

### Method

1. 10 ml of normal venous blood is collected into a siliconized tube containing EDTA.

2. 2.5 ml of Plasmagel is added to the blood and allowed to stand at room temperature for 30 minutes to allow for red cell sedimentation to occur. If the room temperature is below 22°C, allow to sediment at 37°C.

3. The white cell rich plasma and top layer of red cells are removed with a Pasteur pipet and transferred to a siliconized tube (10 × 75 mm).

4. Centrifuge at 1,000 rpm for 10 minutes and all but 0.1 ml of the supernatant plasma is removed and placed in a tube (13 × 100 mm).

5. This platelet-rich plasma is centrifuged at 3,000 rpm for 30 minutes to obtain a platelet-poor plasma. Keep for later use.

6. The original cell button (Stage 4) is resuspended in the residual 0.1 ml of plasma, transferred to a tube (6 × 50 mm) and allowed to resediment for 20 to 30 minutes.

7. The creamy supernatant is transferred to a second tube (6 × 50 mm) and an equal amount of volume of EDTA buffer added.

8. 2.0 ml of the platelet-poor plasma (Stage 5) is placed into a tube (7 × 100 mm) and the leukocyte suspension obtained in Stage 6 layered on the top of the plasma column.

9. The suspension is centrifuged at 1,000 rpm for 2 1/2 minutes to allow the leukocytes to pass through the gradient to form a loose pellet, leaving the platelets above the column of undiluted plasma.

10. The supernatant plasma and the platelet layer are removed to about 5 mm from the bottom of the tube.

11. Resuspend the leukocytes in a diluent consisting of 1 volume EDTA buffer and 3 volumes of platelet-poor plasma.

12. A total leukocyte count is determined on the suspension and the concentration adjusted to approximately 6,000 cells/mm$^3$ with the diluent.

13. 0.02 ml of the patient's serum is placed in a tube (6 × 50 mm).

14. One drop of leukocyte suspension is added with a Pasteur pipet, making sure that the drops are delivered directly into the serum.

15. Mix each tube and incubate at room temperature for 2 hours.

16. With a Pasteur pipet remove the leukocytes to a clean slide and examine for agglutination at 400×.

*Notes*

1. Leukoagglutinins are frequently found as a result of the transfusion of large volumes of blood, especially in disorders such as aplastic anemia and leukemia.

2. The continual transfusion of whole blood and white cells induces an antigen antibody reaction promoted by the white cells; it is known that specific blood groups are present in these cells.

3. Leukocyte antibodies have also been reported in the serum of patients with Hodgkin's disease, disseminated lupus erythematosus and paroxysmal nocturnal hemoglobinuria.

4. The demonstration of leukoagglutinins has practical importance in the investigation of suspected transfusion reactions and in determining the pathogenesis of leukopenic conditions.

## DETERMINATION OF BLOOD VISCOSITY[14]

*Principle.* The time required for a heparinized blood sample to pass between two points of a capillary glass bulb is compared with the time required for distilled water.

### Reagents and Apparatus
1. Viscosimeter: The apparatus consists of a U-shaped capillary tube with one arm approximately 3 inches long and a second arm about 1 inch in length. The end of the longer arm is funnel shaped, enabling blood to be introduced into the tube. The short arm contains a bulb with a mark directly under it (1) and a second mark (2) directly above it.
2. Heparinized venous blood
3. Stopwatch

### Method
1. 5 ml of venous heparinized blood is added through the funnel opening of the capillary stem.
2. The time required for the blood to travel from mark 1 to mark 2 on either side of the bulb is recorded.
3. Steps 1 and 2 are repeated, using distilled water in place of the blood.

*Results.* The viscosity of the blood is expressed as a ratio of the blood movement time to that of distilled water.

*Normal.* The viscosity of blood is normally 4.8 to 5.2 times that of distilled water.

*Note.* Blood viscosity is increased in congestive heart failure. Other conditions which can produce an increased viscosity are polycythemia,

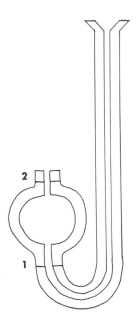

FIG. 7-2. Denning viscosimeter.

lymphatic leukemia, diabetes mellitus, multiple myeloma, pneumonia and myeloid leukemia. Dehydration raises the viscosity by 25 to 30%.

## CHROMOSOMAL CULTURES OF BLOOD AND BONE MARROW[15]

*Principle.* Blood or bone marrow specimens are cultured in a tissue-culturing medium, thus allowing cell division to continue but to be stopped in the metaphase by the addition of colchicine. The cells are then harvested, fixed, stained and the chromosomes photographed. The photographs of the chromosomes are arranged in corresponding pairs.

### Reagents and Apparatus
   1. Sterile whole blood
   2. Sterile culture medium:

|  | *ml* |
|---|---|
| TC 199 Medium* | 7 |
| Phytohemagglutinin M* | 0.1 |
| Autologous sterile plasma | 2 |
| Penicillin (10,000 units per ml) | 0.1 |
| Streptomycin (10 mg per ml) | 0.05 |

* Available from Difco Laboratories, Detroit, Mich.

3. 37°C incubator
4. Centrifuge
5. Graduated sterile pipets—10 ml
6. Graduated sterile pipets—1 ml
7. Sterile micropipets—0.1 ml
8. Sterile micropipets—0.05 ml
9. Heparin (1,000 units per ml)—phenol-free
10. Sterile tubes
11. Colchicine (5 mg. per ml; Colcemid)*
12. 0.37% Sodium citrate
13. Carnoy's fluid:
    50 ml of glacial acetic acid
   150 ml of methyl alcohol
14. Giemsa stain:
    2 ml of stock (p. 111)
    50 ml of distilled water
15. Sterile syringes   10 ml
16. Pasteur pipets
17. Acid-clean slides:

Soak the slides in chromic acid cleaning mixture. Wash in copious volumes of tap water and rinse in distilled water. Store in distilled water in the refrigerator.

### Method (Blood)

1. 10 ml of sterile venous blood is added to 0.1 ml of heparin in a sterile tube. It is allowed to stand at room temperature for 2 hours for the white cell-rich plasma to separate.

2. 1 ml of the plasma is removed with a sterile pipet and added to a culture bottle containing the sterile culture media.

3. The culture is incubated at 37°C for 72 hours.

4. 0.15 ml of colchicine (5 mg per ml) is added to arrest the cell division.

5. Centrifuge at 700 rpm for 5 minutes and discard the supernatant, using a Pasteur pipet.

6. Add slowly, shaking continuously, 4 ml of 0.37% sodium citrate. Gently resuspend the cells with a Pasteur pipet and leave at room temperature for 20 minutes.

7. Centrifuge at 500 rpm for 5 minutes and discard the supernatant, using a Pasteur pipet.

8. Slowly add 5 ml of fresh Carnoy's fluid, shaking the tube constantly. Resuspend the cells during this process. Leave at room temperature for 10 minutes.

---

* Available from Ciba Pharmaceuticals, Summit, N.J.

9. Repeat steps 7 and 8 at least twice.

10. Centrifuge at 500 rpm for 5 minutes after the addition of the last Carnoy's fluid. Discard all the supernatant and resuspend the cells in 1 ml of Carnoy's fluid.

11. Drain the distilled water from the prepared slides, add 2 drops of the fixed cell suspension from 10 to the slide, blow hard directly onto the slide, flame quickly and allow to dry.

12. Stain with Giemsa stain for 15 minutes.

13. Rinse in tap water for 2 to 3 seconds.

14. Rinse in distilled water (pH 6.8) for 5 seconds.

15. Allow to dry overnight and mount.

### Method (Bone Marrow)

1. 0.5 ml of bone marrow is added to the culture media as in 2 above.

2. The culture is incubated at 37°C for 8 to 12 hours.

3. Steps 4 through 15 are carried out as in the blood preparation.

**Results.** There are 22 pairs of autosomes and 2 sex chromosomes in human somatic cells. The chromosomes are arranged serially in descending order according to their lengths. They are classified and distinguished, according to the relative position of their centromeres, under seven major group headings. The centromere is the nonstaining part of the chromosome. Its position may be median (mesocentric) or near the end (acrocentric) of the chromosome.

### Notes

1. Cells capable of mitosis, obtained from peripheral blood white cells, are mainly lymphocytes. It has been postulated that phytohemagglutinin acts as a stimulus to mitosis, and that this stimulus may be related to its property as an antigen.

2. Immature cells from leukemic peripheral blood do not appear to depend on the action of phytohemagglutinin for enhancement of mitosis. It has been found that the percentage of abnormal cells in mitosis increases when leukemic cells are cultured without phytohemagglutinin.

## THE EFFECTS OF DRUGS ON HEMATOLOGY RESULTS[16]

*Red Cell Counts and Hemoglobin Determinations.* Over 50 different drugs or drug groups are known to cause anemia; they include aminosalicylic acid, chloramphenicol, mepacrine, acetophenazine maleate, amphotericin B, nitrites, novobiocin, oleandomycin, penicillin, phenylbutazone, phenobarbital, radioactive agents, sulfonamides, thiocyanates, excessive vitamin A, and prolonged use of mercurial diuretics.

*Leukocytes.* Elevated total white counts have been reported due to barbiturates, atropine, erythromycin, and streptomycin, etc.

Eosinophilias have been reported due to aminosalicylic acid, ampicillin, cephalothin, cloxacillin, digitalis, epinephrine, gold compounds, hydantoin derivatives, iodides, kanamycin, methicillin, methyldopa, etc.

Leukopenia has been reported resulting from the administration of over 90 different drugs: they include antineoplastic agents, bismuth, chloramphenicol, corticosteroids, furosemide, gold compounds, hydralazine, indandione derivatives, mefenamic acid, mepacrine, mercurial diuretics, methocarbamol, oleandomycin, oxacillin, paraldehyde, phenylbutazone, pyrazole derivatives, quinine, radioactive agents, ristocetin, sulfonamides, thiazide diuretics, and the prolonged use of vitamin A.

*Platelets.* Drug-induced thrombocytosis is rare. Thrombocytopenia has been reported due to the action of the following drugs: amphotericin B, antimony compounds, antineoplastic agents, arsenicals, chloramphenicol, gold salts, mefenamic acid, methyldopa, phenylbutazone, quinidine sulfate, quinine, salicylates, smallpox vaccine, oral hypoglycemic agents, ristocetin, etc.

*Bleeding Time.* Elevated bleeding times can be the result of dextran, pantothenyl alcohol and derivatives, and streptokinase-streptodornase administration.

*Coagulation Time.* Elevated times can be due to the action of anticoagulants (Dicoumarol, etc) or to the excessive use of tetracyclines. Decreased times have been reported following the administration of corticosteroids and epinephrine, etc.

*Prothrombin Time.* Increased prothrombin times can follow the administration of antibiotics, oral anticoagulants, hydroxyzine, methylthiouracil, phenyramidol, phosphorus, oral contraceptives, salicylates, sulfonamides, vitamin A, etc.

Shortened times have been reported due to the action of barbiturates, oral contraceptives, and vitamin K.

*Sedimentation Rate.* Elevated results due to drug action have incriminated dextran, methyldopa, penicillamine, trifluperidol, and vitamin A.

## QUALITY CONTROL

Accuracy and precision are two terms often misunderstood and poorly defined. Accuracy is the closeness of the test value to the true value; precision is the spread between replication or the variation within the analytic method (reproducibility). In hematological testing, the production of precise cell counts using an electronic counter cannot be used to assess accuracy unless frequent calibrations of centrifuges for centrifugal force and photometers for wavelength adjustments are made to ensure accuracy.

In any competent laboratory, range and correlation are also important. Range can be defined as the spread between the highest and lowest measurements in a series. It covers every measurement, including the outer limits which bracket all the data. Correlation is the agreement between different methods of analysis performed on a single sample expressed as a ratio.

Three basic elements are needed in the establishment of a test method to ensure accuracy and precision: calibration, standardization, and control. Calibration is the process of relating a measurement instrument to primary physical constants. Any test method should be recalibrated regularly, regardless of its simplicity. Such period recalibration is important to ensure that no changes have taken place which would invalidate the initial calibration. Standardization establishes the response of a test method to known standard materials. Standards are usually highly purified materials of known composition. Analysis of standards relates to a definite test response to an absolute empirical value.

A control is defined as a known material whose physical and chemical composition more closely resembles the unknown test specimen than the standard. It is used to challenge the test system by checking on performance of the system against known materials closely relating to the unknown. Controls whose absolute values are unknown can only measure precision and cannot measure accuracy.

### Sources of Error in Hematology

*Methods of Sampling.* There is a marked difference in blood count results obtained from capillary blood and venous blood. Massaging the finger is found to reduce the count by 5% and, when a poor venipuncture is made, the resulting blood count varies from 17 to 26% higher than the true value.

*Preservation.* Insufficient and incorrect anticoagulants and a source of hematological error. Insufficient mixing of blood with the anticoagulant is also a common fault.

*Technical Error.* Improperly calibrated spectrophotometers, inaccurate pipets, use of poor standards which have evaporated and deteriorated, unstable electrical current, and unmatched or dirty cuvets are examples of potent sources of instrumental error.

*Personal Error.* Personal errors can arise from inaccurate pipeting, inaccurate use of the spectrophotometer, incomplete mixing of the blood and solutions in the various stages of the technique, inaccurate reading of optical densities and other apparatus due to bias, fatigue or carelessness, and from inaccuracies in transcribing and recording results.

TABLE 7-3. Comparison Between a Standard[17] and a Control.

| | STANDARD | CONTROL |
|---|---|---|
| Composition | Completely known | Known with a reasonably high degree of reliability |
| Stability | Considerable | Moderate |
| Physical properties | Completely known | Closely resembles unknown specimens |
| Reactivity | Well defined | Similar to unknown specimens |
| Verification | By several different methods | By replicates of one method |
| Information yielded | Accuracy and precision under ideal conditions | Accuracy and precision under actual conditions |

**Definitions[17]**

Chance is an uncontrolled factor in all tests. Once it becomes predictable it is termed probability.

The precision of a probability estimate will depend on the size of the sample taken, and its accuracy increases as the number of tests increase. A basic mathematical tool, used for the investigation of the frequency (the number of tests producing identical results) of a set of results is the bell-shaped curve. It is constructed by making a series of measurements and plotting them with the frequency on the vertical (ordinate) and the magnitude or the horizontal (abscissa). If the graph is symmetrical it is said to follow a gaussian distribution. In such situations, the predictability of the test results for that particular set of circumstances can be calculated.

Approximately 68% of the test values will fall within ± 1 standard deviation from the mean; 95% of the values will fall between ± 2 standard deviations from the mean; 99.7% of the test values will fall between ± 3 standard deviations.

The standard deviation is defined as the degree to which test data tend to vary about the average value. Another way of expressing the test results in terms of percentage deviation from the mean is to calculate the coefficient of variation. This enables a comparison to be made between variations of methods using a common unit, percentage the coefficient of variation is calculated by dividing the mean value into the standard deviation and multiplying by 100.

Most laboratory observers incorrectly assume that test data is usually gaussian in distribution, when in fact it is skewed in form. The acuteness or asymmetrical shape of the curve is most important in the decision to use or not to use the standard formula

$$SD = \sum \frac{d^2}{n-1}$$

in calculating quality control data. If possible, a better and more accurate way of determining such data is to use a cumulative frequency calculation, which takes into account any alterations in the shape of the curve. Cumulative standard deviations are accurate only if the data are based on large numbers of determinations. In such cases, it is possible to determine where the 5th percentile and the 95th percentile estimates are (or any other percentiles) for any set of tests. Cumulative estimations are, however, difficult for the average laboratory to calculate and are best left to statisticians and computers.

## Errors Introduced by Hematological Equipment and Reagents

### Hemocytometer
1. Irregular cellular distribution in the counting chamber
2. Incorrectly setting up the hemocytometer, so that the coverslip is not forming a chamber having a depth of 0.1 mm
3. Dirty counting chamber
4. Bias in counting the cells

### Pipet
1. Dirty and inaccurately calibrated pipets
2. Contaminated diluting fluids

### Electronic Counting Apparatus
1. Inaccuracies in any autopipets used
2. Incorrect setting of the threshold and fluctuations in the electric current
3. Electronic malfunction of the equipment
4. Air leaks in the manometer or dirty mercury, both of which will produce faulty electrical contacts (Coulter counter)
5. Foaming due to saponin or detergent residue
6. Incomplete red cell hemolysis when determining white blood counts
7. Contaminated diluting fluid
8. Accumulation of cell debris and hematin in the wash valve of the counting module (SMA4)
9. Faulty alignment of the cuvet (SMA4)

10. Incorrect phasing (SMA4)
11. Poor mixing of whole blood samples (SMA4)

*Hematocrits*
1. Variation in the diameter of the capillary tube
2. Slow centrifugal speeds due to worn electrical brushes
3. High hematocrits resulting from insufficient centrifuging time
4. Improperly sealed capillary tube
5. Errors in reading the final packed cell volume
6. Poor mixing of blood sample, especially when using electronic methods (YSI apparatus)
7. Fibrin clots present in poorly mixed blood samples

*Clot Timing Procedures*
1. Removing the tube from the waterbath too quickly, resulting in a coagulation mixture cooling to room temperature
2. Failure to see fibrin formation at the correct time
3. Faulty timing devices
4. Dirty plastic cups or dirty glass tubes

## Calibration of Pipets

*Reagents and Apparatus*
1. Tuberculin syringe, well-greased
2. Analytical balance
3. Mercury
4. Thermometer
5. Small weighing bottle
6. Narrow rubber tubing—1 inch in length
7. Sahli pipets—3

*Method*
1. The rubber tubing is fitted over the end of the tuberculin syringe and the top of a Sahli pipet is attached to the other end of the tubing.
2. The weight of the weighing bottle is carefully determined to 4 decimal places.
3. Mercury is allowed to reach room temperature and the syringe-pipet assembly is held so that the pipet tip is just below the mercury meniscus.
4. The syringe plunger is slowly withdrawn until the mercury reaches the 20 cu mm mark.
5. The mercury pool is quickly removed and the mercury in the pipet is expelled into the previously weighed weighing bottle.
6. The weight of the bottle and mercury is determined.
7. The temperature of the room is determined.

*Calculation*

$$\text{Volume of mercury} = \frac{\text{weight of mercury at } T_1}{\underbrace{\text{room temperature} - \text{volume factor at } T_1}_{\text{density}}}$$

when $T_1$ is room temperature.

## Inherent Errors in Manual Counting

1. Random distribution of cells in the counting chamber conform to certain absolute theoretical distributions. The standard error of such a distribution is given by the formula $\sigma = \pm \sqrt{m}$, where m is the mean number of cells in the area. This is termed Poisson distribution.

2. In practice, $\sigma = \pm 0.92 \sqrt{m}$, but this difference is often neglected in favor of the mathematically more simple $\sigma = \pm \sqrt{m}$.

3. If a counting chamber is filled with standard particles so that the mean particle count is 400, 95% of the counts made on this suspension will be within the range of 360 to 440 (i.e., 2 standard deviations):

$$m \pm 2 \sqrt{m}$$
$$400 \pm 2 \sqrt{400} = 400 \pm 2 \times 20$$

4. In 66% of the total counts made, the number of particles will range from 380 to 420 (i.e., 1 standard deviation):

$$400 \pm \sqrt{m} = 400 \pm 20$$

5. In 99.7% of the counts made, the number of particles will range from 340 to 460 (i.e., 3 standard deviations):

$$400 \pm 3 \sqrt{m} = 400 \pm 60$$

7. One method of expressing the inherent error of a count is to calculate the coefficient of variation (V) $V = \sigma/m$. The inherent error can be reduced by counting more particles, either by determining counts in duplicate or triplicate or by increasing the total counting area under surveillance.

TABLE 7-4. Density Factors.

| TEMPERATURE °C | 1 ML OF MERCURY IN GRAMS | 1 ML OF WATER IN GRAMS |
|---|---|---|
| 20 | 13.547 | 0.9972 |
| 21 | 13.545 | 0.9970 |
| 22 | 13.543 | 0.9968 |
| 23 | 13.541 | 0.9966 |
| 24 | 13.539 | 0.9964 |
| 25 | 13.537 | 0.9961 |

8. The error of the hemocytometer should also be taken into consideration. The error of the ruled area does not normally exceed ±2%, but the manufacturing tolerance of the depth of the chamber is frequently ±5%.

The error of the chamber depth does not depend only on the manufacturing tolerance but also on the coverglass. Thin coverglasses may bend if they are pressed on the chamber; in fact, poor quality covers may already be curved.

In addition, the smallest particle of dust on the bars of the chamber can cause slight inclinations of the coverglass.

Finally, there is the risk of scratches, which can increase the already existing errors considerably.

## Methods of Checking Hematology Quality

### Replicate Testing

1. Determine a hematological test at least 11 times on the same sample of blood.
2. Calculate the mean of the 11 results.
3. From each of the results, subtract the mean calculated in 2. This is the difference d.
4. Square the differences from the mean. This is $d^2$.
5. Calculate the sum of all the squares ($\Sigma d^2$).
6. 1 standard deviation $- \pm \sqrt{\Sigma d^2/n - 1}$, where n is the number of determinations used.

### Duplicate Testing

1. Determine one hematological test in duplicate on at least 11 different samples.
2. Subtract the differences between each pair of results. This is d.
3. Square these differences. This is $d^2$.
4. Calculate the sum of all the squares ($\Sigma d^2$).
5. 1 standard deviation $= \pm \sqrt{\Sigma^2 d/2n}$, where n is the number of specimens.

### Shorthand Checking of Results

1. Hemoglobin (gm) $\times$ 3 = hematocrit (%) ± 2 (i.e., 10 $\times$ 3 = 20 ± 2). When the hemoglobin is 10 g, the hematocrit should fall between 28 and 32%.
2. Hematocrit (%) + 6 (±3) = the first two figures of the red cell count (i.e., 30 + 6 (±3) = 33 − 39). When the hematocrit is 30%, the expected total red cell count should be in the range of 3,300,000 to 3,900,000 cu mm.

*Use of Absolute Indices to Check Hemoglobin, Hematocrit and Red Cell Count*

1. Select all adult hematocrits over 36%. Make sure that the red cell counts and hemoglobins are available.

2. Determine the MCV, MCHC and MCH on at least 11 such samples.

3. Calculate the mean of each of these indices.

4. Subtract the mean from the value of each of the samples (for all 3 indices). This is value d.

5. Square the differences from the mean. This is $d^2$.

6. Calculate the sum of the squares ($\Sigma d^2$).

7. Calculate one standard deviation, as previously described on page 355, for each of the indices.

8. The MCHC should produce 1 standard deviation below 0.5. The MCH should produce 1 standard deviation below 0.7. The MCV should produce 1 standard deviation below 2.0.

Plus and minus 2 standard deviations defines the range within which 95% of replicate determinations will fall. If a test is repeated on a patient and the difference is more than 2 standard deviations between the results, there is only one chance in twenty that this difference occurred as a test variable. Conversely, if a test is repeated and the difference in results is within the calculated 2 standard deviations, there is no clinical significance in the difference.

## Moving Standard Deviations

Moving two standard deviations (M2SD) is a technique used for calculating two standard deviations derived from the sum of the differences from the mean value. This sum, when divided by the M2SD constant, gives a value that approximates the conventional ± 2 standard deviations. M2SD eliminates the need for squaring the differences from the mean value, totaling these differences, dividing by the number of tests, extracting the square root to obtain the standard deviations, and multiplying by 2 for the ± 2SD value.

### Method

1. Record the control value for the test daily for 5 days.

2. Enter, daily, the difference of the test value from the control value (d).

3. Total these differences at the end of the 5-day period (Eed)

4. Divide this total by 2 to give the ± 2SD for that week $\frac{Ed}{2}$

5. The following week, steps 1 to 3 are repeated and the total of the differences for the past two weeks calculated. This figure is divided by 2 to give the standard deviation for the last two weeks.

6. Steps 1 to 5 are continued indefinitely, producing (a) the standard deviation for any one week (b) the cumulative or moving standard deviation for that period of time.

7. The weekly and M2SD are plotted on linear graph paper. When the daily values vary too far from the mean value in either direction, an increase in the weekly 2SD will result indicating reevaluation in technique, reagents, or equipment.

TABLE 7-5. Staggered Moving Controls.

| TEST | MON | TUES | WED | THUR | FRI | SAT | SUN |
|------|-----|------|-----|------|-----|-----|-----|
| Hemoglobin gms/dl | 11.9 | 12.7 | 12.5 | 12.6 | 12.6 | | |
| RBC $\times 10^6/mm^3$ | 4.0 | 4.1 | 4.1 | 4.1 | 3.9 | | |
| WBC $\times 10^3/mm^3$ | 3.0 | 3.1 | 3.1 | 2.9 | 2.9 | | |
| Hct % | 33 | 38 | 38 | 39 | 37 | | |
| Platelets $\times 10^3/mm^3$ | 291 | 229 | 242 | 248 | 264 | | |
| Hemoglobin | | 12.9 | 12.8 | 12.9 | 12.9 | 12.9 | |
| RBC | | 4.7 | 4.6 | 4.6 | 4.6 | 4.6 | |
| WBC | Start | 11.5 | 11.7 | 11.0 | 10.2 | 9.7 | |
| Hct | → | 41 | 42 | 43 | 42 | 42 | |
| Platelets | | 342 | 380 | 380 | 387 | 374 | |
| Hemoglobin | | | 15.1 | 15.3 | 15.4 | 15.4 | 15.3 |
| RBC | | | 4.6 | 4.7 | 4.7 | 4.7 | 4.4 |
| WBC | | Start | 8.7 | 9.2 | 8.6 | 7.0 | 6.8 |
| Hct | | → | 42 | 43 | 43 | 44 | 43 |
| Platelets | | | 257 | 253 | 250 | 225 | 230 |
| Hemoglobin | 13.7 | | | 14.7 | 14.5 | 14.7 | 14.6 |
| RBC | 4.9 | | | 5.2 | 5.0 | 5.1 | 5.1 |
| WBC | 11.4 | | Start | 12.5 | 12.5 | 12.2 | 12.0 |
| Hct | 42 | | → | 43 | 43 | 43 | 42 |
| Platelets | 260 | | | 310 | 306 | 295 | 271 |
| Hemoglobin | 15.2 | 16.3 | | | 16.3 | 16.3 | 16.3 |
| RBC | 5.0 | 5.0 | | Start | 5.0 | 5.0 | 5.1 |
| WBC | 6.2 | 5.8 | | → | 7.0 | 7.0 | 6.5 |
| Hct | 46 | 45 | | | 45 | 45 | 45 |
| Platelets | 270 | 272 | | | 280 | 256 | 280 |
| Hemoglobin | 13.1 | 13.8 | 14.0 | | | 14.2 | 13.7 |
| RBC | 4.4 | 4.3 | 4.5 | | Start | 4.7 | 4.3 |
| WBC | 3.5 | 3.4 | 3.0 | | → | 4.0 | 4.0 |
| Hct | 41 | 41 | 42 | | | 42 | 41 |
| Platelets | 250 | 240 | 219 | | | 245 | 297 |
| Hemoglobin | 7.7 | 8.9 | 8.9 | 8.9 | | | 8.9 |
| RBC | 3.2 | 3.0 | 3.0 | 3.1 | | | 3.1 |
| WBC | 4.7 | 4.7 | 4.5 | 4.5 | | Start | 4.9 |
| Hct | 28 | 28 | 29 | 28 | | → | 28 |
| Platelets | 370 | 410 | 380 | 350 | | | 402 |

**Staggered Testing (Staggered Moving Controls)**

*Method*

1. Determine all routine hematology tests (except the sedimentation rate and coagulation tests) on a sample of freshly drawn EDTA anticoagulated blood. Store at 4°C.

2. On day 2, repeat the tests carried out on the first day. Obtain another sample of blood from a different individual and carry out the same set of tests. Store all samples at 4°C.

3. On day 3, repeat all tests carried out on the bloods from days 1 and 2, and obtain and test a third fresh sample from a different patient. Store all samples at 4°C.

4. Continue to test one freshly obtained blood every day, while retesting the previously tested samples for up to 5 days. At the end of the fifth set of tests, discard the first blood sample.

5. This system can be carried out over a 5- or a 7-day week in any laboratory.

6. An example of the results are shown in Table 7-5:

*Interpretation*

1. Shifts in test values are compared for the same set of blood samples. If all samples show similar trends (i.e., reduced by the same percentage), the test values are left and the calibration not adjusted (e.g., platelets usually show a drop of value between 5-10% per day).

If the test results are erratic beyond the normal standard deviations for that test, compare those remaining test values for the same day.

2. In the examples shown, hemoglobins appear approximately 1 g lower on Monday than on other days. This would indicate a miscalibration on Monday. Platelets and total white cell counts show characteristic fluctuations but generally tend to drop in value the older the blood. Despite this drawback, the values obtained from serial testing, can be used to estimate whether the drop is greater than normal, and when this is so, the necessary restandardization can be carried out.

*Information from Quality Control Worksheets*

1. The precision of the individual technologist or group of technologists can be calculated from the standard deviation.

2. The mean of any estimation, if sufficiently large samples are taken, is a guide to the normal range in any one laboratory.

3. If the average MCHC is calculated at 29.5% and 2 standard deviations equal 0.6, the precision of the work is excellent, although the average MCHC is much below that normally expected. If such results are consistent, they can be used as a guide to detect technical faults in any particular method. For example, an MCHC of 29.5% would suggest

that hemoglobins are estimated at approximately 2 g lower than the true figure or hematocrit values are about 5% high. The spectrophotometer should be checked with a series of standards, and a tachometer should be used to check the speed of the centrifuge.

4. Valuable clinical information can be obtained from accurately computed quality control worksheets. These figures can be interpreted to the clinician and evaluated so as to clarify whether a series of tests reflects a patient's true condition or whether the results are within the laboratory range of technical error. For example, if a patient is reported to have a hemoglobin drop of 1.0 g, the laboratory should be able to interpret this result in the light of its own standard deviation for the test. If one standard deviation for the test has been calculated at 0.1 g, there is a 95% chance that the patient would have a hemoglobin difference of only ±0.2 g on a repeat test. The difference of 1.0 g would be considered clinically significant.

### *Quality Control in Cellular Morphology*

Morphology, unlike a numerical calculation, is difficult to control. The reports are subjective and, therefore, hard to reproduce. The best control is to have a group of technologists, trained by the same person in the department, reporting all morphologies. Failing this, the senior technologist should review all abnormal blood smears before releasing the reports to the wards. The terms "slight," "moderate" and "marked" mean different things to different observers. All that needs to be stated about most aspects of morphology is that a particular feature is unusual in its pattern of maturation, or that a certain value is increased or decreased. There are, however, a number of ways to bring about a semblance of control. Red cell size can be easily estimated by the use of an eyepiece micrometer, calibrated against the rulings of a counting chamber. The term anisocytosis means little and can be confusing to the doctor. A better system would be to use the terms microcytosis and macrocytosis more freely. Hypochromia should never be reported if the MCHC is above 31%, providing an accurate control is enforced daily on the MCHC complex. The term poikilocyte is much misused. Unless true poikilocytosis is present, a better way to describe the cells would be in more definite terms, as ovalocytes or burr cells. Well-made blood smears also can be prepared to control quantitative counts. The following is a rule of thumb:

| AVERAGE LEUKOCYTES PER HIGH-POWER FIELD | ESTIMATED TOTAL LEUKOCYTE COUNT |
| :---: | :---: |
| 2-4 | 4,000- 7,000 |
| 4-6 | 7,000-10,000 |
| 6-10 | 10,000-13,000 |
| 10-20 | 13,000-18,000 |

| AVERAGE PLATELETS PER HIGH-POWER OIL IMMERSION FIELD | ESTIMATED PLATELET COUNT/MM³ |
|---|---|
| 2-4 | 50,000-100,000 |
| 4-6 | 100,000-150,000 |
| 6-10 | 150,000-250,000 |
| 10-20 | 250,000-500,000 |

In situations where there is an excess of 4 per cent nucleated red cells seen in the differential smear, the total white cell count should be corrected by the following formula to give the "corrected white count:"

$$\frac{\text{Total white count} \times 100}{100 + \text{nucleated red cells}} = \text{corrected white count}$$

### Use of Controls in Differential White Cell Counts and Reticulocyte Counts

These two tests are probably the most poorly controlled of any hematological investigation. Unlike most quantitative tests, no absolute standards are available. In their place, controls to assess reproducibility are used, but they do not provide verification for accuracy in these subjective tests.

#### Method

1. Ten well-made blood smears and reticulocyte smears are made, numbered and stained on day 1.

2. The technologists are instructed to determine one differential count and one reticulocyte count by their normal method, every day for 10 days.

3. An assessment of both the overall laboratory performance and of individual technologist's performances can be judged by calculating standard deviations for each group.

Using such a method it is possible to detect particular weaknesses in the ability of any staff to detect or recognize individual cells.

### Quality Control in Coagulation Procedures

Coagulation tests can be controlled in a manner similar to other tests. Particularly important is the rigid control of the one-stage prothrombin time and the partial thromboplastin time tests. These tests can be checked using commercial standards, but they should also be controlled by replicate and duplicate testing (see p. 355). One series of tests that is rarely checked is the bleeding and clotting time. The most satisfactory way to establish a normal range in the laboratory is to carry out enough tests on known normal subjects and then to establish the normal range. An example of such a procedure would be to determine 20 bleeding times in duplicate on patients with no hemorrhagic history, taking care to select examples from all age groups and from both sexes. The laboratory normal can be calculated from these results.

## REFERENCES

1. Wintrobe, M. M.: The erythrocyte sedimentation test. Internat. Clin., Ser., *46*, *2*: 34, 1936.
2. Westergren, A.: Studies of the suspension stability of the blood in pulmonary tuberculosis. Acta Med. Scand., *54*: 247, 1921.
3. Landau, A.: Microsedimentation; its serviceability and significance in pediatrics; the use of modified apparatus with simplified technic; also serviceable in ambulant practice. Am. J. Dis. Child., *45*: 681, 1933.
4. Davidsohn, I.: Serologic diagnosis of infectious mononucleosis. JAMA, *108*: 289, 1937.
5. Davidsohn, I., Stern, K., and Kashiwagi, C.: Antisheep agglutinins in infectious mononucleosis. Experimental investigations. Am. J. Clin. Pathol., *21*: 1101, 1951.
6. Sadoff, L., and Goldsmith, O.: False positive infectious mononucleosis spot test in pancreatic carcinoma. JAMA, *218*: 1297, 1971.
7. Phillips, G. S.: False positive Monospot test results in rubella. Letters to the Journal. JAMA, *222*: 585, 1972.
8. Horwitz, C. A., Polesky, H., Stillman, T., Ward, P. C. J., Henle, G., and Herle, W.: Persistent haemagglutination for infectious mononucleosis in rheumatoid arthritis. Br. Med. J., *1*: 591, 1973.
9. Mollison, P. L.: Blood Transfusion in Clinical Medicine. ed. 5, p. 105. Philadelphia, F. A. Davis, 1972.
10. Heinle, R. W., Welch, A. D., Scarf, V., Meacham, G. C., and Prusoff, W. H.: Studies of excretion (and absorption) of $Co^{60}$ labeled vitamin $B_{12}$ in pernicious anemia. Trans. Ass. Am. Phys., *65*: 214, 1952.
11. Valentine, W. N., and Beck, W. S.: Biochemical studies on leukocytes; phosphatase activity in health, leukocytosis and myelocytic leukemia. J. Lab. Clin. Med., *38*: 39, 1951.
12. Dausset, J., Nenna, A., and Brecy, H.: Leukoagglutinins; leukoagglutinins in chronic idiopathic or symptomatic pancytopenia in paroxysmal nocturnal hemoglobinuria. Blood, *9*: 696, 1954.
13. Amos, D. B., and Peacocke, N.: Leukoagglutination technique. Histocompatibility Testing. Publication 1229. Washington, D.C., National Academy of Sciences—National Research Council, 1965.
14. Denning, A., du P., and Watson, J. H.: A simple form of clinical viscosimeter. Lancet, *2*: 89, 1906.
15. Goh, K.: Disease-A-Month. Human Cytogenetics. p. 5. Chicago Year Book Publications, 1965.
16. Elking, M. P., and Kabat, H. F.: Drug induced modifications of laboratory test values. Am. J. Hosp. Pharm., *25*: 485, 1968.
17. Simmons, A.: Basic Hematology. p. 264. Springfield, (Ill.) Charles C Thomas, 1973.

# 8

# *Basic Immunohematology*

Immunology is the science which deals with natural and acquired resistance to disease. When this is applied to red cells, white cells, and platelets, the term immunohematology is used. For the student to understand the subject and to be able to work in a hospital blood bank, he should be conversant with the basic theory of antigen-antibody reactions. If these fundamentals are understood, they will serve as the foundation for work in blood banks and will also act as an extra measure of quality control.

## CLASSIFICATION

### Antigens

The term "antigen" is used commonly to describe a protein, glycoprotein or polysaccharide (substance) which can induce a specific immunological response in the form of an antibody, which can interact with a specific antigen of like chemical specificity, or immune cells in vivo or in vitro. An antigen which is capable of inducing a de novo immune response is an "immunogen," and "immunogenicity" defines its capacity to stimulate the formation of antibodies. Normally, a host will respond immunologically to foreign immunogens, but will not respond against its own potentially immunogenic cells and soluble components. Immunocompetent cells are able to distinguish between "self" and "nonself," a breakdown in this mechanism leading to the formation of autoantibodies.

The human blood group antigens or red cells are present in an alcohol-soluble form. They are polymorphic in their differences among groups of humans and are termed "isoantigens." As such there are very fine immunological characteristics of a particular group or a specific individual, and they are usually poor antigens when compared with other species.

Antigens are usually large organic molecules having a rigid chemical structure. They can be proteins or large polysaccharides but are rarely lipid in form. Occasionally, antigens are composed of all three moieties, and this is more often found in the structure of cell surface antigens. In such forms, the lipid or protein carrier may add to the necessary size and the polysaccharide fraction present in the form of side chains confers the immunologic specificity.

**Antibodies**

Antibodies are specific proteins produced by the lymphoid tissue as a result of stimulation with an antigen. These proteins are found in the globulin fraction of plasma or serum. Various physiochemical tests, such as ultracentrifugation, diffusion, and immunoelectrophoresis have shown that there are many different forms of antibody globulins. These forms are grouped together under the term immunoglobulins and are referred to as Ig forms. Five recognized globulin classes have been described: IgG, IgM, IgD, IgA, and IgE.

The IgG molecule is composed of four chains held together by disulfide bonds; two of the chains are "light", and two "heavy". The light chains of all immunoglobulins are identical and may be one of two different forms, $\kappa$ or $\lambda$; the difference being in their amino acid composition (Fig. 8-1). The heavy chains, unlike the light chains, differ for every class of immunoglobulin. Table 8-1 illustrates the differences in molecular structure.

Other common properties and differences between the IgG and IgM globulins are shown in Table 8-2.

In addition to the division of antibodies into their immunoglobulin classes, a further breakdown is possible based upon their in vivo reaction.

TABLE 8-1. Serological and Structural Composition of the Immunoglobulins.

| CLASS | HEAVY CHAINS | LIGHT CHAINS | SEROLOGICAL CHARACTERISTICS | ABILITY TO FIX COMPLEMENT |
|-------|-------------|--------------|----------------------------|---------------------------|
| IgG | $\gamma$ | $\kappa\lambda$ | Usually incomplete | Yes |
| IgM | $\mu$ | $\kappa\lambda$ | Usually complete | No |
| IgE | $\epsilon$ | $\kappa\lambda$ | ? | ? |
| IgA | $\alpha$ | $\kappa\lambda$ | Usually incomplete | No |
| IgD | $\delta$ | $\kappa\lambda$ | ? | ? |

TABLE 8-2. Common Properties and Differences Between IgG and IgM Globulins.

| PROPERTIES | IgG | IgM |
|---|---|---|
| Reaction (media) | Macromolecular media (albumin) | Saline |
| Optimal (reactive) temperature | 37°C | 4-20°C |
| Type | Frequently immune | Frequently naturally occurring |
| Sedimentation constant | 7S | 19S |
| Reduced by 2 ME (mercapto-ethenol) | No | Yes |
| Placental transfer | Yes | No |
| Approximate molecular weight | 150,000 | 900,000 |
| Electrophoretic mobility | $\gamma$ | Between $\gamma$ and $\beta$ |

## Factors Influencing Red Cell Agglutination

Agglutination is controlled by a combination of at least 3 factors.
1. The length of the antibody molecule
2. The electrical charge at the red cell surface
3. The position of the combining site on the red cell surface

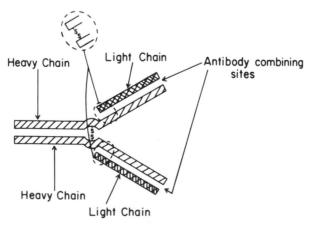

FIG. 8-1. Schematic of an IgG molecule.

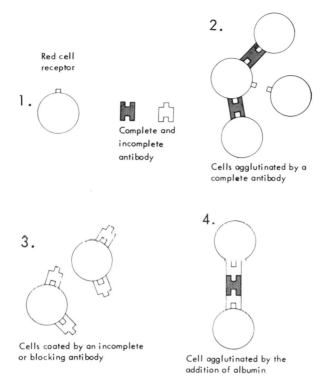

FIG. 8-2. The action of complete and incomplete antibodies.

Figure 8-2 is a schematic representation of the binding actions of complete and incomplete antibodies.

Most complete antibodies, being IgM in form, possess molecular lengths approximating 1000 Å; incomplete antibodies, mainly IgG in form, have lengths of about 250 Å. If red cells are suspended in a saline media having IG incomplete antibodies, they tend to attach themselves to the red cell combining sites, but the cells are situated too far from each other for the antibody to make a molecular bridge between the cells, and agglutination does not occur. If the antibody is an IgM-complete form, the longer antibody molecule will more easily complete the cell-antibody bridge and form red cell agglutinates.

## The Effect of Zeta Potential

The surface red cell charge is also an important factor in the determination of agglutination by IgG and IgM molecules. It is known that the surface of the cells is negatively charged, due in part to the presence of sialic acid residues. Since like charges repel, the cells are naturally kept apart from each other by this electrical repulsion. The suspending media also play a part in the electrical repulsion of the cells. Cations travel in a constant configuration around each red cell and become part of the kinetic unit of the cell. The edge of this cation cloud traveling with the cell is termed the slipping plane, and the electrical potential at this point is known as the zeta potential. This electrical potential is decreased when the cells are suspended in a high molecular weight fluid such as albumin. Such suspending media have increased dielectric constants (relative measure of its charge-dissipation character) and result in the lowering of the effective charge at the slipping plane, which finally results in the cells coming closer together. High molecular weight suspending solution therefore reduce the zeta potential sufficiently to enable IgG antibody molecules to make red cell-antibody bridges and so cause agglutination.

Another way of effectively reducing the zeta potential is to remove some of the red cell's negative surface charge. This is usually accomplished by the use of enzymes, such as trypsin, papain, ficin, bromelin and neuraminidase. However, the removal of proteins from the red cell surface by these enzymes also may play a role by increasing the accessibility of some antigens. In this process, however, some specific antigenic determinants are denatured. Antigenic receptor sites for M, N, S, $Fy^a$ and $Fy^b$ are all damaged by enzyme action, and consequently the use of enzymes in the detection of antibodies to these antigens is not recommended.

### The Position and Number of Antigen Sites

Although the antibody length and the dielectric constant of the suspending solution are important in the red cell antigen-antibody reaction, a third factor also contributes to the mechanism of the reaction. The fact that IgG anti-A will agglutinate saline-suspended red cells, whereas IgG anti-Rhesus will not, suggests that the number of antigen sites may be an important factor in the determination of agglutination, since the number of antigenic cell determinants for A is about a hundred times greater than for the Rh sites. Estimates for the quantitations of the ABO sites are as follows:

$A_1$ sites   $0.81\text{-}1.17 \times 10^6$
$A_2$ sites   $0.24\text{-}0.29 \times 10^6$
B sites   $0.75 \times 10^6$

The number of D ($Rh_0$) sites situated on red cells of the following phenotypes were reported as follows[2]:

CcDee       $9.9\text{-}14.6 \times 10^3$
ccDee       $12.0\text{-}20.0 \times 10^3$
ccDEe       $14.0\text{-}16.6 \times 10^3$

| CCDee | $14.5\text{-}19.3 \times 10^3$ |
|-------|--------------------------------|
| CcDEe | $23.0\text{-}31.0 \times 10^3$ |
| ccDEE | $15.8\text{-}33.3 \times 10^3$ |

In the Kell system the numbers of Kell antigen sites are believed to be as follows[3]:

| KK | $6.1 \times 10^3$ |
|----|-------------------|
| Kk | $3.5 \times 10^3$ |

Additionally, it can be postulated that in the more weakly reacting blood group systems, the antigen sites, while being fewer in number occupy positions on the cell surface that are more inaccessible to penetration by the antibody. In such cases, it is possible that red cells will not agglutinate even when they are relatively close together, if the antibody cannot reach the surface antigen by virtue of the latter's physical position. If such antigens were to be situated at the surface in a more accessible location, agglutination would occur.

Steric hindrance is another physicochemical effect which must be considered when dealing with antigen-antibody reactions. If red cells are subjected to a serum containing two antibodies having antigenic determinates in close proximity to each other, the antibodies will compete for space in reaching their individual receptor sites. The net result could be mutual blocking ending in neither molecule being bound to the red cell.

Alternatively, if one antibody is present in far greater strength than the other antibody, the stronger antibody would "outcompete" the weaker molecule for the combining site space. This would result in the likelihood of only one antibody type attaching itself to the cell surface.

### Antigen-Antibody Equilibrium

Other factors responsible for red cell antigen-antibody reactions concern the nature of the bond once it is made on the cell surface. Antigen and antibody do not form covalent bonds. The complementary nature of the structures on the antigen and antibody enable the antigenic determinants to come into close apposition with the antibody binding site. They can be held together by relatively weak intermolecular bonds. The reaction between antigen (Ag) and antibody (Ab) is reversible and may be expressed as

$$\text{Ab} + \text{Ag} \underset{K_2}{\overset{K_1}{\rightleftharpoons}} \text{AbAg}$$

where $K_1$ and $K_2$ are rate constants for the forward and reverse reactions.

According to the law of mass action

$$\frac{[AbAg]}{[AB] \times [Agg]} \frac{K_1}{K_2} = K$$

where [Ab] [Ag] and [AbAg] are the concentration of Ab, Ag and the combined product AbAg, and K is the equilibrium constant. At equilibrium

$$\frac{[AgAb] \; eq}{[Ab] \; eq} = K \; [Ag] \; eq$$

so that the higher the equilibrium constant, the greater the amount of antibody combining with antigen at the equilibrium state. When the equilibrium constant is high, the antigen-antibody band is stronger and will be less easily broken. Thus, IgG molecules have 2 binding sites, while most IgM molecules possess 10 sites. In comparison, most IgM molecules, especially of the ABO groups, are more avid in reactivity.

**Factors Affecting the Equilibrium Constant**

The equilibrium constant (EC) is affected by pH, ionic strength, and temperature. The EC is believed to be highest between pH ranges of 6.5 to 7.4, and the rate of association of antibody with antigen is increased, as previously shown above by the lowering of the ionic strength of the suspending media. Temperature effects can be differentiated into two reactions: their effect on the equilibrium constant, and their effect on the rate of reaction. For warm reacting IgG molecules, lowering the temperature to 4°C does not perceptibly increase the equilibrium constant, but it does greatly slow down the reaction rate.

**Time**

The effect of time on the strength of the reaction depends upon the equilibrium constant; that is the association and dissociation rate of the antigen-antibody. In most instances, the attachment of the antibody to red cells continues over long time periods; but there comes a time when the dissociation rate becomes greater than the association rate, causing the agglutination to disperse. If the association rate governs the dissociation rate, it becomes apparent that antibodies of high binding capacity but low titer will be undetected when prolonged incubation periods are employed. This takes place because by the end of the incubation period, the reaction will have come to equilibrium below the level of antibody detection. If a short incubation period is used with antibodies having low binding constants, there will be insufficient time for the reaction to reach completion. Most blood group antigens possess relatively high binding constants so that incubation periods of up to 1 hour are optimal for the maximal detection of the reactions.

## MECHANISMS OF INHERITANCE

The nucleus of the cell contains pairs of similar chromosomes, each carrying a number of genes responsible for specific inherited characteristics. The genes of any particular chromosome are thought to be constant in number and position. They exist in pairs, similar in type, but not necessarily identical. Such genes, which are unable to exist together in the same chromosome, but occupy the same position in corresponding chromosomes of the pair, are termed *allelomorphs*. An example of allelomorphic characters can be shown in the Kell blood group system. This system consists of two antigenic substances, K and k, each of which causes the production of its own specific antibody, anti-K and anti-k. Red cells that are agglutinated by only anti-K have the antigenic makeup of only K, whereas cells agglutinated by only anti-k have the antigen makeup of only k. Those cells that are agglutinated by both anti-K and anti-k will have antigens to both these sera. Cells having only the antigen K are termed *homozygous* K-positive; cells having only the antigen k are termed homozygous k-positive and those having both these antigens are known as heterozygous K-positive. The homozygous K-positive cell has, by definition, two genes, KK. This is known as the *genotype* and can be considered as the allocation of genes to any one chromosome or the genetic makeup of that chromosome. The heterozygous K-positive cell has the genetic makeup of Kk. This makeup is the phenotype or the observed genetic makeup, and does not consider the possibility of the presence of a second gene that is suppressed or recessive to the stronger or dominant gene. Common examples of dominant, recessive and codominant genes are to be found in the ABO

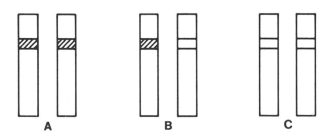

Fig. 8-3. Kell blood group systems. (*A*) Homozygous Kell positive; (*B*) heterozygous Kell positive; (*C*) homozygous cellano (k) positive (Kell negative).

blood group system. The gene A is dominant to the gene O in a cell having the genotype AO. Such a cell would be grouped as type A. In an AB cell, both the genes A and B are observed and are codominant (i.e., neither is suppressed).

## COMPLEMENT CLASSICAL PATHWAY OF ACTIVATION

Antigen-antibody activity frequently is mediated by the complement system. Among the actions initiated by the system, the ability to effect lysis on the cells participating in the reaction, is the most important from a practical blood banking aspect. Complement is a normal component of serum, and is composed of a mixture of $\alpha_2$ and $\beta$ globulins fractions, which become activated in a cyclic pathway, not unlike the cascade theory of blood coagulation, to finally weaken the red cell membrane and cause hemolysis. Two different pathways are believed to be concerned in the cycle. The classical pathway is summarized in Figure 8-4.

### Classical Complement Pathway

The initial reaction in the cycle is the activation of the C1 component. This has three fractions which are noncovalently linked by a calcium bond. The subgroup C1q recognizes and binds to the Fc region of the antibody molecule, showing a preference for IgG and IgM immunoglobulins, with the exception of IgG4.

Aggregation increases C1 binding in direct proportion to the size of the aggregates. The two remaining subunits C1r and C1s make up with C1r and calcium the bound C1 fraction known as $\overline{C1}$. The C1s fraction mediates the attachment of many C4 units, apprximately 5% of which attach to the red cell membrane. Each C4 unit becomes bound to a C2 unit by a magnesium bond forming a bound $C\overline{42}$ unit (C3 convertase). This is able to cleave C3 and liberate a fragment having anaphylatoxin activity. In addition to cleavage of C3, the interaction of C42 and C3 results in the formation in the fluid phase or on the cells of a new proteolytic enzyme C423, which is able to cleave C5 and release a low molecular weight fraction C5a.

After the cleavage of C5, the remaining sequence of the pathway is concerned with insult to the cell membrane, by the action of C5 through C9. These components must attach to the target cell membrane in order to effect membrane damage. When C5 attaches to the cell membrane, a swelling results and ultrastructural lesions appear without evidence of a permeable defect. The C6 and C7 units also become active and are believed to be present on the cell surface in a triangular arrangement.

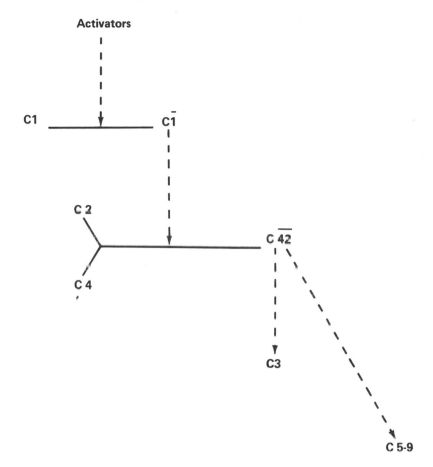

FIG. 8-4 Classical compliment pathway. (After Cooper, N.R.: Progress in Transfusion and Transplantation. A.A.B.B. Washington, 1972)

The effect of C6 and C7 on the cell membrane is unclear, but the complex C567 appears to additionally modify the surface and provide a binding site for the unit C8. This furnishes additional binding sites for 6 C9 molecules, which puncture the cell membrane lysing the red cell[5]. The specific mode of action of the terminal stages of complement activity is unclear, but it has been suggested that hydrophobic interactions with membrane lipids may play an important role[6].

### Alternative Pathway of Activation

This pathway is summarized in Figure 8-5.
The C3 activator pathway converges with the classical C142 pathway

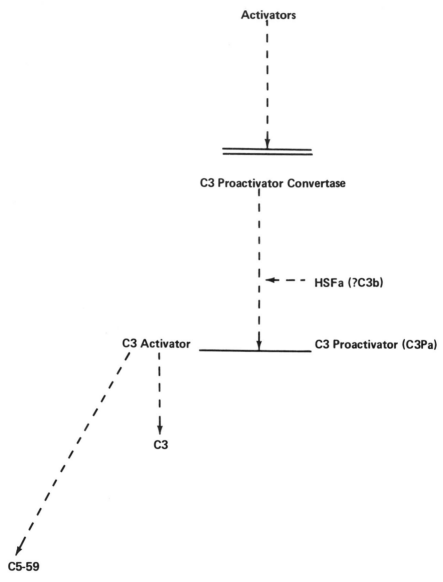

Fig. 8-5. Alternative pathway of activation. (After Cooper, N.R.: Progress in Transfusion and Transplantation., Washington, 1972)

at the C3 stage. Complement activation by this alternate route occurs on addition of various aggregated immunoglobulins or immune complexes to serum. It can also be activated by addition of serum of any of a variety of naturally occurring plant and bacterial polysaccharides including inulin, zymosan, agar, and bacterial endotoxins. Other means of activation include that following cobra serum addition and the action of a C3 fragment termed HSFa. It is believed that this fragment enables the C3PAse enzyme to attack and cleave C3Pa and thus initiate the pathway.[7]

## General Considerations

All blood groups, with the exception of the Lewis system, are permanent characteristics. The antigenic polysaccharides comprising these groups can be identified by their behavior with corresponding antibodies in neutralization, agglutination, lysis or by precipitation. Two unresolved theories exist as the to exact nature of a specific antigen-antibody reaction. The one-to-one theory holds that each antigen consists of a single substance responsible for the formation of a single specific antibody; whereas the mosaic theory postulates that some antigens are mixtures of different factors, each of which is antigenic. The resulting antibody formed is a mixture of antibodies directed at the different factors of the mosaic. Blood group substances are found in the red cells, urine, semen, gastric juice, plasma, saliva and amniotic fluid.

## The Nature of Human Antibodies

*Definitions. Heteroagglutinins* are antibodies which react with red cells from a different species of animal (e.g., anti-M serum derived from rabbits reacts with M-positive human cells). *Natural antibodies* exist without the exposure of the host to the usual antigenic stimulus, and *immune antibodies* result from such a stimulus. There are 3 main routes of immunization: transfusion, pregnancy, and intramuscular injections of blood.

### Factors Governing Immunization
1. The antigenic potential of the particular blood group substance involved. For example, anti-A and anti-D are strongly antigenic, anti-Fy and anti-Jk produce only relatively weak antibodies.
2. The simultaneous introduction of other antigens may result in competition for the antigenic stimulus. In such cases, either no immunization occurs or antibodies will be produced only against the strongest antigens. The more similar the antigenic structure of the individual blood to that of the recipient, the greater the chance of immunization to any

remaining antigenic difference. An example of this phenomenon is the increased incidence of Rhesus immunization of mothers with Rhesus-positive husbands of compatible ABO groups, (e.g., mother O Rhesus-negative, father O Rhesus-positive).

3. The number of previous exposures to the antigen. The chance of becoming immunized becomes greater with repeated stimulation.

4. The route of injection. Direct transfusion produces greater degrees of immunization.

5. Inherited characteristic. Certain individuals are more prone to form antibodies.

6. The interval between exposures to the antigen. Spaced exposures are likely to produce greater sensitization.

### Factors Affecting Blood Group Reactions

1. The degree of agglutination varies with the age of the donor.

2. The reactivity of the cells decreases with increasing age of the specimen. For example, although a Lewis blood group substance is relatively thermostable, a Kell blood group substance is thermolabile.

3. The degree of agglutination varies with the blood group system involved. The ABO blood system produces strong agglutination; the agglutination with the Lewis groups is weak.

4. The condition of storage influences agglutinability. Blood stored in citrate-phosphate-dextrose solution retains its agglutinability for approximately 28 days at 4°C. Heating the cells at 56°C for 10 minutes damages some antigens but does not affect all of them (e.g., the D antigen is destroyed, whereas the c antigen retains much of its agglutinability).

5. The degree of agglutination depends on the proportions of antigen and antibody brought together. Excess of antigen in the presence of little antibody can cause absorption of the antibody onto the cell without antigenic agglutination.

6. Agglutination is changed by partial digestion of the cell surface by proteolytic enzymes such as trypsin, papain, ficin, bromelin. The removal of sialic acid residues, however, is the primary action of these enzymes and results in the reduction of the red cell's zeta potential. Some blood group systems are inactivated and destroyed by these enzymes (the MNS, Kell and Duffy systems).

7. If a cell is homozygous for a blood factor, it sometimes gives a stronger reaction in a particular antiserum than does a corresponding heterozygous cell (for example, EE vs Ee, MM vs MN). This is known as a dosage phenomenon.

8. The influence of other antigens can also affect other blood group reactions. Some cells produce weaker or stronger reactions with specific antisera, the strength of the reactions being influenced by the presence

or absence of other antigens. For example, E cells that lack the antigen D produce stronger reactions with anti-E than E cells that have the D antigen. The D antigen partly suppresses the E antigen and also the antigen-antibody reaction. Heterozygous A cells (AO) produce stronger reactions with anti-A than do AB cells with the same antiserum. The anti-B suppresses this antigen-antibody reaction.

### Serum Factors

1. The manufacturer's instructions should always be followed when using commercial antisera.

2. The antiserum may be specific only at certain dilutions (prozone effect), or it may act only in specific media. High protein antisera and saline antisera are examples of this phenomenon.

### Reaction Factors

1. Choice of technique. Complete antibodies agglutinate cells in isotonic saline. Incomplete antibodies fail to agglutinate a saline suspension of cells, but agglutinate when suspended in a macromolecular medium whose molecular weight approximates that of human plasma, such as dextran, PVP, gum acacia, gelatin.

2. The speed of the reaction: (1) slide method; (2) tube technique; and (3) centrifuge method.

### Personal Factors

1. The technologist *must* understand the principle of the test and the technique being used.

2. All materials used should be specific, the sera avid and the cells fresh.

3. No shortcuts should be allowed. Incubation time should be carefully followed and the technologist should possess scrupulous honesty.

### THE USE OF THE PASTEUR PIPET[8]

### Method

1. With the hand held palm down and the fingers extended, the pipet with rubber bulb is placed, point upward, between the middle and ring fingers (see Fig. 8-6, 1).

2. The middle finger is rolled upward and outward over the ring finger and the hand is turned clockwise through 90°.

3. The pipet should then be in the correct working position with the bulb between the thumb and index finger (see Fig. 8-6, 2).

4. In order for agglutination reactions to be read microscopically, a portion of the sedimented cells is transferred to a slide and spread in a thin film. To do this, the rubber bulb is squeezed and the stem of the pipet inserted in the tube until its tip is just above the cell layer.

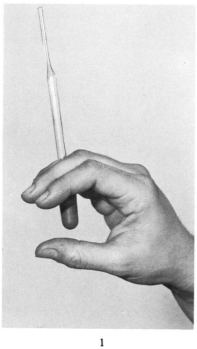

1

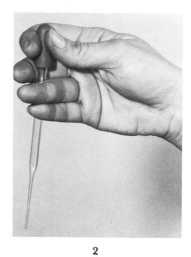

2

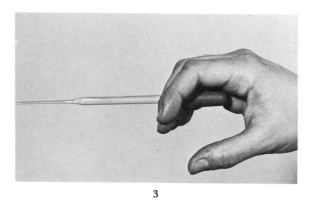

3

FIG. 8-6. The use of the Pasteur pipet.

5. A small volume of the cells is withdrawn into the stem, with care taken to avoid the introduction of air bubbles.

6. The cells are gently expelled onto one end of a slide and, with the hand held palm down and the pipet stem balanced between the middle and ring fingers, the tip of the pipet is allowed to point in a horizontal plane away from the technologist.

7. The stem of the pipet is slowly brought up against the cells and the cell layer allowed to make contact with the pipet. The pipet is immediately drawn away in a quick sweeping motion, allowing the cell button to be spread in a thin film.

## REFERENCES

1. Economidou, J., Hughes-Jones, N. C., and Gardner, B.: Quantitative measurements concerning A and B antigen sites. Vox Sang, *12*: 321, 1967.
2. Rochna, E., and Hughes Jones, N.C.: The use of purified $I^{125}$ labeled anti-γ globulin in the determination of the number of antigen sites on red cells of different phenotypes. Vox Sang., *10*: 675, 1965.
3. Hughes-Jones, N.C., and Gardner, B.: The Kell system studies with radioactively labeled anti K. Vox Sang., *21*: 675, 1965.
4. Hughes-Jones, N. C., Gardner, G, and Telford, R.: The effect of pH and ionic strength on the reaction between anti-D and erythrocytes. Immunology, *7*: 72, 1964.
5. Kolb, W. P., Haxby, J. A., Arroyave, C. M., *et al.*: Molecular analysis of the membrane attack mechanism of complement. J. Exp. Med., *31*: 549, 1972.
6. Inove, K., and Kinsky, S. C.: Fate of phsopholipids in liposomal model membranes damaged by antibody and complement. Biochemistry, *9*: 4767, 1970.
7. Muller-Eberhard, H. J., and Götze, O.: C3 proactivator convertase and its mode of action. J. Exp. Med., *135*: 1003, 1972.
8. Dunsford, I., and Bowley, C. C.: Techniques in Blood Grouping. p. 34, ed 2, vol. 1. Springfield, (Ill.), Charles C Thomas, 1967.

# 9

# *Blood Bank Methodology*

## PREPARATION OF FOUR PER CENT WASHED CELLS

*Method*

1. A saline suspension composed of 1 ml whole blood is made in a tube (12 x 75 mm). The cells are mixed by inverting the tube, and the mixture centrifuged at 3,600 rpm for 30 seconds in a Serofuge.

2. The supernatant saline is decanted and the cells rewashed at least two additional times.

3. The cells are resuspended in saline and finally recentrifuged at 3,600 rpm for 2 minutes.

4. The supernatant saline is completely removed by decantation followed by draining the tubes over a wad of absorbent paper.

5. 0.2 ml of the washed packed cells are added to 4.8 ml of 0.85% saline in a 13 x 100 mm tube. The tube is well mixed and the cells used at this concentration.

## STANDARDIZATION OF AGGLUTINATION READINGS

*Method*

1. Remove the tubes from the centrifuge. Do not agitate the cell button.

2. Turn the tube so that the cell button is on the top side of the tube and the diluent cuts across the center of the cells.

3. Agitate the cell button by gently flexing the wrist. The cells must be completely removed from the bottom of the tube before a reading is made.

4. The degree of agglutination is graded as follows:

4+: One large clump with a clear background
3+: Several large clumps with a clear background

378

2+: Medium-sized well dispersed clumps with a clear background

1+: Many small clumps with a turbid reddish background

w (±) : Minute clumps with a turbid reddish background or microscopic aggregates

−: Negative; no agglutination

## METHODS OF DETECTING ANTIGENS AND ANTIBODIES

### Tube Technique (for Use with Complete Antibodies)

*Principle.* Serum is added to a saline suspension of cells in a tube. After allowing sufficient time for the reaction to take place, the sedimented cells are microscopically examined for agglutination.

#### Reagents and Apparatus

1. Cells: Approximately 2 drops of whole blood is added, from a standard Pasteur pipet held vertically, to 2 ml of isotonic saline. If the pipet is held at an inclined angle, the drops delivered are larger and will vary with the angle of the pipet.

2. Tubes—10 × 75 mm

3. 20°C or 37°C Waterbath, depending on the optimal temperature of the blood group system being investigated

4. Pasteur pipets

5. Test serum

6. 5% Saline suspension of appropriate cells

7. Microscope

#### Method

1. 1 Volume of serum is added to 1 volume of a 5% saline suspension of cells. The serum-cell suspension is mixed and incubated at the desired temperature for 45 to 60 minutes.

2. The cells are examined microscopically, using a 10× objective *without centrifugation*. This is accomplished by gently tipping an aliquot of the cells onto a glass slide or by removing the cells carefully with a Pasteur pipet (see p. 375).

### Tube Technique (for Use with Incomplete Antibodies)

*Principle.* Visible agglutination is obtained in one of two ways: by suspending red cells in a macromolecular medium in a tube, or by adding a saline suspension of red cells, whose surfaces have been partly digested by enzymes, to the serum in a tube.

### Reagents and Apparatus

1. Red cells: The cells are suspended in bovine albumin or in their own serum to make a 5% suspension *having a total protein of approximately 15%.*

2. Other reagents and apparatus as described in the above technique.

### Method

1. Steps 1 and 2 are carried out as in the above technique, using albumin suspensions of red cells in place of the saline suspension.

## The Use of Papain (One-Stage Method)[1]

*Principle.* The zeta potential of a cell suspension reduced by the action of enzymes by the removal of sialic acid residues from the cell surface. Saline suspensions of enzyme-suspended cells react in a visible manner with some incomplete antibodies, but the effect is variable because the proteolytic effect of the enzyme enhances some reactions and inhibits others.

### Reagents and Apparatus

1. M/2 Cysteine: 0.79 g of L-cysteine hydrochloride is added to 10 ml of distilled water.

2. Buffer pH 5.4:

    a. 9.08 g of potassium dihydrogen phosphate anhydrous is added to 1 liter of distilled water.

    b. 11.88 g of disodium hydrogen phosphate dihydrate is added to 1 liter of distilled water.

964 ml of solution a is added to 36 ml of solution b to obtain a buffer of pH 5.4.

3. Papain: 2 g of papain* is ground with 100 ml of buffer pH 5.4. The mixture is filtered and 10 ml of M/2 cysteine is added. The total volume is then diluted to 200 ml with buffer, the papain mixture is incubated for 1 hour at 37°C, distributed into small tubes and stored frozen at −20°C. The solution is stable for 4 months.

4. Pasteur pipets

5. Tubes—10 × 75 mm

6. 37°C Waterbath

7. Test serum

8. 5% Saline suspension of appropriate cells.

### Method

1. 3 Volumes of enzyme solution is added to 1 volume of test serum.

2. An equal volume of a 5% saline suspension of cells is added to the enzyme-serum mixture.

---

\* Available from Merck, Sharpe and Dohme as Papayotin.

3. Incubate the cells-serum mixture for 2 hours at 37°C and observe for macroscopic agglutination *without* centrifugation.

## Two-Stage Method[2]

### *Reagents and Apparatus*
1. Papain stock solution: 1 g of papain is ground with 100 ml of 0.85% saline. The suspension is filtered through a Whatman 1 filter paper and the supernatant stored in 1 ml aliquots at −20°C. The enzyme is stable at this temperature for 6 months.
2. Buffer. Double phosphate M/15, pH 7.4:
    a. 9.08 g of anhydrous potassium dihydrogen phosphate is dissolved in distilled waer and the volume made up to 1 liter.
    b. 9.47 g of anhydrous disodium hydrogen phosphate is dissolved in distilled water and the volume made up to 1 liter. Before mixing the 2 phosphate solutions, allow to warm up to room temperature.
    c. 20 ml of M/15 potassium dihydrogen phosphate is added to 80 ml of M/15 disodium hydrogen phosphate.
    d. 10 ml of this stock buffer (pH 7.4) is added to 90 ml 0.85% saline.
3. Papain working solution: 9 ml of buffered saline is mixed with 1 ml of stock papain solution. The working papain solution should be prepared on the day of its intended use.
4. Tubes—10 × 75 mm
5. 37°C Waterbath
6. Test serum and cells
7 Pasteur pipets
8. Pipets—0.1 and 0.2 ml

### *Method*
1. Approximately 1.0 ml of cells are washed 3 times in a large volume of isotonic saline.
2. 0.1 ml of the washed packed cells are placed in a tube together with 0.2 ml of papain working solution.
3. Incubate the cell-enzyme mixture at 37°C for 30 minutes, agitating it frequently.
4. Separate the cells by centrifugation, and rewash 3 times in saline.
5. Dilute the cells so as to obtain a 2% saline suspension.
6. Two volumes of test serum are then placed in a tube with 1 volume of papain-treated cells.
7. The cell suspension is mixed and incubated at 37°C for 15 to 30 minutes.
8. The tube is examined for agglutination or hemolysis using either the ×4 microscope objective or with a hand lens. *Do not centrifuge.*

9. If no agglutination is present, convert the test to the antiglobulin test.

## The Use of Bromelin[3]

*Principle.* As in the papain method described on page 380.

### Reagents and Apparatus

1. Bromelin: 0.5 g of bromelin powder is added to 90 ml of saline and the mixture is buffered by the addition of 10 ml of the phosphate buffer described under the one-stage method. Sodium azide at a concentration of 0.1% can also be added as a bactericidal agent. The enzyme is stored frozen at −20°C in small aliquots and is stable for 4 to 5 months at this temperature.

2. 5% Saline suspension of appropriate cells
3. Test serum
4. Tubes—10 × 75 mm
5. Pasteur pipet
6. Centrifuge

### Method

1. 2 Volumes of test serum is added to 1 volume of a 5% suspension of cells.

2. 1 Volume of bromelin is added to the serum-cell mixture in a tube (10 × 75 mm) and the whole is incubated at room temperature for 5 to 15 minutes.

3. The tube is centrifuged at 1,000 rpm for 1 minute and the sedimented cells are gently dislodged and observed for macroscopic agglutination.

## The Use of Trypsin[4]

*Principle.* As in the papain method described on page 380.

### Reagents and Apparatus

1. Stock buffer:

a. 11.88 g of disodium hydrogen phosphate dihydrate is dissolved in 1 liter of distilled water.

b. 9.08 g of anhydrous potassium dihydrogen phosphate is dissolved in 1 liter of distilled water.

76.8 ml of solution a is added to 23.2 ml of solutio b to produce a buffer of pH 7.3.

2. Buffered saline: 1 volume of stock buffer prepared in 1 is added to 9 volumes of normal saline.

3. Trypsin: 1 g of crude trypsin is added to 100 ml of buffered saline

and shaken to mix. Undissolved material is removed by Seitz filtration and the filtrate stored in small aliquot at −20°C. At this temperature it is stable for 5 months.

4. Pasteur pipets
5. 37°C Waterbath
6. Centrifuge
7. 2% Saline suspension of appropriate cells
8. Test serum

*Method*

1. 1 Volume of buffered trypsin solution is added to 10 volumes of a 2% saline suspension of cells; the enzyme-cell suspension is mixed and incubated for 10 minutes at 37°C.

2. The cells are washed 3 times in normal saline and suspended to make a 2% saline suspension.

3. 1 Volume of serum is added to 1 volume of the enzyme-treated cells and incubated for 15 minutes at 37°C.

4. The contents of the tube are centrifuged at 1,000 rpm for 1 minute and the sedimented cells gently dislodged and observed for macroscopic agglutination.

**The Use of Ficin[5]**

*Principle.* As in the papain method described on page 380.

*Reagents and Apparatus*

1. Stock buffer pH 7.3:

    a. 5.14 g of sodium dihydrogen phosphate is dissolved in 1 liter of distilled water.

    b. 4.45 g of disodium hydrogen phosphate is dissolved in 1 liter of distilled water.

1 volume of solution a is added to 4 volumes of solution b to produce a buffer of pH 7.3.

2. Stock ficin solution: 1 g of ficin is added to 100 ml of buffer and shaken to mix. The ficin solution is distributed in aliquots and stored at −20°C. At this temperature the enzyme is stable for 5 months.

3. Working ficin solution: This is prepared fresh immediately prior to use by diluting 1 volume of stock solution with 4 volumes of saline.

4. Pasteur pipets
5. Tubes—10 × 75 mm
6. 37°C Waterbath
7. Centrifuge
8. 5% Saline suspension of washed cells
9. Test serum

*Method*

1. 1 volume of working ficin is added to 1 volume of cells and the mixture is incubated for 15 minutes at 37°C.

2. The cells are washed once with saline and resuspended in the residual saline; 1 volume of serum under test is added to the treated cells, mixed, and centrifuged at 1,000 rpm for 1 minute.

3. The sedimented cells are gently dislodged and examined for macroscopic agglutination.

*Notes*

1. Ficin-treated cells can be stored at 4°C for 24 hours.

2. The enzyme is dangerous to handle and care should be taken to avoid contact of the powder with eyes or skin.

3. Of the four enzymes listed, trypsin is generally considered the least sensitive, papain and bromelin rather more sensitive, and ficin the most sensitive.

## General Comments on Enzyme Use

1. With any enzyme technique, it is very important to adhere rigidly to the directions in order to obtain comparable results. Factors which can cause variation in specificity and titer are:

    a. Concentration of the enzyme

    b. pH

    c. Incubation time of treatment

    d. Temperature

2. The use of controls is of utmost importance. Normal serum as a negative control should be used to show that overtreatment has not resulted causing nonspecific agglutination. A positive control of standardized dilute anti-D should be used as the positive control to demonstrate that the treatment is adequate.

3. Serum should be added to the tubes before the enzyme-treated cells. If the cells are added first, the antibody causes the cells to stick to the glass and so prevent or reduce agglutination.

4. Trypsin: Concentration of trypsin used can vary from 0.004% to 0.2%. Above this concentration, nonspecific agglutination appears. Trypsin does not enhance titers of naturally occurring antibodies from the ABO system but does enhance the activity of nonspecific cold agglutinins and of autoantibodies present in acquired hemolytic anemia.

5. Bromelin: This enzyme does not require activation, and hence pretreatment of red cells is unnecessary. The technique is similar to Low's papain method in that the enzyme is added directly to the serum-cell mixture, but differs in that it requires only a 15-minute

incubation period at room temperature. Like other enzymes, bromelin enhances the sensitivity of serological tests to the point that nonspecific cold agglutinins are easily demonstrated.

6. Papain: In the Low's method, L-cysteine is used to overcome the effect of papain inhibitors in normal serum. The optimal pH for papain reactions is between 5 and 7.

7. Serological tests using enzymes are most valuable in detecting very low concentrations of certain antibodies, although this sensitivity has disadvantages. The major problem associated with enzyme use is the enhancement of cold nonspecific antibodies of no clinical importance.

Enzymes should not be used as the only test for compatibility, because certain blood group antibodies may not be detected with these procedures. Antibodies easily missed belong to the MN, Duffy, Kidd, and Kell systems. Nevertheless, exception to these observations exist, and some Kell, Kidd, and Duffy antibodies have been detected with enzyme use. (See Table 9-1, pp. 386 and 387.)

Listed below are examples of some antibodies which, while not detected with routine enzyme tests, may be detected with the antiglobulin reaction or enzyme-treated cells. Such antibodies include, anti-S, anti-s, anti-K, anti-k, anti-Js$^a$, anti-Lu$^a$, anti-Lu$^b$ and some examples of anti-Fy$^a$, anti-Fy$^b$, anti-Jk$^a$ and anti-Jk$^b$.

8. Reactions of anti-Le$^a$, anti-Le$^b$, and anti-P, are stronger with enzyme-treated cells. Some examples of Lewis antibodies which fail to hemolyze untreated cells may lyse enzyme-treated cells.

### Tube-Centrifuge Technique

*Principle.* This is similar to the classical tube technique, except that the incubation time is shorter and the cell-serum mixture is centrifuged, thus accelerating and enhancing the reaction

#### Reagents and Apparatus
1. As in the tube technique described on page 379.
2. Serofuge centrifuge*

#### Method
1. Step 1 of the classical tube technique described on page 379 is carried out, except that the incubation time is shortened to 15 minutes.
2. The tube is *centrifuged* for 1 minute and the button of cells gently broken up by tapping the tube.
3. The cells are examined under the 10× objective for agglutination.

---

* Available from Clay-Adams Co., New York, N.Y.

TABLE 9-1. The Effect of Enzyme Treatment on Antibodies of Various Blood Group Systems.

| Antibody | Saline | Enzymes + Albumin | Antiglobulin Test (AGT) | Enzymes | Enzymes AGT | Comment |
|---|---|---|---|---|---|---|
| Natural A and B | ++ | ++ | 0 | ++ | + | Little or no enhancement by enzymes |
| Immune A and B | 0 | + | +++ | +++ | ++++ | Some enhancement by enzymes |
| Saline, Rhesus | ++ | ++ | ++ | ++ | ++ | Enzymes show no improvement |
| Incomplete, Rhesus | 0 | ++ | ++++ | ++++ | ++++ | Enzymes show great enhancement |
| M | ++ | ++ | 0/++ | 0 | 0 | Trypsin may enhance |
| N | ++ | ++ | 0/++ | 0 | 0 | Trypsin may enhance |
| S | 0 | 0 | ++ | 0 | +++ | Trypsin may enhance |
| s | 0 | 0 | ++ | 0 | ++ | |
| $Mi^a$, $V^w$ | +++ | + | ++++ | 0 | ++++ | |
| $P_1$ | ++ | ++ | ++ | +++ | +++ | Slight enhancement |
| $P+P_1+p^k(Tj^a)$ | ± | ± | +++ | +++ | | |
| $P+P_1+p^k$ fresh | hem | | | hem | | |
| $Le^a$ fresh | ++/hem | ++ | ++++ | ++++/hem | ++++ | |
| $Le^a$ | 0 | 0 | 0/++ | 0/+ | ++++ | |

|  |  |  |  |  |  |
|---|---|---|---|---|---|
| Le^b | ++/hem | ++ | ++++ | ++++/hem | ++++ |
| Le^b fresh | 0 | 0 | 0/+++ | 0/+ | ++++ |
| K | 0 | 0 | +++ | 0 | +–+ |
| k | 0 | 0 | +++ | 0 | +++ |
| Fy^a | 0 | 0 | +++ | 0 | 0/+++ |
| Fy^b | 0 | 0 | +++ | 0 | 0/++ |
| JK^a (fresh) | 0 | ++ | ++++ | ++ | ++++ |
| JK^a | 0 | 0 | ++– | 0 | ++++ |
| JK^b (fresh) | 0 | ++ | ++++ | ++ | ++++ |
| JK^b | 0 | 0 | +++ | 0 | ++–+ |
| Lu^a | +++ | + | ++ | 0/+ | 0/++ |
| Lu^b | +++ | + | ++ | 0/+ | 0/++ |
| Di^a | 0 | 0 | +++ | 0 | +++ |
| Js^a | 0 | 0 | +++ | 0 | +++ |
| Xg^a | 0 | 0 | +++ | 0 | 0 |
| I | ++ | ++ |  | +++ |  |

Some examples may react in enzyme-AGT test (Fy^a, Fy^b)

Some examples may react in enzyme-AGT test (Lu^a, Lu^b)

* This chart is not designed to express the degree of agglutination usually produced by antigen-antibody reactions in the various media, but is an indication of the augmentation or diminution of reactivity when influenced by enzymes.

## Albumin Replacement Method (Sheffield Technique)

*Principle.* This is similar to the classical tube technique used to detect complete antibodies, except that agglutination is enhanced by the substitution of the saline supernatant with albumin.

### Reagents and Apparatus
1. 2% Saline suspension of cells as described in the classical tube technique on page 379.
2. Test serum
3. Pasteur pipets
4. 20°C or 37°C Waterbath, depending on the optimal temperature of the blood group system being investigated
5. 22% Bovine albumin
6. Tubes—10 × 75 mm
7. Microscope

### Method
1. 1 Volume of saline suspension of cells is added to 1 volume of serum.
2. The mixture is incubated at 37°C for 45 minutes, and the supernatant saline-serum layer is carefully removed with a Pasteur pipet without disturbing the sedimented cells.
3. An equal volume of 2% albumin is carefully layered onto the cells, taking care *not to mix* the albumin with the cells.
4. The tube is reincubated for an additional 15 to 30 minutes, and the sedimented cells are carefully removed and read microscopically for agglutination.

## Slide Method

*Principle.* A concentrated cell suspension is mixed with serum on a slide. The mixture is left for 1 to 2 minutes and the slide slowly tilted to loosen the agglutinates. A slow circular rolling motion of the slide will make the agglutinates form into large masses.

### Reagents and Apparatus
1. Anticoagulated whole blood or 50% cells suspended in their own serum
2. Antiserum
3. Slides
4. Microscope
5. Applicator stick

*Method*
1. 1 Drop of whole blood is added to 1 drop of serum on a clean slide.
2. The cells and serum are mixed with an applicator stick; the slide is gently rocked back and forth and examined both macroscopically and microscopically for agglutination.

*Note.* This is the most rapid technique of demonstrating antigen-antibody reaction. The method has a disadvantage in that it is of use only when potent avid sera are used. If left for a long time at room temperature, the mixture can dry on the slide and give false-positive results.

**Chown Capillary Method**

*Principle.* Cells are allowed to settle through a column of serum in a capillary tube. Agglutinations are read macroscopically or with a hand lens.

*Reagents and Apparatus*
1. Capillary tube—9 cm long, internal diameter 0.4 mm
2. Viewing box
3. Avid antiserum
4. Patient's cells in their own serum
5. Incubator

*Method*
1. Sufficient serum is taken into the tube by capillary attraction to occupy a column of approximately 1.5 cm.
2. Keeping the serum-filled end of the tube down to prevent the introduction of air bubbles, the tube is dipped into the cell suspension and about 2 cm of cells is taken up by capillarity.
3. The tube is inverted and the lower end placed in modeling clay in an inclined position on the viewing box with the cells on top of the serum.
4. The capillary tube is incubated at 37°C for 15 to 30 minutes and examined with a hand lens for agglutination.

*Notes*
1. The advantage of this technique is that it uses only a very small quantity of antiserum.
2. The viewing box consists of an oblong box containing two 25-watt lamps to provide heat and light, surmounted by a length of opal glass 8 cm high that is inclined backward at an angle of 45°. A strip of vinyl putty or modeling clay is placed along the lower edge of the glass.

## Clerical Errors

1. Blood samples can be mislabled or tubes can be inaccurately labeled as to antiserum or the patient's name.

2. Mislabeling blood units; the use of only the patient's name and a failure to always incorporate the patient's hospital number, ward, and the doctor's name. In many institutions, the date of birth of the patient is used in place of the patient's age.

3. Errors in labeling the correct blood type and other accessory information, such as antibody titer, VDRL and indirect Coombs' results.

## Technical Errors

### Causes of False-Negative Results

1. The omission of serum from the tube

2. The use of serum that is weak due to improper storage, incomplete thawing after storage at −20°C, or the use of out-of-date serum.

3. Allowing insufficient time for the reaction to take place. Always read the positive control prior to reading the test.

4. The use of incorrect techniques to detect the suspected antibody (e.g., saline suspension of cells with a high protein antiserum).

5. The use of a concentrated red cell suspension, resulting in the absorption of the antibody into the red cell surface without causing agglutination.

6. The use of old stored red cells that have lost viability or the ability to react with a given antiserum.

7. The reading of hemolysis as a negative reaction. Any antigen-antibody reaction that results in any degree of hemolysis should be read as a positive reaction. The antibody is then a hemolysin and not an agglutinin.

8. Poor technique in removing cells from the tube and in spreading the cells on the slide, resulting in the dispersion of weak agglutinates. Students, in particular, should pay attention to the removal of cells from the tube and to their careful spreading.

9. Prozone effect: The failure of the serum to give a visible reaction against a constant volume of red cells, although a visible reaction takes place when the serum is further diluted. Always read titrations from the highest dilution down to the most concentrated tube to avoid prozone.

### Causes of False-Positive Results

1. The use of sera contaminated with bacteria or with other sera.

2. The use of nonspecific sera. Occasionally it is possible for antibodies, which were thought to have been absorbed, to reappear after

prolonged storage; this is due to incomplete absorption (e.g., the presence of anti-A in an anti-D serum derived from a Group B donor).

3. The presence of rouleaux formation or pseudoagglutination. The red cells resemble a pile of coins, the phenomenon being due to high globulin levels in the patient's serum. The effect can be removed by the addition of 1 drop of 1.5% saline to the agglutinates in the tube. Rouleaux formations will disperse, whereas true agglutination will remain (see p. 399).

4. The presence of "plasma clots," resulting in the use of anticoagulated blood or freshly drawn clotted blood that has had insufficient time to completely coagulate. This difficulty can be overcome by the addition of 10 units of thrombin to 1 ml of whole blood or by allowing the blood to completely clot at 37°C.

5. The presence of Wharton's jelly in cord blood samples. This can be removed by washing the cells 3 or 4 times in clean 37°C saline.

6. Huebener Thomsen phenomenon. This is a panagglutination caused by a bacteria-infected sample of red cells. Panagglutination of this type can be removed by using fresh cell suspensions.

7. The presence of autoagglutinins associated with the patient's clinical condition.

8. Nonspecific warm and cold agglutinins. These can be removed by selectively absorbing the antibody from the serum with selected cells at the appropriate temperature.

9. Saline contaminated with foreign red cells or dirty tubes will be potent sources of false-positive reactions.

## THE USE OF CONTROLS

1. *Positive and negative controls should always be set up simultaneously with each test.* Positive controls are used to demonstrate that the sera are active; negative controls show that they are specific in nature.

2. When setting up the controls, the positive tube should be adjusted so that a *weak* reaction is apparent. This demonstrates that the reagents used in the test will detect weak antibodies or antigen receptors.

3. The use of absorption controls is frequently overlooked in classroom exercises. Their use ensures that any serum that has had anti-A or anti-B absorbed from it remains specific.

4. The autoagglutinin control should be *routinely* set up to ensure that the patient's cells and serum do not react together.

5. Group O serum (anti-AB) from an O blood should *always* be used when ABO-typing. This serves as an additional check on the anti-A and anti-B used; also this antiserum is more sensitive than anti-A to the weaker subgroups of A.

## THE PREPARATION OF ANTIGLOBULIN-POSITIVE
## CONTROL CELLS

*Principle*. Antiglobulin control cells are used to demonstrate that the test has been carried out correctly. If the procedure has been adequately performed, free antiglobulin serum is present in the tube following a negative reaction. A previously sensitized and adequately washed cell suspension should therefore be agglutinated when added to the mixture. If the antiglobulin serum is omitted from the tube, or if it is partially neutralized by virtue of inadequate saline washing, agglutination of the control-coated cells will not take place.

*Reagents and Apparatus*
1. Group O Rhesus-positive cells
2. Anti D serum—high protein
3. Centrifuge (Serofuge)
4. 0.85% Saline
5. Tubes—16 × 100 mm

*Method*
1. 3 ml of anticoagulated Group O Rhesus-positive blood is placed in a tube (16 × 100 mm) and the tube filled with saline, centrifuged, and decanted.
2. A 2% saline suspension of the washed cells are made and 1 volume of commercial anti-D serum added to 9 volumes of the 2% cell suspension.
3. The mixture is mixed and incubated at 37°C for 30 minutes.
4. The cells are washed 3 times in saline and completely drained after the last wash.
5. Sufficient saline is added to make approximately a 6% suspension of cells.
6. The coated cells are checked for sensitivity by adding 1 drop to 1 drop of antiglobulin serum in a tube (12 × 75 mm), centrifuging for 15 seconds at 3,600 rpm and macroscopically examining for agglutination.

## DIRECT ANTI-HUMAN GLOBULIN TEST (DIRECT COOMBS' TEST)

*Principle*. Anti-human globulin may be obtained from various animals after injection with human serum or plasma. When this antiserum is added to red cells that have been coated with an incomplete antibody, agglutination takes place. The coated cells are washed in saline to remove any excess of the uncombined globulin, which, if present, will neutralize the anti-human serum and produce a false-negative result.

The anti-human globulin possesses the property of combining more easily with unbound serum globulin than with serum globulin bound to the red cells; 1 volume of anti-human globulin is neutralized by 1 volume of globulin in 4,000 volumes of saline.

### Reagents and Apparatus

1. Anti-human globulin serum
2. Tubes—10 × 75 mm
3. Centrifuge
4. Clean fresh saline
5. Anticoagulated blood or red cells from clotted blood; test and normal control

### Method

1. A 2% saline suspension of red cells is prepared and washed at least 3 times in saline to remove any traces of free serum protein.

2. 1 Volume of washed red cells is added to 1 volume of antigamma and nongamma globulin (broad spectrum Coombs') serum.

3. The contents of the tube are mixed and centrifuged at 1,000 rpm for 1 minute.

4. The sedimented cells are gently dislodged and observed for macroscopic agglutination.

5. Steps 1 to 4 are repeated, using normal cells in place of test cells. *This is the negative control.*

6. Steps 1 to 4 are repeated, using saline in place of the Coombs' serum. *This is also a negative control.*

7. Steps 1 to 4 are repeated, using weakly coated red cells in place of test cells. *This is the positive control.* These cells are made up by adding 1 drop of a 5%-saline suspension of Rhesus-positive (D) cells to 1 drop of a 1:16 albumin dilution of a high protein slide test anti-D. The cell-serum mixture is incubated for 15 minutes at 37°C, washed 3 times in saline and used as the positive control in the above test. Alternatively, the procedure listed on page 392 can be used.

**Results.** Agglutination of the test cells and the presence of adequate controls indicate that the cells are coated with an antibody of unknown specificity.

### Notes

1. The direct Coombs' test is used to detect antibodies that have coated the test cells in vivo, and is an important tool in the detection of erythroblastotic infants and sensitized cells in patients with hemolytic anemia.

### Differential Antiglobulin Tests

#### Method of Preparation of Anti-IgG Reactive Coombs' Reagent

1. Dilute 1 volume of "broad spectrum" Coombs' serum with 1 volume of naturally occurring anti-Le$^a$
2. Incubate for exactly 10 minutes at 37°C.

#### Anti-IgG Controls

1. Positive control: A saline suspension of Rhesus-positive cells are added to high protein reactive anti-D.
2. Negative control: The same cells used in the positive control are washed in saline and used uncoated.

#### Anti-Complement Controls

1. Positive: Le$^{a+}$ red cells are added to a 1:1 dilution of naturally occurring anti-Le$^a$ serum (fresh or fresh-frozen).
2. Negative: The same cells used in the positive control are washed in saline and used uncoated.

(**Note:** All the controls should be tested against broad spectrum and anti-IgG Coombs' sera.)

#### Method

1. The patient's or panel cells to be tested are washed 3 times in saline.
2. The cells are aliquoted into 2 tubes, and broad spectrum Coombs' reagent and anti-IgG reagent added to each respectively.

#### Interpretation

1. Positive results with broad spectrum Coombs' and anti-IgG Coombs' sera indicate that IgG antibodies are present on the cells tested.
2. Positive results with broad spectrum Coombs' and negative results with anti-IgG Coombs' sera indicate that a complement requiring antibody is present on the cells tested.
3. Positive results with broad spectrum Coombs' and a weakened reaction with anti-IgG Coombs' sera indicate that both IgG and complement are likely present on the cells being tested.

(**Note:** When carrying out the above tests, commercially prepared complement-sensitized red cells and IgG-sensitized cells may be used*)

#### Method of Preparation of Anti-Complement Reactive Coombs' Reagent

1. Dilute 1 volume of broad spectrum Coombs' serum with 3 volumes saline.

---

*Available from Gamma Biologicals, Houston, Texas.

2. Add 1 volume of Rh immune globulin (Rhogam, etc) and mix well.

3. Incubate for exactly 10 minutes at 37°C.

(**Note:** Make up fresh prior to use.)

*Controls.* Anti-IgG and anti-complement controls should be made up and used as in the preparation and use of anti-IgG Coombs' serum.

### Interpretation

1. Positive results with broad spectrum Coombs' and anti-complement Coombs' sera indicate that complement is present on the cells tested. IgG antibodies may also be present and this may be verified by the use of anti-IgG Coombs' reagent.

2. Positive results with broad spectrum Coombs' serum and negative results with anti-complement Coombs' serum indicate IgG on the cells tested.

3. Positive results with broad spectrum Coombs' serum and weakened reactions with anti-complement Coombs' serum indicate that both IgG and complement are likely present on the cells tested.

Complete or saline antibodies are absorbed onto the cell surface when suspended in a saline medium, causing visible agglutination.

Incomplete antibodies also attach themselves to the cell surface but do not agglutinate in a saline medium. When they are attached, they prevent agglutination of the cells by saline-reacting antibodies and are known as "blocking" antibodies.


## INDIRECT ANTI-HUMAN GLOBULIN TEST

### (INDIRECT COOMBS' TEST)

*Principle.* This modification of the direct test detects the presence of incomplete antibodies in the serum of sensitized patients. The serum under investigation is added to appropriate cells and is incubated at 37°C to allow the cells to become coated with the serum antibody. After this sensitization has taken place, the coated cells are washed as in the direct test, and anti-human globulin serum is added. The difference between this test and the direct test is that in the former the *cells* are being tested for the antibody coating, whereas in the direct test the patient's *serum* is being tested for the presence of the antibody.

*Reagents and Apparatus.* As in the direct Coombs' technique described on page 393.

### Method

1. A 5% saline suspension of red cells is prepared and 2 volumes of this is added to 2 volumes of test serum.

2. The cells and serum are mixed and incubated at 37°C for 30 to 60 minutes.

3. The cells are centrifuged at 1,000 rpm for 1 minute, gently dislodged and observed for macroscopic agglutination. If the test is negative, the following steps are carried out.

4. The button of cells is washed 3 times in clean saline and resuspended in the residual saline following the last washing.

5. 1 drop of anti-human globulin serum is added to the washed cells, mixed and centrifuged at 1,000 rpm for 1 minute.

6. The button of cells is gently dislodged and examined macroscopically for agglutination.

7. A negative control is set up, using saline in place of serum, and steps 1 to 6 are repeated.

8. Steps 1 to 6 are repeated, using the coated red cells prepared as described on page 392.

*Results.* Agglutination in step 3 above indicates the presence of a saline antibody. Failure of the cells to agglutinate in step 3, with the presence of agglutination or hemolysis in step 6, indicates the presence of an immune (incomplete) antibody.

*Notes*

1. It is *essential* that the supernatant saline be removed completely after each centrifugation, either by a Pasteur pipet or by pouring off and removing the last drop from the rim of the tube with clean absorbent material or with a flick of the wrist.

2. It is equally essential that the cells be resuspended by sharply tapping the tube with the finger.

## EDTA TWO-STAGE ANTIGLOBULIN TEST[6]

*Principle*

EDTA is added to stored serum chelating the calcium ions necessary for the binding of the Clq, Clr, Cls complex to form Cl. Using this chelated serum, antigen-antibody complexes are formed, but CI is unable to attach to the antibody-combining site, and it is removed with the antibody by washing. Fresh compatible serum is added, enabling the antibody complex to bind.

*Reagents and Apparatus*

1. EDTA solution: 4 g of dipotassium EDTA and 0.3 g of sodium hydroxide are dissolved in distilled water and made up to 100 ml. The final pH should approximate 7.0 to 7.4.

2. Patient's serum

3. Fresh compatible normal serum

4. Centrifuge (Serofuge)

5. Test cells

### Method

1. 0.1 ml of EDTA solution is added to 1 ml of serum and the mixture left at room temperature for 10 minutes.

2. The test cells are washed in 0.85% saline and 4 volumes of the EDTA-serum mixture is added to 1 volume of dry packed cells.

3. The cell-serum mixture is incubated at 37°C for 1 hour.

4. The cells are thoroughly washed 3 times in saline, making sure to completely resuspend between washings.

5. After the third washing, the saline is completely drained from the tube and 2 volumes of fresh compatible serum added.

6. The mixture is incubated at 37°C for 15 minutes and step 4 is repeated.

7. Drain the residual saline from the tube and add 2 volumes of antiglobulin serum to the cell button.

8. Mix well and centrifuge at 3,600 rpm for 15 seconds.

9. The cell button is gently dislodged and examined both macroscopically and microscopically.

### Causes of False-Positive Coombs' Reactions

1. Incomplete cold agglutinins. Cells, from clotted blood that have been stored in a refrigerator will frequently have naturally occurring cold agglutinins adsorbed on their surfaces. Such cells should be washed in warm saline, and the Coombs' serum should be brought to room temperature before use.

2. Colloidal silica derived from glass tubes is a source of false-positive reactions. Saline that has been autoclaved in certain types of glass containers or certain detergents that cause leaching of silicates have been shown to cause false-prositive results.

3. Bacterial contamination. The most common source is the use of contaminated cell specimens from the pilot tubes attached to blood transfusion bags or bottles. Contaminated serum may also cause the same difficulty.

4. Nonspecific species antibodies in the Coombs' serum

5. Inadequate cell washing. Coombs, et al.,[7] and Dunsford, et al.[8] have described a condition in which the anti-human globulin serum, although free from anti-species agglutinins, may clump red cells that have not been completely separated from their surrounding plasma or serum. The antiglobulin serum reacts with the plasma proteins, precipitating and enmeshing the red cells. The importance of adequate and proper cell washing before the addition of Coombs' serum is strongly emphasized.

6. Another difficulty is the appearance of "graininess." When a serum is being investigated to determine an antibody, the cells to which it is sensitized should be washed at least *twice* before being incubated with the serum. Even if the cells are subsequently washed well before the addition of the antiglobulin serum, the final reaction will often be weak and difficult to interpret.

7. Reticulocytes may react with antiglobulin serum due to the $\beta$-globulin transferrin in the cell reacting to the $\beta$-globulin component of the serum.

8. Overcentrifugation.

### Causes of False-Negative Coombs' Reactions

1. The neutralization of antiglobulin by traces of serum. There are five sources of unwanted globulin: incompletely washed cells; dirty glassware; dirty stoppers; contaminated saline; and the technologist's fingers used in the mixing of the cells. The test cells should be adequately washed at least 3 times with a minimum of 10 volumes of saline each time. Resuspending the cells *should not* be done by holding the fingers over the tube. A clean stopper should be used.

2. The use of aged red cells. Fresh cells give the best results; those stored in saline may hemolyze and, if this does not take place, the antibody coating of the cells may be released in a few hours. Sensitized cells from clotted blood stored at 4°C will sometimes give a negative reaction.

3. Overcentrifugation. Although agglutination can occur immediately upon the addition of the antiglobulin serum, it is recommended that the mixture be allowed to stand for 5 minutes so that the interaction may be possible before the tube is centrifuged. If spinning is begun too soon or if high speeds are used, there may be insufficient contact between the antigen and the antibody for a reaction to take place and false-negative results will be produced.

4. Deteriorated antiglobulin serum. Poor storage and contamination may result in loss of potency of the serum.

5. Elution of the antibody from the red cells may take place if the test procedure is delayed or interrupted.

6. A cell suspension that is either too weak or too heavy will not produce optimal coating with the antibody.

7. Complement-dependent antibodies will not be detected if plasma is used for the test. Anticoagulated blood is devoid of calcium which is either removed as calcium salts or chelated and of magnesium. Both of these ions are needed in the activation of complement (see p. 370).

8. The omission of the antiglobulin sera

9. Incorrect incubation time

## THE PROBLEM OF ROULEAUX FORMATION

*Principle.* Rouleaux formation is exhibited by a serum that possesses the property of forming pseudoagglutination with red cells. The pseudoagglutination of the cells resembles a stack of coins end on end.

There are two major causes of rouleaux formation in serums: (a) the exogenous administration of solutions to patients or (b) an intrinsic patient protein abnormality secondary to an underlying disease state.

The intravenous administration of dextran fibrinogen or polyvinylpyrrolidone may cause serum to produce marked rouleaux formation which may persist for up to 36 hours after the infusion. Dextrans usually produce rouleaux formation when the molecules are large and exceed a molecular weight of 60,000, but low molecular weight dextrans can cause rouleaux formation when crossmatches are carried out using enzyme methods.[9] Fibrinogen has the greatest influence on rouleaux formation, the large asymmetrical molecules being most active in its formation.

Extreme rouleaux is associated with many diseases exhibiting hyperproteinemia and hyperglobulinemia. These diseases include multiple myeloma, macroglobulinemia, cryoglobulinemia, Boeck's sarcoid, cirrhosis, and hyperfibrinogenemia secondary to infections. The microscopic difference between rouleaux formation and mixed field true agglutination is shown in Figures 9-1 and 9-2.

### Methods of Proceeding with Rouleaux Formation

#### Method 1[10]

1. Centrifuge the serum-cell mixture when rouleaux formation is suspected.
2. Remove the serum and replace with an equal volume of 0.85% saline.
3. Mix and recentrifuge
4. Resuspend the cell mixture and observe for agglutination.

*Result.* Rouleaux formation will disperse, but true agglutination will remain.

#### Method 2[11]

1. 2 volumes of patient's serum are placed in each of 2 sets of 5 labeled tubes.
2. Saline is added to both sets of tubes as follows:

| Tube | 1 | 2 | 3 | 4 | 5 |
|---|---|---|---|---|---|
| Saline (volumes) | 0 | 1 | 2 | 3 | 4 |

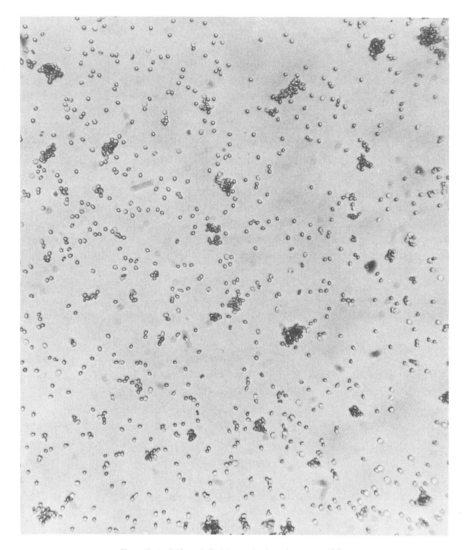

Fig. 9-1. Mixed field agglutination. (×430)

3. Two volumes of a 2% saline suspension of patient's washed cells are added to 1 set of tubes, and the same volume of a 2% saline suspension of donor's red cells to the second set of tubes.

4. Compatibility tests are completed and the results of each set of tubes compared.

**Results.** Compatibility is indicated if the set of tests with donor's cells

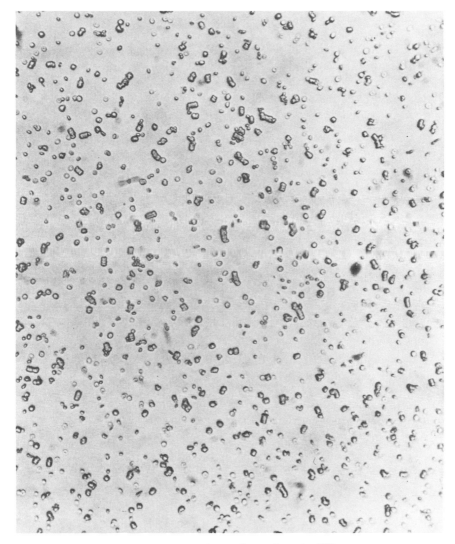

FIG. 9-2. Rouleaux formation. (×430)

is negative at the same or lower tube number than the corresponding set with patient's cells.

### Notes

1. The cell suspension *should not* be mixed on the slide to break up the rouleaux. This practice has been recommended to break up pseudoagglutination, and it has been suggested that true agglutination

will quickly reform. This is not true, however; mixing the suspension is a poor method to differentiate true agglutinates from rouleaux.

2. If difficulty is encountered in typing a blood, due to rouleaux, the cells should be washed 3 times in clean saline and used.

### Detection of Penicillin and Cephalosporin Antibodies[12]

1. Fresh Group O cells are thoroughly washed 3 times in saline.

2. $1 \times 10^6$ Unit (600 mg) of K-benzyl penicillin G is dissolved in 15 ml of barbital buffer pH 9.6.

3. The penicillin is added to 1 ml of the washed packed cells and incubated at room temperature for 1 hour.

4. The cells are rewashed as in step 2 and used in the test.

### Preparation of Cephalothin (Keflin)-"Coated" Cells

1. Fresh Group O cells are washed as in step 1 above.

2. 400 mg of Keflin is dissolved in 10 ml of barbital buffer pH 9.6 and added to 1 ml of the washed packed cells.

3. The mixture is incubated at 37°C for 2 hours and the cells washed as in step 4 above.

#### Method (When the patient has a positive-direct antiglobulin test)

1. An eluate prepared from the patient's cells is prepared either by the ether or the heat methods.

2. The eluate and the patient's serum are tested against the same untreated and treated cells.

3. Set up serial dilutions of the patient's serum from 1:1 to 1:64. Do not titrate out the eluate, but use as obtained.

4. Incubate 1 volume of a 2% saline suspension of drug-treated and untreated cells to 2 volumes of eluate and to each serum dilution.

5. Incubate at room temperature for 15 minutes, centrifuge (Serofuge) at 3,600 rpm for 30 seconds, and examine an aliquot for microscopic agglutination.

6. Resuspend the cells, and reincubate at 37°C for 30 minutes. Recentrifuge and examine for microscopic agglutination.

7. Wash all cell suspensions 4 times in saline and add 1 drop of antiglobulin serum to each tube. Centrifuge at 3,600 rpm for 1 minute and examine with a low power hand lens for agglutination.

#### Results

1. IgM penicillin antibodies will agglutinate saline-suspended penicillin-treated cells but not untreated cells. IgG penicillin antibodies will react in the same way by the indirect antiglobulin test.

2. Keflin-treated cells can absorb proteins nonspecifically, causing all

normal serum to produce a positive-indirect antiglobulin test if incubated with the drug for extended time periods. The reaction does not occur when the normal protein is diluted out to more than 1:20. The eluate test does not cause such problems due to the low protein found in this material.

## Differentiation Between IgG and IgM Antibodies

*Principle.* IgM antibodies when treated with 2-mercaptoethanol, result in the disintegration of the disulfide bonds of the antibody molecule and the loss of serological activity. IgG antibodies are unaffected by this treatment.

### Reagents and Apparatus
1. 0.1M 2-Mercaptoethanol (in phosphate buffer pH 7.4) (2 ME)
2. Phosphate-buffered saline pH 7.4
3. Tube style dialyzing membrane
4. String

### Method
1. Six tubes are set up as in Table 9-3. (The 2 ME should be carefully handled, preferably under an exhaust hood.)
*Key:* Tubes 1 = Test, 2 = Patient control, 3 = Positive test, 4 = Positive test control, 5 = Negative test, 6 = Negative-test control.
2. All tubes are incubated at 37°C for 2 hours.
3. Cut 6 dialyzing membranes, each 6 inches long, and soak in a small volume of buffer.
4. Tie one end of each membrane and fill each with the incubated samples.
5. Tie the other end (leave a long string attached) and place the sacs in 1 liter of phosphate-buffered saline pH 7.4 and dialyze overnight.
6. Place the contents of the sacs in labeled tubes and set up a series of titrations of the diluents against commercial pooled O cells.
7. Determine the saline and antiglobulin titer of each diluent tested by standard technique (pp. 134, and 149).

TABLE 9-2.

| TUBE | 1 | 2 | 3 | 4 | 5 | 6 |
|---|---|---|---|---|---|---|
| Patient's serum (ml) | 1 | 1 | — | — | — | — |
| 2 ME (ml) | 1 | — | 1 | 1 | 1 | — |
| Known IgM (strong cold agglutinin, ml) | — | — | 1 | 1 | — | — |
| Anti D (ml) | — | — | — | — | 1 | 1 |
| Phosphate buffer (ml) | — | 1 | — | 1 | — | 1 |

*Notes.* The test is of value when the serum of a pregnant patient contains an antibody rarely associated with hemolytic disease of the newborn. In such situations, the test is useful in determining which form of antibody exists, IgG or IgM.

## Preservation of Red Cells by Freezing

*Principle.* When rare red cells are found (Lu$^a$ positive, KK, U-negative), it is a good practice to preserve them until they can be used in the detection of an antibody. Red cells may be preserved by freezing them in a solution of ACD. Alsever's solution or a normal saline suspension may be used.

### Reagents and Apparatus
1. Normal saline
2. −20°C Deep freeze
3. Glycerol-citrate solution: 6 volumes of 5% trisodium citrate is added to 4 volumes of glycerol.

### Method
1. A saline suspension of cells is centrifuged at 2,000 rpm for 5 minutes and the supernatant saline removed.
2. An equal volume of glycerol-citrate solution is added to the packed cells at room temperature.
3. The cells and citrate mixture is inverted to mix and divided into 1-ml aliquots.
4. The volumes are stored in the deep freeze until ready for use. To recover the frozen cells, the following steps are carried out.
5. The tube of frozen cells is thawed in a 37°C waterbath.
6. 16% Glycerol-citrate mixture is added to the thawed cells, mixed well, and centrifuged at 3,000 rpm for 3 minutes.
7. The supernatant is removed and the cells washed, using 8%, 4% and 2% glycerol-citrate mixtures in turn.
8. After the final washing in 2% glycerol-citrate, the cells are re-washed 3 times with normal saline and made up to a 5%-saline concentration for use.

## REFERENCES

1. Löw, B.: A practical method using papain and incomplete Rh antibodies in routine Rh blood grouping. Vox Sang., 5: 94, 1955.
2. Technical methods and procedures. p. 112, 1970. Washington, D.C. American Association of Blood Banks, 1970.
3. Pirofsky, B., and Magnum, M. E., Jr.: Use of bromelin to demonstrate erythrocyte antibodies. Proc. Soc. Exper. Biol. Med., *101*: 49, 1959.

4. Morton, J. A., and Pickles, M. M.: Use of trypsin in the detection of incomplete anti-Rh antibodies. Nature, *159*: 779, 1947.
5. Allen, N. K.: Hyland Reference Manual of Immunohematology. p. 83. Los Angeles, Hyland Laboratories, 1963.
6. Polly, M. J., and Mollison, P. L.: The role of complement in the detection of blood group antibodies: special reference to the antiglobulin test. Transfusion, *1*: 9, 1961.
7. Coombs, R. R. A., Saison, R., and Joysey, V. C.: A circumstance in which the phenomenon of co-agglutination could complicate the anti-globulin sensitization test by stimulating agglutination. Br. J. Exp. Pathol., *36*: 179, 1955.
8. Dunsford, I., Cowen, J., and Malone, R. H.: The Coombs' Test. J. Med. Lab. Tech., *9*: 137, 1951.
9. Selwyn, J. G., Seright, W., Donald, J., and Wallace, J.: Matching blood for receipients of dextran. Lancet, *2*: 1032, 1968.
10. Gralnick, M. A.: Rouleaux. *In* Seminars on problems encountered in pretransfusion tests. p. 79. Washington, D.C. AABB, 1972.
11. Kuhns, W. J., and Bailey, A.: Use of red cells modified by Papain for detection of Rh antibodies. Am. J. Clin. Pathol. *20*: 1967, 1950.
12. Garratty, G.: Detection of antibodies to penicillin and cephalosporins by passive agglutination technics. p. 50. *In* Seminar on problems encountered in pretransfusion tests. AABB, 1972.

# 10

## *Blood Groups*

Many excellent texts on genetics and blood groups exist, but the bare skeleton of the basic properties of the common blood group systems is presented here in order to introduce the student to, and refresh the graduate technologist with, some of the more common properties of the system.

### ABO SYSTEM

*Properties*. The system consists of four basic groups having naturally occurring antibodies. These antibodies react in the cold most strongly at 4°C, but, because of the interference of nonspecific cold antibodies, they are best demonstrated at room temperature. The system has a wide thermal range and antigen-antibody reactions also take place at 37°C, although in a weaker form. The immune antibodies of this system react best at 37°C and are often demonstrated as hemolysins and not as agglutinins. Immune antibodies have the power of fixing complement, and fresh serum is usually hemolytic unless neutralized by either A or B group-specific substance. Stimulation of immune anti-A or anti-B may be provoked by the injection of prophylactic bacterial vaccines.

*Variants*. Anti-A serum from a B blood usually contains two different antibodies which act on group A cells. Anti-A agglutinates $A_1$ cells, $A_2$ cells, $A_1B$ cells and $A_2B$ cells; anti-$A_1$ agglutinates only $A_1$ cells and $A_1B$ cells. Weaker forms of A exist ($A_3$, $A_4$, $A_0$), but these groups have only minor clinical significance. The difference in these subgroups is explained theoretically by assuming that the basic ground substance of the system is a polysaccharide termed H. According to this theory, both groups A and B are mutations of the original H group, and the difference in the apparent antigenic strength of each group is due to quantitative differences in the amount of H substance present. From Figure 10-1 it can be seen that Group O blood possesses more H substance than do $A_4$ bloods; these, in turn, have more H substance than do $A_3$, $A_2$, $A_2B$, $A_1$

TABLE 10-1. Natural Agglutinins in the ABO Blood Group System.

| BLOOD GROUP | AGGLUTINOGENS ON CELLS | AGGLUTININS FREQUENTLY PRESENT IN PLASMA | AGGLUTININS RARELY PRESENT IN PLASMA |
|---|---|---|---|
| $A_1$ | A | Anti-B | Anti-H |
| $A_1B$ | $A_1$, B | None | Anti-H |
| $A_2$ | $A_2$ | Anti-B | Anti-$A_1$ (1–2%) |
| $A_2B$ | $A_2$, B | None | Anti-$A_1$ (25–30%) |
| B | B | Anti-A | Anti-H |
| O | None | Anti-A and Anti-B | None |

and $A_1B$ cells in that order. The reactions between the subgroups of A and anti-A, anti-$A_1$ and anti-H are shown in Table 10-3. Anti-H does not react with $A_1$ cells, because there is little H substance on the cells; but as the subgroups become weaker, more H substance is present and the reaction of anti-H becomes stronger. Very rarely, red cells occur that are not agglutinated with either anti-A, anti-B or anti-H. These are known as the Bombay blood groups. Such cells are thought to be formed under the influence of a suppressor gene and are characterized by reactions resembling those of Group O cells. The plasma contains anti-A and anti B, but the cells do not react with anti-H (as do Group O cells), or with anti-$A_1$ or anti-B. Differentiation is based on the presence of anti-H in the plasma and a lack of H substance on the cells.

Normal Group O cells have no anti-H in the plasma and possess H

TABLE 10-2. Properties of the Common ABO Blood Groups.

| Genes | $A_1$ | $B_1$ | O | | | |
|---|---|---|---|---|---|---|
| Genotypes | AA | BB | AB | OO | AO | BO |
| Frequency | | Caucasian | | | Negroid | |
| | 0–43% | B–9% | | 0–51% | B–17% | |
| | $A_1$–34% | $A_1$B–3% | | $A_1$–21% | $A_1$B–1% | |
| | $A_2$–10% | $A_2$B–1% | | $A_2$–6% | $A_2$B–3% | |
| Optimal temperature | | | 4–20°C | | | |
| Natural or immune forms | Usually natural antibodies are found Occasionally immune forms are seen | | | | | |
| Type of antigen-antibody reaction | Agglutination, occasionally hemolysis | | | | | |
| Clinical importance | Cause of severe and fatal transfusion reactions Cause of ABO hemolytic disease of the newborn Medicolegal | | | | | |

| BLOOD TYPE | A$_1$ | A$_2$ | A$_3$ | A$_4$ | O |
|---|---|---|---|---|---|
| H SUBSTANCE CONVERTED to A SUBSTANCE | +++ | +++ | ++ | + | ∓ |

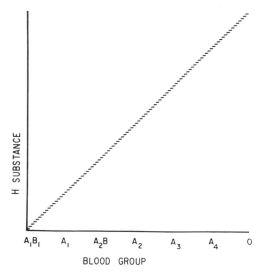

FIG. 10-1. H substance in the individual ABO groups.

TABLE 10-3.  Reactions Between Anti-A, A$_1$ and H and
Group A Variants.

| GROUP | ANTISERA | RESULTS |
|---|---|---|
| A$_1$ | Anti-A | +++ |
| | Anti-A$_1$ | +++ |
| | Anti-H | − |
| A$_2$ | Anti-A | +++ |
| | Anti-A$_1$ | − |
| | Anti-H | + |
| A$_3$ | Anti-A | + |
| | Anti-A$_1$ | − |
| | Anti-H | ++ |
| A$_x$ | Anti-A | − |
| | Anti-A$_1$ | − |
| | Anti-H | +++ |

TABLE 10-4. Subgroups of A and Their Reactions.

| | FORWARD-TYPING ANTISERA | | | | | BACKTYPING CELLS | | | | SALIVA IF SECRETOR |
|---|---|---|---|---|---|---|---|---|---|---|
| GROUP | ANTI-A | ANTI-A$_1$ | ANTI-B | ANTI-A,B | ANTI-H | A$_1$ | A$_2$ | B | 0 | |
| A$_3$ | w/+ | 0 | 0 | +++ | ++ | 0 | 0 | ++++ | 0 | A and H Substance |
| A$_4$ | w/+ | 0 | 0 | ++ | ++++ | + | 0 | ++++ | 0 | H Substance |
| A$_x$ | o/w | 0 | 0 | +/++ | ++++ | w | o/w | ++++ | 0 | H Substance |
| A$_m$ | o/w | 0 | 0 | o/w | ++++ | 0 | 0 | ++++ | 0 | A and H Substance |
| A$_{el}$ | 0 | 0 | 0 | 0 | ++++ | 0 | 0 | ++++ | 0 | H Substance |
| A$_{end}$ | +(1%) | 0 | 0 | +(1%) | ++++ | 0 | 0 | ++++ | 0 | H Substance |

+/w = variable weak reaction
o/w = weak to negative reaction
w = weak reaction

substance on the cells. Anti-O is an antibody related to anti-H and confusion exists as to the exact difference between them. The antibody reacts with both A$_u$ cells and O cells but is not capable of being neutralized by secretor saliva containing H substance.

*Subgroups.* There are several forms of the A antigen that differ both qualitatively and quantitatively. These weak A determinants are of clinical importance in that if not detected they could result in blood being transfused to a Group O individual, causing a transfusion reaction. If a patient having a weak subgroup is transfused Group A blood, a mild reaction could be possible if the patient possessed anti-A$_1$.

The commoner subgroups of A and their characteristic reactions are shown in Table 10-4.

A subgroup of B analogous to subgroup A$_2$ does not exist but weak forms of the B group have been described. They are, however, not clinically important and are rarer than the A subgroups. The serological characteristics of some of the B variants are shown in Table 10-5.

*Secretors.* Approximately 80% of the population *secrete* a *water-soluble* form of ABH substance in their saliva, tears and other body fluids. Group A people secrete A substance and H substance, Group B people secrete B substance and H substance; and Group O people secrete only H substance. The secretion of these substances is controlled by a

TABLE 10-5. Subgroups of B and Their Reactions.

| | FORWARD-TYPING ANTISERA | | | | | BACKTYPING CELLS | | | SALIVA IF SECRETOR |
|---|---|---|---|---|---|---|---|---|---|
| GROUP | ANTI-A | ANTI-A$_1$ | ANTI-B | ANTI-A,B | ANTI-H | A | B | O | |
| B | 0 | 0 | ++++ | ++++ | 0 | ++++ | 0 | 0 | B and H substance |
| B$_3$ | 0 | 0 | w | w/+ | ++++ | ++++ | 0 | 0 | B and H substance |
| B$_x$ | 0 | 0 | o/w | o/+ | ++++ | ++++ | 0 | 0 | H substance |
| B$_g$ | 0 | 0 | w/+ | w/+ | +++ | ++++ | 0 | 0 | B and H substance |
| B$_m$ | 0 | 0 | 0 | o/w | ++++ | ++++ | 0 | 0 | B and H substance |
| B$_m^h$ | 0 | 0 | + | + | 0 | ++++ | 0 | 0 | B and H substance |

0/w = weak to negative reaction
w = weak reaction
w/t = weak to 1 plus reaction

TABLE 10-6. Differences Between the Bombay Group and
Normal Group O Cells.

| BOMBAY | | NORMAL GROUP O CELLS | |
|---|---|---|---|
| CELLS CONTAIN | SERUM CONTAINS | CELLS CONTAIN | SERUM CONTAINS |
| Absence of H substance | Anti-A₁ Anti-B Anti-H | H substance | Anti-A Anti-B |

TABLE 10-7. Reactions Between Bombay and Normal Group O Cells.

| | SERA | | | | CELLS | | | |
|---|---|---|---|---|---|---|---|---|
| GROUP | ANTI- A | ANTI- B | ANTI- H | ANTI- O | A₁ | A₂ | B | O |
| Bombay | — | — | — | — | + | + | + | + |
| O | — | — | + | + | + | + | + | — |

dominant gene (Se), which is independently inherited from the Lewis blood group gene. Twenty per cent of the population possess an *alcohol-soluble* form of ABH substance and are termed *nonsecretors* (se). It has been found that all nonsecretors are type Le$^{(a+)}$.

## RELATIONSHIP BETWEEN THE LEWIS SYSTEM, SECRETOR, AND H

Lewis substances are not produced by the red cells and are not true blood group substances. The Lewis material is primarily acquired secondarily from the plasma, and as secreted substances they are influenced by the secretor gene.

The Lewis system is inherited by means of two genes Le and le. The Le (Lewis-positive) gene determines or converts precursor substance to Le$^a$ substance while the le gene (Lewis-negative) cannot convert precursor substance. In the presence of both H and secretor genes (Se), the Le$^a$ substance is converted to Le$^b$ substance, but usually the conversion is not completely effective, and small quantities of Le$^a$ substance remain. Thus, all Le$^{(a-b+)}$ individuals secrete Le$^a$ and Le$^b$ and ABH substances in their saliva. The anomaly of the individuals secreting Le$^a$ in the saliva, but being Le$^{a-}$ in their red cell type, is a function of the incompleteness of the conversion of the Le$^a$ to Le$^b$. The small amount of Le$^a$ not converted is found in the secretions rather than on the cells, since there is insufficient Le$^a$ material to satisfy both the secretions and the cells.

In individuals inheriting the Le gene, H gene but not the secretor gene (se/se), the final product is influenced by the absence of the Se gene. Since the H/se gene combination cannot convert Le$^a$ to Le$^b$, the end result is always a Le$^{(a+b-)}$ red cell and Le$^a$ secretions. The ABO genes reacting with H substance produced from the H gene results in a normal ABO red cell expression. A summary of the genetic pathways of the three systems is shown in Table 10-8.

Individuals who are Lewis-negative (le le) cannot convert precursor substance to Le$^a$ substance and irrespective of their H or secretor gene status cannot form Le$^b$. Consequently, such persons are always Le$^{(a-b-)}$ in both secretions and in red cell type.

Persons who are Bombay blood group (O$^h$) can be divided into two groups: Lewis-positive (Le) and Lewis-negative (le le). In either situation, the Bombay individual lacks the H gene and cannot convert any Le$^a$ substance even if it is produced to Le$^b$. The Bombay Lewis-positive individual therefore produces Le$^a$ substance in both secretions and on the red cells, but does not secrete any ABH substance because of the lack of H substance. The Bombay Lewis-negative (le le) individual not producing any Le$^a$ substance cannot even secrete Le$^a$ substance and is always Le$^{(a-b-)}$ in both secretions and in cell type. Thus, all Le$^{(a+)}$ individuals are nonsecretors. Conversely, ABH secretion depends on the H and Se genes, so that all Le$^{(b+)}$ individuals must be secretors. ABH secretions, however, can proceed in persons lacking an Le gene; thus, Le$^{(a-b-)}$ persons may be secretors or nonsecretors.

Lewis types and secretor status can be summarized as follows:

Le (a+b−) cells are found in nonsecretors
Le (a−b+) cells are found in secretors
Le (a−b−) cells are usually found in secretors

## ABO Blood Typing

*Principle.* Anti-A, anti-B and anti-AB (Group O serum) are delivered into separate tubes and a 2% saline solution of red cells is added to each. The mixtures are left at room temperature for 4 or 5 minutes, centrifuged, and the cells observed for macroscopic agglutination. This procedure detects the cell antigens and the group is confirmed by testing the serum for naturally occurring antibodies. Such confirmation is carried out by adding fresh A$_1$, B and O cells to the test serum, and following the same procedure as for the detection of the antigens.

TABLE 10-8. Stages in the Production of ABH and Lewis Blood Group Substances and Their Relationship to Secretor Status.

| | PRECURSOR SUBSTANCE | PRECURSOR SUBSTANCE | PRECURSOR SUBSTANCE | PRECURSOR SUBSTANCE | PRECURSOR SUBSTANCE | PRECURSOR SUBSTANCE |
|---|---|---|---|---|---|---|
| Lewis gene | Le | Le | Le | le | le | le |
| Lewis substance | Le$^a$ | Le$^a$ | Le$^a$ | Precursor* substance | Precursor* substance | Precursor* substance |
| Hh genes | H | H | hh | hh | H | H |
| Secretor genes | Se | se | Se or se | Se or se | se | Se |
| Lewis substance | Le$^b$ and small quantity of Le$^a$ | Le$^a$ | Le$^a$ | Precursor substance | Precursor substance | Precursor substance |
| ABO genes | ABO | ABO | ABO | ABO | ABO | ABO |
| ABH substance | ABH substance | ABH substance | none | none | ABH substance | ABH substance |
| Final product | AHB secretor, secretes Le$^b$ and small amounts of Le$^a$ material. Cells type as L$_t$$^{(a-b+)}$ and express ABO types | ABH nonsecretor secretes Le$^a$ material. Cells type Le$^{(a+b-)}$ and express ABO types | ABH nonsecretor secretes Le$^a$ material. Cells type Le$^{(a+b-)}$ but do not express ABO types Bombay O$^h$ | ABH and Lewis nonsecretor Cells type Le$^{(a-b-)}$ but do not express ABO types Bombay O$^h$ O$^h$ | ABH and Lewis nonsecretor Cells type Le$^{(a-b-)}$ and express ABO types | ABH secretor, Lewis nonsecretor Cells type Le$^{(a-b-)}$ and express ABO types |

* Lewis substance cannot be formed from precursor substance in Lewis-negative (le le) individuals. Hence, precursor substance is carried over.

TABLE 10-9. Genetics of Secretion.

| Genotype | Se/Se | Se/se | se/se |
|----------|-------|-------|-------|
| Phenotype | Secretor | Secretor | Nonsecretor |

### Reagents and Apparatus

1. Anti-A, anti-B, anti-AB
2. Tubes—10 x 75 mm
3. Pasteur pipets
4. 2% Saline suspension of test cells—washed 3 times
5. Centrifuge
6. Test serum
7. Fresh 2% saline suspension of $A_1$ cells, B cells and O cells

### Method

1. 1-Volume samples of anti-$A_1$, anti-B, anti-AB and saline are added to 4 tubes, respectively.

2. 1 Volume of a 2% saline suspension of test cells is added to each tube and the contents mixed well.

3. The tubes are left at room temperature for 4 to 5 minutes and centrifuged at 1,000 rpm for 1 minute.

4. The cells are resuspended by gently tapping the tube and are examined macroscopically for agglutination.

5. 1 Volume of test serum is added to each of 4 tubes (10 × 75-mm).

6. 1-Volume portions of fresh 2% saline suspensions of $A_1$ cells, B cells, O cells and patient's test cells are added to the 4 tubes, respectively.

7. Repeat steps 3 and 4.

**Results**. The results are shown in Table 10-10.

TABLE 10-10. Cell-Serum Reactions in the ABO Blood Group System.

| ANTISERA WITH TEST CELLS | GROUP A | GROUP B | GROUP AB |
|--------------------------|---------|---------|----------|
| Anti-A | + | − | + |
| Anti-B | − | + | + |
| Anti-AB | + | + | + |
| Saline | − | − | − |
| **CELLS WITH TEST SERUM** | | | |
| $A_1$ Cells | − | + | − |
| B Cells | + | − | − |
| O Cells | − | − | − |
| Test Cells | − | − | − |

**Notes**

1. Anti-AB and saline tubes are set up in addition to the anti-A and anti-B tubes. The anti-AB serum is used as an extra check on the anti-A and anti-B, and also as an additional precaution to detect the weaker subgroups of A. The saline blank tube is used to provide a negative control for the cells.

2. In the reverse typing (the detection of the naturally occurring antibodies), fresh cells should always be used, because the reactivity of cellular antigens decreases on storage at 4°C.

3. An autoagglutination control tube can be set up to eliminate false-positive reactions that may occur in some forms of hemolytic anemia. In such cases, the blood types as AB, but the autoagglutination control tube provides the technologist with the necessary evidence to reject these results. (See p. 413 for methods of retyping.)

***Discrepancies Between Results of Cell and Serum Grouping.*** Discrepancies are shown in Table 10-11.

## Typing of Subgroups of A

***Principle.*** Anti-A serum from group B blood frequently contains two antibodies that act on Group A cells: $\alpha$, which agglutinates $A_1$, $A_2$, $A_1B$ and $A_2B$ cells, and $\alpha_1$, which agglutinates only $A_1$ and $A_1B$ cells. If anti-A serum containing these two antibodies is added to fresh $A_2$ cells, the $\alpha_2$ is taken up by the cells, which agglutinate and leave behind the $\alpha_1$, which will react with $A_1$ cells. An alternative method is to use anti-$A_1$ lectin derived from the seeds of *Dolichos biflorus*.

***Reagents and Apparatus***
1. 10% Saline suspension of red cells
2. Unabsorbed anti-A
3. Absorbed anti-$A_1$ or lectin anti-$A_1$
4. Tubes—10 x 75 mm

TABLE 10-11. Discrepancies Between Results of Cell and Serum Grouping.

| RED CELLS | | | SERUM | | | |
|---|---|---|---|---|---|---|
| ANTI-A | ANTI-B | ANTI-AB | $A_1$ CELLS | B CELLS | O CELLS | INTERPRETATION |
| + | + | + | + | − | − | $A_2B$ with anti-$A_1$ |
| + | − | + | + | + | − | $A_2$ with anti-$A_1$ |
| + | − | + | + | + | ± | $A_1$ with anti-O or H |
| + | + | + | + | + | ± | $A_1B$ with anti-O or H |

5. Centrifuge
6. Pasteur pipets

*Method*

1. 1 Volume of 10% saline cell suspension is added to 1 volume of anti-$A_1$ serum.

2. An equal volume of cell suspension is added to a second tube containing 1 volume of anti-A serum.

3. The cell-serum suspensions are mixed and centrifuged at 1,000 rpm for 1 minute. The sedimented cells are gently dislodged and observed for macroscopic agglutination.

*Results.* $A_1$ and $A_1B$ cells are agglutinated by both the anti-A and the anti-$A_1$ sera. $A_2$ and $A_2B$ cells are agglutinated by both the anti-A and the anti-$A_1$ sera. $A_u$ and $A_uB$ cells are agglutinated by the anti-A serum, but not by the anti-$A_1$ serum.

## Detection of Immune Forms of Anti-A and Anti-B

*Principle.* When a blood group-specific substance is added to a serum containing a mixture of naturally occurring and immune antibodies, it *absorbs the naturally occurring antibodies,* leaving the immune forms.

*Reagents and Apparatus*

1. Blood group-specific substances A and B
2. Test serum
3. Tubes—10 x 75 mm
4. Centrifuge
5. Pasteur pipets
6. $A_1$ Cells, B cells
7. 37°C Waterbath

*Method*

1. 3 Volumes of A blood group substance is added to a tube containing 1 volume of test serum.

2. 3 Volumes of B blood group substance is also added to 1 volume of the test serum.

3. The tubes are allowed to stand at room temperature for 15 to 30 minutes, and 1 volume of the absorbed serum from each tube is transferred to another tube.

4. 1 Volume of a 5% saline suspension of A cells is added to one tube, and 1 volume of a like suspension of B cells is added to the second tube.

5. The cells and sera are mixed and allowed to stand at room temperature for 10 minutes.

6. Both tubes are centrifuged at 2,000 rpm for 1 minute and examined macroscopically for agglutination. If no agglutination is evident, it indi-

cates that naturally occurring anti-A and/or anti-B have been neutralized by the group-specific substance. If agglutination is present, steps 1 to 6 are repeated, using 6 volumes of group-specific substance.

7. If neutralization is satisfactory, the tubes in 6 are incubated at 37°C for 1 hour and the cells are washed 4 times in large volumes of saline.

8. 1 Drop of anti-human globulin serum is added to each tube, which is then centrifuged at 1,000 rpm for 1 minute. The sedimented cells are gently dislodged and observed for macroscopic agglutination.

*Results.* If no agglutination is present, immune anti-A and anti-B are absent. If the anti-human globulin test is positive, an immune antibody is present.

*Notes.* Positive and negative controls should be set up for the anti-human globulin test as described on page 393.

### Detection of ABO Secretor Status

*Principle.* Secretor status is regulated by a dominant gene for the characteristic (see p. 409). A secretor secretes a water-soluble substance in his body fluids, and usually investigations are carried out using the saliva of the subject. Saliva is collected and placed in a boiling waterbath to destroy enzyme activity that would inactivate ABH substances. It is centrifuged and added to anti-$A_1$, anti-B or anti-H serum. If the saliva is obtained from a secretor, it will neutralize the corresponding antisera (i.e., anti-H neutralized by H substance from a Group O individual, anti-A neutralized by A secretor substance from a group A individual, etc.)

*Reagents and Apparatus*
1. Anti-H (obtained from the seeds of *Ulex europeans*), anti-A or anti-B
2. Test saliva
3. 2% Saline suspension of Group O cells, A cells or B cells.
4. Tubes—10 × 75 mm
5. Centrifuge
6. Boiling waterbath
7. Saline

*Method*
1. 10 ml of test saliva is collected and the enzyme activity is destroyed by placing in a boiling waterbath for 10 minutes.
2. The specimen is centrifuged and the supernatant fluid collected.
3. Set up a row of tubes as shown in Table 10-12.
4. The appropriate antisera is diluted by adding 0.3 ml of the antiserum to 1.2 ml of saline.
5. 0.1 ml of the diluted antisera is added to each of the 9 tubes and

TABLE 10-12. Saliva Dilution for Detection of ABO Secretor Status.

| Tube | Saline (ml) | Saliva (ml) | Final Dilution |
|------|-------------|-------------|----------------|
| 1 | 0.1 | 0.1 | 1:2 |
| 2 | 0.1 | 0.1 of total of tube 1 | 1:4 |
| 3 | 0.1 | 0.1 of total of tube 2 | 1:8 |
| 4 | 0.1 | 0.1 of total of tube 3 | 1:16 |
| 5 | 0.1 | 0.1 of total of tube 4 | 1:32 |
| 6 | 0.1 | 0.1 of total of tube 5 | 1:64 |
| 7 | 0.1 | 0.1 of total of tube 6 | 1:128 |
| 8 | 0.1 | 0.1 of total of tube 7 | 1:256 |
| 9 | 0.2 ml | | Control |

Discard 0.1 ml from tube 8.

mixed well. The tubes are allowed to remain at room temperature for 10 minutes.

6. 0.1 ml of a 2% saline suspension of the appropriate cells is added to each of the tubes, mixed and allowed to remain at room temperature for 5 to 10 minutes.

7. The tubes are centrifuged at 1,000 rpm for 1 minute and the sedimented cells are dislodged and observed for macroscopic agglutination.

*Results.* Saliva from a secretor contains H substance, which, if present, will neutralize anti-H and inhibit agglutination of Group O cells. Likewise, saliva from a secretor containing a substance will neutralize anti-A and inhibit agglutination of Group A cells; saliva from a B individual if a secretor will neutralize anti-B; and that from AB persons will neutralize both anti-A and anti-B.

## DISCREPANCIES IN ABO TYPING

### Cell Grouping

1. Weak missing antigens may be due to rare alleles of either A or B (see Tables 10-3 and 10-5). More common discrepancies are shown in Table 10-11.

2. If results of the routine typing include any combination of the following (Table 10-13):

Proceed by

a. Washing the patient's red cells 3 times in large volumes of saline.

b. Repeating the typing on the washed cells using anti-A, anti-A$_1$, anti-B, anti-A,B, and anti-H. Include Group O adult and cord cells and an autocontrol in the backtyping.

TABLE 10-13.

| FORWARD TYPING* | | BACKTYPING | |
| --- | --- | --- | --- |
| ANTI-A | ANTI-B | A CELLS | B CELLS |
| O/w | O | O | ++++ |
| or O | O/w | ++++ | O |

* Anti-A,B should always be used in routine typing.


    c. Incubating all tubes at 4°C, and if necessary, repeating parts (a) and (b) and reincubate at 20°C

    d. Reading all weak or apparently negative results microscopically.

    3. Mixed field agglutination patterns are sometimes characteristic of chimera. This is an individual possessing more than one population of red cells. Genetic mosaicism due to dispermy (fertilization of an ovum with 2 nuclei by 2 sperm) and chimeric twins produce dual populations of cells for the extent of their lives, while transfusion-induced chimerism is a transient phenomenon arising as a result of a massive transfusion of Group O red cells into a Group A patient. An example of a twin chimera is: In such examples, a transplacental transfusion (graft) from a fraternal

| | GROUP |
| --- | --- |
| Mother | AB |
| Father | O |
| Twin A | A |
| Twin B | AB |

twin to another may establish a line of cells in the recipient twin which are genetically dissimilar to his own. Thus, Twin B is naturally a Group B individual to whom A cells have been grafted. In such cases, Twin B would have two cell populations A and B, and not one, AB, as is at first apparent.

    4. Polyagglutinability.

    5. B-like antigen may be acquired by Group A patients secondary to underlying diseases, (carcinoma of the colon or pelvic areas, leukemia, etc). The red cells absorb a B-like polysaccharide, usually derived from *Escherichia coli* or *Proteus vulgaris,* which reacts with some anti-B sera.

    6. The "innocent bystander effect." This is caused by an antibody to a compound or drug, Forming a complex with that substance and the complex attaches itself to the red cell (see Detection of Drug-induced antibodies, p. 402.

    7. An acriflavin antibody has been reported[1] in a patient's serum that combined with the dye used in most commercial anti-B sera. The

complex attaches itself to the patient's cells resulting in agglutination of those cells when mixed with acriflavin-tinted anti-B, irrespective of the presence of the B antigen.

8. A similar mechanism can result in individuals having antibodies against phenacetin, paracetamol, paraphenacetidin and methacetin.

9. Anti-caprylate antibody in an individual's serum can combine with sodium caprylate used as a stabilizer of commercial bovine albumin, to produce false-positive agglutination whenever the albumin is used in testing.

10. Some typing serums and bovine albumins may be contaminated by antibodies against human γ-globulins. These antibodies when they come into contact with red cells which are already sensitized with other antibodies, may act as anti-antibodies (e.g., rheumatoid factor).

### Serum Grouping

Unexpected antibodies are the commonest cause of apparent dinorep ant results in the backtyping of the ABO groups.

1. Rouleaux formation should be suspected if the autocontrol is positive at room temperature and at 37°C but negative after the antiglobulin test. The problem with the appearance of rouleaux formation is the probability of its marking true agglutination due to specific cold agglutinins such as anti-Le$^a$, anti-M, and anti-P. The causes of rouleaux and the dispersing methods that can be used are found on page 399.

2. Autoanti-I may cause strong agglutination in all backtyping cells and in all panel cells. The agglutination is usually stronger at colder temperatures (4°C and 20°C) but may also be found after 37°C incubation. Since almost all adult cells are I-positive, confirmation can be made by showing negative results using cord cells.

3. Anti-H specificity. In the sequence of events leading to the development of A or B antigens, a precursor substance is converted to H substance through the addition of fructose by the action of fucosyl transferase. Individuals possessing A or B genes elaborate transferases which act to add further sugars to the molecule to determine A or B specificity. Although the A gene end product, N-acetyl-d-galactosamine, attaches to the same sugar molecule as the H gene, the terminal specificity appears to be mainly A with little H. The B gene end product, d-galactose, produces similar expressions of H, and the combined AB gene likewise shows the greatest reduction of H reactivity.

4. Cold-specific antibodies. The cells used for backtyping possess antigenic determinants for cold antibodies such as M, P, Le$^a$, etc. Discrepancies may also be the result of occasional warm antibodies, anti-D, anti-E, anti-C and anti-Kell have all been known to react in this way.

Other antibody reactions found in this type of discrepancy are shown in Table 10-11 (p. 414).

5. Anti IA, IB. Antibodies with these specificities have been found secondary to patients with autoimmune diseases and diseases of the reticuloendothelial system. The presence of such antibodies can be differentiated by their reaction against an interaction product of the genes for I and A (or I and B) but not against the separate products I and A. An IA antibody does not react against adult I-positive cells, unless they are also Group A, nor does it react with cord A cells (I-negative). The antibody is also uninhibited by soluble group-specific substances.

6. Weak agglutinins. The presence of weak agglutinins in the backtyping serum can be secondary to underlying diseases such as hypogammaglobulinemia and chronic lymphocytic leukemia. If the backtyping cells fail to agglutinate, repeat the tests using fresh $A_1$, $A_2$, $B_1$, and O adult and cord cells and an autoagglutinin control. Incubate at room temperature for 30 minutes, and carry out antiglobulin tests on all negative results.

## THE LEWIS SYSTEM

The interaction of the Lewis system with secretor status and its association with the ABO blood groups is discussed on page 410. The common properties of the Lewis system are shown in Table 10-14.

At least four antibodies can be differentiated in this system. Anti-Le$^a$ is commonly found, occasionally accompanied by anti-Le$^b$. More frequently the antibody reacts with Le$^{(a-b+)}$ cells due to the small amount of unconverted Le$^a$ substance present in these cells (see p. 412). Anti-Le$^b$ exists in two forms, anti-Le$^{bH}$ and anti-Le$^{bL}$. The differentiation between these two antibodies is shown in Table 10-15.

Anti-Le$_x$ often reacts with sera from Le$^{(a-b-)}$ individuals containing a mixture of anti-Le$^a$ and anti-Le$^b$. The existence of this antibody as something different from a mixture of anti-Le$^a$ and anti-Le$^b$ is still unresolved, although it has been reported that anti-Le$^x$ reacts wtih most cord cells. This would appear to characterize the antibody as being distinct from a mixture of the two other forms.

Other rare forms of Lewis antibodies are anti-Le$^c$ and anti-Le$^d$. Anti-Le$^c$ reacts with Le$^{(a-b-)}$ cells from individuals of genotype le le, se se and is inhibited by saliva from the same persons. Anti-Le$^d$ reacts with Le$^{(a-b-)}$ cells from individuals of genotype le le, Se se, or le le, Se Se.

Lewis antibodies are frequently found in individuals who have never been transfused or received other antigenic stimuli and are also more commonly found in women during their reproductive period. The antigens often become weaker during pregnancy and females of type Le$^{(a-b+)}$ may lose their antigenicity and type as Le$^{(a-b-)}$ during this period. The

TABLE 10-14. Common Properties of the Lewis System.

| Genes<br>Genotypes | Le, le<br>$Le^{(a-b+)}$ | $Le^{(a-b-)}$ | |
|---|---|---|---|
| $Le^{(a+b-)}$ | | | |
| Frequency | CAUCASIAN (%) | NEGROID (%) | NEWBORN (%) |
| $Le^{(a+b-)}$ | 22 | 22 | 0 |
| $Le^{(a-b+)}$ | 72 | 55 | 0 |
| $Le^{(a-b-)}$ | 6 | 22 | 100 |

| | |
|---|---|
| Optimal temperature | 4-20°C<br>Occasional immune forms react at 37°C |
| Natural or immune forms | Usually natural antibodies found<br>Occasionally immune forms seen |
| Type of antigen-antibody | Agglutination and occasionally hemolysis (anti-$Le^b$) |
| Technique best for detection | Most antibodies react at 4-20°C in saline and albumin<br>Some antibodies react at 37°C in saline, albumin, by the antiglobulin test, and by enzyme techniques |
| Immunoglobulin type | IgM<br>Rare IgG |
| Clinical importance | Of little importance<br>Occasional transfusion reaction reported |
| Secretor status | $Le^{(a+b-)}$ nonsecretor of ABH substance, secretor $Le^a$<br>$Le^{(a-b+)}$ secretor of ABH, $Le^a$ and $Le^b$ substances<br>$Le^{(a-b-)}$ 80% secrete ABH substance<br>20% nonsecretors |

antibodies are not known to cause hemolytic disease of the newborn for two reasons. First, a majority of infants have not taken up the antigens from the plasma to the cells at this stage of maturation and invariably type as $Le^{(a-b-)}$, and second, the antibodies are of the IgM form and do not cross the placental barrier.

Both anti-$Le^a$ and anti-$Le^{bL}$ can cause transfusion reactions. The blood of choice in patients having both of these antibodies is $Le^{(a-b-)}$, and is more easily obtained from Negro populations. In patients with

TABLE 10-15. Reaction Differences Between Anti-$Le^{bH}$ and Anti-$Le^{bL}$.

| CELLS | ANTI-$Le^{bH}$ | ANTI-$Le^{bL}$ |
|---|---|---|
| O $Le^{(b+)}$ | +++ | +++ |
| $A_2Le^{(b+)}$ | +++ | +++ |
| $A_1Le^{(b+)}$ | O/w | +++ |
| $Le^b$ substance (saliva) | Neutralized | Neutralized |
| H substance | Neutralized | Not neutralized |

anti-Le$^a$ (a more common situation), Le$^{(a-b-)}$ blood should be transfused, thus avoiding the risk of a reaction with Le$^{(a-b+)}$ blood carrying small amounts of Le$^a$ substance. Patients possessing anti-Le$^b$ can be safely transfused with Le$^{(a+b-)}$ blood.


## MNSs SYSTEM

The MNS system was discovered by injecting human red cells into rabbits, absorbing the resulting immune serum with one sample of human cells and showing that it would still react with other samples.

The system was believed to be simple, but since its discovery, large numbers of blood factors have been found to be associated with it. It promises to surpass many other blood group systems in complexity.

The four antigens, M, N, S and s are controlled by two sets of alleles at closely linked loci. At the first locus are either M or N and at the second locus either S or s. Table 10-16 lists the common properties of the system.

The U antigen is of very high incidence. Nearly all caucasians are U-positive, but U-negative Negroid bloods have been demonstrated. The antigen is still incompletely understood. All samples of S+s−, S+s+, and S−s+ cells are U-positive, but disagreement between apparent U-positive and U-negative samples has been reported in the amorphic situation S−s−. The postulation that there is a mosaicism of the U antigen has been made, resulting in more than one type of U-negative individual. However, the role of the U antigen is still unclear, and the determinant should be considered as being separate and distinct from S and s.

Other rare alleles of the MNSs locus include N$_2$, M$^g$, M$^c$, M$_I$, M$^k$ and M$^v$. Satellite antigens belonging to the system include Hu, He, Mi$^a$, Vw (Gr), Mur, Hil, Vr, Ri$^a$, St$^a$, Mt$^a$, Cl$^a$, Ny$^a$ and Sul.

The common properties of the MNSs system are shown in Table 10-16. The antibodies are naturally occurring, but occasional immune forms can be found. Anti-M and anti-N react well at 20°C in saline and do not exhibit reactions when enzyme techniques are used. Most antibodies (anti-M and anti-N) are IgM in composition, but a few anti-M antibodies are found as immune IgG forms. Most of the forms of these two antibodies neither bind complement nor cause lysis in vitro.

Anti-S and anti-s differ in some of their reactions. Some anti-S sera react in saline and by antiglobulin methods but do not react with enzyme techniques. Anti-s rarely reacts in saline but reacts by antiglobulin methods and enzyme techniques. Anti-S is found both as IgG and IgM forms, the IgG forms occasionally having the ability to bind complement, while the IgM forms do not possess this property. Anti-U mostly react by the antiglobulin and by enzyme techniques, but a few examples reacting by saline and albumin methods at 20°C and 37°C have been reported.

Most of the antibodies directed against the Mi$^a$ (Miltenberger) complex (anti-Gr, Mur, Hil and Mi$^a$) react both by saline techniques at room temperature and by antiglobulin methods. The MNSs system is clinically important in that transfusion reactions due to anti-M, anti-S, anti-s, anti-U, and some of the rarer Mi$^a$ groups occur. Hemolytic disease of the newborn (HDN) due to anti-S, anti s and anti-U occurs, but only rare examples of the disease due to anti-M are known. Anti-N has not been implicated in HDN.

TABLE 10-16. Common Properties of the MNS System.

| Genes | M, N, S, s, U |  |
|---|---|---|
| | M$_1$, M$_2$, N$_2$, M$^g$, M$^c$, M$^v$ | |
| | Hu, He | |
| | Mi$^a$, Gr, Mur, Hil, Vr, Ri$^a$, St$^a$, Mt$^a$, Cl$^a$, Ny$^a$, Sul | |
| Frequency | CAUCASIAN (%) | NEGROID (%) |
| MM | 28 | 26 |
| MN | 50 | 44 |
| NN | 22 | 30 |
| SS | 11 | 3 |
| Ss | 44 | 28 |
| ss | 45 | 69 |
| Optimal temperature | 4-20°C | |
| | Occasionally immune forms react at 37°C | |
| Natural or immune forms | Usually natural antibodies found | |
| | Occasionally immune forms seen | |
| Type of antigen antibody reaction | Agglutination, except some forms of anti-M which cause hemolysis | |
| Technique best for detection | Most anti-M and anti-N antibodies react best at 4-20°C in saline or albumin, not as well with antiglobulin test, and negatively with enzymes | |
| | Anti-S antibodies react best at 20-31°C by saline albumin, and antiglobulin tests but not with enzymes | |
| | Most anti-s antibodies react by antigloublin test and enzyme procedures | |
| | Anti-U reacts best by antiglobulin tests and enzymes but rarely in saline or albumin. | |
| Immungolobulin type | Most anti-M, anti-N, and anti-M$_1$ antibodies are IgM forms | |
| | Most anti-s and anti-U are IgG antibodies | |
| | Anti-Mi$^a$ complexes anti-s usually found both as IgG and IgM forms | |
| Clinical importance | Transfusion reactions have implicated anti-M, anti-S, anti-s, anti-U and anti-Mi$^a$ | |
| | Hemolytic disease of newborn reported due to anti-S, anti-s, anti-U, and rarely anti-M, and anti-M$_1$ medicolegal implication | |
| | Paternity tests | |

## MN Blood Typing

*Principle.* Commercial anti-M and anti-N, produced by injecting rabbits with human N and M antigens, is used. The antisera are added to test cells, incubated at room temperature, and examined for agglutinations.

### Reagents and Apparatus
1. Anti-M and anti-N sera
2. 2% Saline suspension of test cells.
3. Tubes—10 × 75 mm
4. Centrifuge
5. Pasteur pipets
6. Saline
7. M and N control cells

### Method
1. 2 Volumes of 2% saline suspension of test cells is added to each of 2 tubes.
2. 1 Volume of anti-M is added to one tube and 1 volume of anti-N is added to the other tube.
3. Steps 1 and 2 are repeated, using M-positive cells and N-positive cells.
4. The cell-serum suspensions are mixed and left at room temperature for 20 to 30 minutes. They are then examined macroscopically for agglutination.

### Notes
1. *Do not* centrifuge before examining the tubes.
2. If anti-M and anti-N lectin sera are used, the procedure is repeated and the tubes centrifuged at 1,000 rpm for 1 minute before examining for agglutination.

## P SYSTEM

An hypothesis of the genetics of the P system is shown in Table 10-17.

$\dot{p}K$ represents a hypothetical precursor substance which is acted on successively by a gene Y converting $\dot{p}^k$ to $\dot{p}$, and by $P_1$ and $P_2$ converting $\dot{p}$ to $PP_1$ and P respectively; p is considered an amorph which makes no conversion of $\dot{p}$ substance.

The gene y is also considered an amorph, making no conversion of $\dot{p}^k$ substance which then becomes exposed to the action of $P_1$ and $P_2$ and these genes convert $\dot{p}^k$ into $P^kP_1$ and $P^k$ respectively.[2]

A comparison of the P system with the ABO system is shown in Table 10-18.

The reactions of the P blood group system are shown in Table 10-19 and the common properties of the system in Table 10-20.

TABLE 10-17. Hypothetical Interpretation of the Genetic Background of the P System.[2]

| GENES | SUBSTANCE | GENES | ANTIGEN |
|---|---|---|---|
| | | $P_1P_1$ or $P_1P_2$ or $P_1p$ | $PP_1$ |
| YY or Yy | | | |
| | $\dot{P}$ | $P_2P_2$ or $P_2p$ | $P$ |
| $\dot{P}K$ | | pp | $\dot{p}$ |
| yy | | | |
| | | $P_1P_1$ or $P_1P_2$ or $P_1P$ | $P^kP_1$ |
| YY | $\dot{p}K$ | $P_2P_2$ or $P_2p$ | pK |
| | | pp | $\dot{p}K$ |

TABLE 10-18. The P and ABO Systems Compared.

| ANTISERA | | | | RED CELL PHENO TYPE | GENOTYPE | ANTIBODIES IN SERUM |
|---|---|---|---|---|---|---|
| ANTI-P+ $P_1$ | ANTI-A+ $A_1$ | ANTI- $P_1$ | ANTI- $A_1$ | | | |
| + | | + | | $P_1$ | $P_1 P_1$, $P_1$, $P_2$, $P_1\overline{p}$ | None |
| | + | | + | $A_1$ | $A_1 A_1$, $A_1$, $A_2$, $A_1 O$ | None |
| + | | O | | $P_2$ | $P_2P_2$, $P_2p$ | Sometimes anti-$P_1$ |
| | + | | 0 | $A_2$ | $A_2A_2, A_2, A_2O$ | Sometimes anti-$A_1$ |
| 0 | | 0 | | P | pp | Anti-P+$P_1$+$p^k$ |
| | 0 | | 0 | 0 | 0 | Anti-A+$A_1$ |

TABLE 10-19. Common Reactions of the P Blood Group System.

| CELL PHENOTYPE | REACTIONS WITH | | | |
|---|---|---|---|---|
| | ANTI-$P_1$ | ANTI-P | ANTI-$PP_1P^k$ | ANTI-$P^k$ |
| $P_1$ | + | + | + | 0 |
| $P_2$ | 0 | + | + | 0 |
| $P_k$ | 0 | W | 0 | 0 |
| $P_1$ | + | 0 | + | + |
| $P_2{}^k$ | 0 | 0 | + | + |

TABLE 10-20. Common Properties of the P Blood Group System.

| Genes | $P_1 P_2 \bar{p}$ | CAUCASIAN (%) | NEGROID (%) |
|---|---|---|---|
| Frequency | $P_1$ ($P_1$, $P_1P_2$, $P_1p$) | 79 | 94 |
| | $P_2$ ($P_2P_2$, $P_2p$) | 21 | 6 |
| | p (pp) | Rare | Rare |
| | $p^k$($P_1^k$, $P_2^k$) | Rare | Rare |

| | |
|---|---|
| Optimal temperature | 4-20°C |
| | Rare antibodies reacting at 37°C |
| Natural or immune forms | Natural |
| Type of antigen-antibody reaction | Hemolysis and agglutination |
| Technique best for detection | Most anti-$P_1$ antibodies react at 4°C in saline and albumin, the reaction becoming progressively weaker as temperature increases to 20°C and 37°C |
| | Occasional anti-$P_1$ antibodies react by enzyme methods and antiglobulin test |
| | Most anti-P sera react best at 20-37°C in saline, at 4-37°C in albumin, by antiglobulin test and enzymatic methods |
| | Anti-PP$_1$, P$^k$ (anti-Tj$^a$) antibodies react similarly as anti-P |
| Immunoglobulin type | Mostly IgM |
| | A few examples of IgG forms of anti-PP$_1$P$^k$ (Tj$^a$) reported |
| Clinical importance | Anti-PP$_1$P$^k$ (Tj$^a$) and anti-P responsible for transfusion reactions |
| | PP$_1$ P$^k$ (Tj$^a$) rarely implicated in hemolytic disease of newborn |

# RHESUS BLOOD GROUP

*Properties.* The Rhesus blood group is one of the most complicated systems. The finding of so many antibodies characterizing different antigens has led to difficulties in nomenclature and symbolization. Two theories have been proposed to explain the inheritance of the Rhesus factors. Weiner theorizes that there are multiple alleles occurring at a single locus on a chromosome, each controlling the appearance of characteristic antigens. Rh-Hr factors are transmitted by a series of 8 allelic pairs, giving rise to 36 phenotypes. Weiner proposes that the gene be symbolized as a unit controlling an agglutinogen (a red cell antigen), which may have multiple blood factors. The Fisher-Race postulation is that there are closely linked genes on the same chromosome, which are inherited as a unit. Each gene determines a corresponding antigen, which is identified by a specific antiserum. (See Fig. 10-2 and Table 10-21.)

According to this theory, genes on a chromosome are not linked, although they are in close proximity to each other. This factor is used to

| CHROMOSOME | AGGLUTINOGEN | BLOOD FACTOR | ANTIBODY |
|---|---|---|---|
| WEINER'S THEORY | $R^Z$ SINGLE GENE | $Rh_Z$ | Rh⁰ rh' rh'' | ANTI Rh₀ ANTI rh' ANTI rh'' |

| | ANTIGEN | | |
|---|---|---|---|
| FISHER- RACE THEORY | D C E CLOSELY LINKED GENES | D C E | ANTI D ANTI C ANTI E |

FIG. 10-2. Weiner's and Fisher-Race postulates.

explain the occurrence of rare genotypes by means of crossing over. This process is a separation and exchange of genes situated some distance from each other and it is thought to take place during meiosis, when the number of chromosomes is reduced. (See Fig. 10-3.)

A third nomenclature free of genetic interpretation has been suggested.[3] This system uses numbers assigned to the antigens in the sequence of their discovery and permits the representation of the reac-

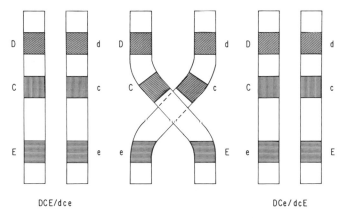

DCE/dce                    DCe/dcE

FIG. 10-3. Fisher-Race theory of crossing over.

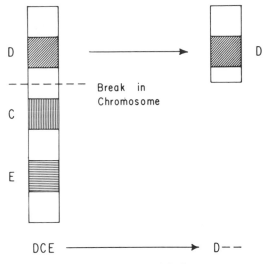

FIG. 10-4. Gene deletion.

tions of the cells with the antisera. Table 10-22 illustrates the comparisons of the three different nomenclatures.

The interpretation of the Weiner and Fisher-Race systems can be facilitated by the use of the following rules.

1. R denotes the presence of $Rh_0$ (D), r reflects its absence.

2. The superscript 1 or ′ (prime) signifies the determinant rh′ (C); 2 or ″ (double prime) signifies the determinant rh″ (E).

3. Usually when rh′ (C) is present, hr″ (e) is also present; and rh″ (E) is usually accompanied by hr′ (C).

*Antigens.* The five commonest antigens of the system are $Rh_0$ (D), hr′ (c), rh′ (C), rh″ (E) and hr″ (e). Of the variants, the most important is $Rh_0$

TABLE 10-21. Comparison of the Weiner and Fisher-Race Genotypes.

| GENES | | | |
|---|---|---|---|
| FISHER-RACE | WEINER | AGGLUTINOGEN | FACTORS |
| CDe | $R_1$ | $Rh_1$ | $Rh_0$, rh′, hr′, rh; |
| cde | r | rh | hr″, hr′, hr |
| cDE | $R_2$ | $Rh_2$ | $Rh_0$, hr″, rh′ |
| cDe | $R^0$ | $Rh_0$ | $Rh_0$, hr″, rh; |
| Cde | r′ | rh′ | rh′, hr″, rh; |
| cdE | r″ | rh″ | rh″, hr′ |
| CDE | $R_z$ | $Rh_z$ | $Rh_0$, rh′, rh″ |
| CdE | $r^y$ | $rh_y$ | rh′, rh″ |

TABLE 10-22. A Comparison of the Three Rhesus Nomenclatures.

| WEINER | FISHER-RACE | NUMERICAL |
|--------|-------------|-----------|
| $Rh_o$ | D | Rh1 |
| $Rh_o$ | $D^u$ | Rhw1 |
| rh' | C | Rh2 |
| rh" | E | Rh3 |
| hr' | c | Rh4 |
| hr" | e | Rh5 |
| hr | f (ce) | Rh6 |
| $rh_i$ | Ce | Rh7 |
| $rh^{w1}$ | $C^w$ | Rh8 |
| $rh^x$ | $C^x$ | Rh9 |
| $hr^v$ | V ($ce^s$) | Rh10 |
| $rh^{w2}$ | $E^w$ | Rh11 |
| $rh^G$ | G | Rh12 |
| $Rh^A$ | — | Rh13 |
| $Rh^B$ | — | Rh14 |
| $Rh^C$ | — | Rh15 |
| $Rh^D$ | — | Rh16 |
| $Hr_o$ | — | Rh17 |
| Hr | — | Rh18 |
| $hr^s$ | — | Rh19 |
| — | VS ($e^s$) | Rh20 |
| | $C^G$ | Rh21 |
| — | CE | Rh22 |
| — | $D^{WIFI}$ | Rh23 |
| — | $E^T$ | Rh24 |
| — | LW | Rh25 |
| $hr^A$ | Deal | Rh26 |
| — | cE | Rh27 |
| $hr^h$ | Harper-Comacho | Rh28 |

($D^u$), originally referred to as a weak $Rh_o$ (D). This antigen occasionally causes confusion because some examples are agglutinated by some $Rh_o$ (D) antisera and not by others. Two different grades of the antigen are known. The first is detected only by the antiglobulin test and the second is distinguished from ordinary $Rh_o$ (D) only by the fact that agglutination in saline is brought about by only a proportion of complete anti-$Rh_o$ (D) sera.

The original form of the antigen was shown to be inherited. A true $Rh_o$ ($D^u$) (so-called low grade) is the direct product of an inherited gene. Therefore, this form of antigen can be passed on to future generations. Ordinarily it can be detected only by the antiglobulin test after first sensitizing the cells with anti-D sera. The high grade form of the antigen reacts weakly with either complete or incomplete anti-$Rh_o$ (D) and only seldom requires the use of the antiglobulin test for its detection. This form is due to a gene interaction brought about by position effects of other Rh determinants. Thus, a gene controlling rh′ (c) in the transposition may suppress the $Rh_0$ (D) antigen on the opposite chromosome. Cells of genotype $R_1$ r′ (CDe/Cde) or $R_1$ rY (CDe/CdE) may give weak results with anti-$Rh_0$ (D) and appear as $R,R′$ (CD$^u$e/Cde) or $R_1$rY (CD$^u$e/CdE). This "high grade" variation is not passed on to future generations since its development depends upon the rare r′ (Cde) or rY (Cd) chromosomal arrangement.

It is doubtful whether $Rh_0$ (D$^u$) can elicit an immune response, and although individuals with the antigen have been reported as forming anti-$Rh_0$ (D) if transfused with $Rh_0$ (D)-positive blood, the occurrence is extremely rare and is not fully accepted. Consequently an $RH_0$ (D$^u$)-positive individual should be considered $Rh_0$ (D)-positive as a blood donor, and can be transfused either $Rh_0$ (D)-positive or -negative blood when a recipient.

The determinant rh$^G$ (G) was discovered when red cells were found to react to anti-$Rh_0$rh′ (CD) but not to anti-rh′ (C) or anti-$Rh_0$ (D). This antibody is in reality anti-rh′ (C) + anti-$Rh_0$ (D) + anti-rh$^G$ (G) and explains the inability to separate the anti-rh′ (C) and anti-$Rh_0$ (D) from some $Rh_0$rh′ (CD) serums by selective absorption.

More unusual antigens referred to as "gene interaction antigens" are also found in the Rhesus system. The antigen hr (f) detects a product expressed on the cell when the determinants hr′ (c) and hr″ (e) are on the same chromosome. Other similar antigenic expressions are CE, rh$_i$ (Ce) and hr$^v$ (ce$^8$). This antigen ce$^8$ is also referred to as V. It differs from hr (f) or (ce) by exhibiting a higher frequency among Negroes than Caucasians. As hr (f), it is only found in individuals who have hr′ (c) and hr″ (e) on the same chromosome. Most examples of anti-hr$^v$ (ce$^8$) or (V) have been formed by individuals or rh rh (cde/cde) genotype indicating the possibility that hr (f) or (ce) and hr$^v$ (ce$^8$) are alleles on the same chromosome.

A possible genetic pathway for the Rhesus blood group system was proposed by Race[4]. The theory postulates the conversion of a precursor substance to a second form ordinarily mediated by a gene called X′r if present in either the homozygous or heterozygous forms. The recessive gene X°r when present in the homozygous form is believed to block the conversion of precursor substance 1 to substance 2 resulting in the amorphic type $Rh_{NULL}$ (---/---). Since this genotype merely halts the metabolic production of the substrate which the LW and CDE genes convert and does not affect the presence of those genes, they are passed on and expressed in the offspring. It appears that there is a reduced amount of precursor substance 2 in the heterozygote X°r genotype. Since this is a weakening of the Rh antigens but not the LW antigens when X°r is heterozygous, it is possible that either the requirements for

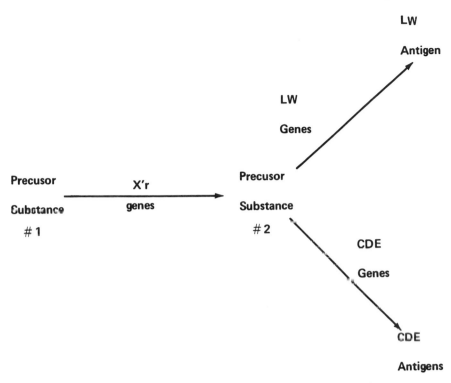

FIG. 10-5. Postulated pathway producing Rh antigens.[4]

the LW gene use less substance 2 than the CDE genes, or that the LW gene needs are satisfied first. An individual lacking the LW genes (having lw/lw) blocks the conversion of the precursor substance 2 to the LW antigen, resulting in an LW-negative phenotype. Figure 10-5 is a proposed schematic of this genetic postulation.

*Antibodies.* The common properties of the antibodies of the Rhesus system are shown in Table 10-23. With a few minor exceptions, the antibodies are all IgG forms and arise as the result of the immune mechanism. The antibodies are all detected by albumin, enzyme and antiglobulin tests, and are implicated in both transfusion reactions and many in hemolytic disease of the newborn

None of the antibodies of this system possesses the ability to blind complement and consequently does not cause hemolysis in vitro

### Rhesus Blood Typing

*Principle.* Incomplete (high protein, slide) antiserum is mixed with whole blood in a tube and incubated at 37°C.

TABLE 10-23. Common Properties of the Rhesus Blood Group System.

| Genes | D C E c e f G V Ce cE CE $C^w$ $C^u$ $C^x$ $E^w$ $E^u$ $e^s$ $e^i$ | | |
|---|---|---|---|
| | | CAUCASIAN (%) | NEGROID (%) |
| Frequency and genotypes | $R_1r$ $R_1$ $R_0$ | 34 | 24 |
| | $R_1R_1$ | 17 | 3 |
| | rr | 15 | 6 |
| | $R_1R_2$ | 13 | 2 |
| | $R_2R_0R_2r$ | 12 | 12 |
| | $R_0R_0$ $R_0$ r | 2 | 49 |
| | $R_2R_2$ | 2 | 2 |
| | $R_1R_1$ | 1 | 1 |

| | |
|---|---|
| Optimal temperature | 37°C |
| Natural or immune forms | Immune forms |
| Serological behavior | Albumins, antiglobulin test and enzymes |
| | Occasionally saline reacting anti-E and anti-$C^w$ found |
| Immunoglobulins | Most Rh antibodies are IgG; some anti-D, anti-E and anti-$C^w$ are IgM |
| Type of antigen-antibody reaction | Agglutination |
| Clinical importance | Hemolytic disease of newborn |
| | Transfusion reactions, medicolegal (paternity cases, forensic) |

### Reagents and Apparatus

1. Incomplete antisera (anti-C, anti-D, anti-E or anti-c)
2. 2% Test cells in their own serum
3. Tubes—10 × 75 mm
4. 37°C Waterbath
5. Centrifuge
6. Known positive and negative control cells

### Method

1. 1 Volume of incomplete antiserum is added to an equal volume of 2% test cells in their own serum.

2. The cells and serum are mixed, incubated at 37°C for 5 minutes, and centrifuged at 1,000 rpm for 1 minute.

3. Steps 1 and 2 are repeated, using known positive and negative cells in place of the test cells.

4. The sedimented cell button is gently agitated and observed for macroscopic agglutination.

*Results.* Agglutination denotes that the blood is positive for the particular antigen corresponding to the antiserum used.

### Notes

1. Both a known heterozygous-positive blood and a negative blood should be used as controls.

2. Rh typing can also be carried out, using a complete or saline antibody. When this is done, the test and control cells are resuspended in saline and *not* in their own serum. The procedure is repeated as previously described.

3. Slide techniques can be adopted, using incomplete antisera. A major disadvantage of any slide method is the occurrence of false-positive reactions due to drying of the cell-serum mixture and to misinterpretation of agglutination at the periphery of the drop.

4. False-negative reactions should be excluded and are often caused by improper refrigeration of test bloods, contamination, dirty glassware and excessive anticoagulants. In addition, the G factor is known to produce negative reactions with both anti-C and anti-D, but positive reactions with anti-CD. Such variants are characterized by a weak reaction. The commonest variant, $D^u$, may be classified as Rh-negative unless care is taken.

5. To ensure that the $D^u$ variant is absent, anti-human globulin tests should be carried out on all D negative bloods. If a blood sample is $D^u$ positive, it will produce a positive anti-human globulin test, although the tube reaction with anti-D is often negative.

## KELL BLOOD GROUP SYSTEM

This system has three major pairs of allelic characters; K and k, $Kp^a$ and $Kp^b$ and $Js^a$ and $Js^b$ occupying closely linked genetic loci.

The genetic pathways of the system have been postulated by Race and Sanger[5]. A precursor substance is acted upon by an allele X, which converts the precursor material to KL substance necessary for the proper expression of the genes K k $Kp^a$ $Kp^b$ $Js^a$ $Js^b$ and $Ul^a$. The presence of the gene $K^o$ does not convert KL substance, and this is expressed in the type $K^o$ (Peltz).

In the presence of homozygous xx genes the precursor substance does not become fully converted to KL substance leaving mostly precursor substance and traces of KL material. In the presence of the normal Kell genes, this small amount of KL substance is utilized in the formation of only traces of K, k, $Kp^a$, $Kp^b$, $Js^a$, $Js^b$, $Ul^a$ antigens producing the very rare McLeod and Claas types.

The common properties of the Kell system are shown in Table 10-24

Some Kell antibodies possess the ability to bind complement, but nearly all of the antibodies in the system fail to cause in vitro lysis.

### Kell Blood Typing

#### Method
1. Two drops of anti-$Fy^a$ (and/or anti-$Fy^b$) serum is added to each of 3 6 tubes.

TABLE 10-24. Common Properties of the Kell Blood Group System.

| Genes | K k Kpª Kpᵇ Jsª Jsᵇ Ulª K k Kp | | |
|---|---|---|---|

| Frequency and genotype | | CAUCASIAN (%) | NEGROID (%) |
|---|---|---|---|
| | KK | 0.2 | Rare |
| | Kk | 8.6 | 2 |
| | kk | 91.2 | 98 |
| | Kp$^{(a+b-)}$ | Rare | — |
| | Kp$^{(a+b+)}$ | 2 | — |
| | Kp$^{(a-b+)}$ | 98 | — |
| | Js$^{(a+b-)}$ | — | 1 |
| | Js$^{(a+b+)}$ | Rare | 19 |
| | Js$^{(a-b+)}$ | 100 | 80 |

| | |
|---|---|
| Optimal temperature | 37°C |
| Natural or immune form | Immune |
| Serological behavior | Antiglobulin test |
| | Same anti-K, k and Kpª react in saline at 37°C and by enzyme techniques |
| | Most antibodies of system do not react well in albumin at 37°C |
| | Anti-Jsª and Jsᵇ react best by saline antiglobulin method |
| Immunoglobulins | Most K antibodies are IgG but some are IgM in structure |
| | The remainder of the antibodies of this sytem are IgG. |
| Type of antigen-antibody reaction | Agglutination |
| Clinical importance | Hemolytic disease of newborn (due to antibodies to K, k, Kpᵇ and Ku-Jsᵇ rarely) |
| | Transfusion reactions due to antibodies to K, k, Kpª, Kpᵇ, Jsª, and Jsᵇ |

| Nomenclature | FULL NAME | NOMENCLATURES | |
|---|---|---|---|
| | Kell | K | K1 |
| | Cellano | k | K2 |
| | Penny | Kpª | K3 |
| | Rautenberg | Kpᵇ | K4 |
| | Peltz | Kᵒ | K5 |
| | Sutter | Jsª | K6 |
| | Matthews | Jsᵇ | K7 |
| | — | Kʷ | K8 |
| | Claas | KL | K9 |
| | — | Ulª | K10 |

2. Two drops of a 2% saline suspension of patient's cells, Kell-positive cells and Kell-negative cells are added respectively to each tube.

3. The tubes are shaken to mix, incubated at 37°C for 30 minutes, and washed 3 times in 0.85% saline.

4. The saline is thoroughly removed from the last washing by decantation and blotting, and 2 drops of antiglobulin serum added.

5. The tubes are shaken to mix and centrifuged at 3600 rpm for 15 seconds (Serofuge).

6. The cell button is gently agitated and observed for macroscopic agglutination.

## DUFFY BLOOD GROUP SYSTEM

The common properties of the Duffy system are shown in Table 10-25.

### Duffy Blood Typing

#### Method

1. Two drops of antiFy$^a$ (and/or anti-Fy$^b$) serum is added to each of 3 (or 6) tubes.

2. Two drops of a 2% saline suspension of patient's cells, Fy$^a$-positive cells, and Fy$^{a-}$ cells are added respectively to each tube.

TABLE 10-25. Common Properties of the Duffy Blood Group System.

| Genes | | | |
|---|---|---|---|
| Frequency and genotype | Fy$^a$, Fy$^b$, Fy$^x$, Fy$^3$, Fy$^4$, Fy$^5$ | | |
| | | CAUCASIAN (%) | NEGROID (%) |
| | Fy$^{(a+b-)}$ | 17 | 9 |
| | Fy$^{(a+b+)}$ | 49 | 2 |
| | Fy$^{(a-b+)}$ | 34 | 22 |
| | Fy$^{(a-b-)}$ | — | 68 |
| Optimal temperature | 37°C. | | |
| Natural or immune form | Immune | | |
| Serological behavior | Antiglobulin test | | |
| | Rare examples of anti-Fy$^a$ reacting in saline known | | |
| | Treatment of Fy$^{a+}$ cells with enzymes apparently destroys their antigenic receptor sites | | |
| | Fy$^b$ antigen not as susceptible to enzyme action | | |
| Immunoglobulin | IgG | | |
| Type of antigen-antibody reaction | Agglutation (same examples of both anti-Fy$^a$ and Fy$^b$ bind complement but do not cause in vitro lysis) | | |
| Clinical importance | Transfusion reactions | | |
| | Hemolytic disease of newborn. | | |
| Miscellaneous | Anti-Fy$^4$ reported to react with Fy$^{(a-b-)}$ | | |
| | Fy$^{(a+b-)}$ and Fy$^{(a-b+)}$ cells | | |
| | Fy 4 believed to be allele of Fy$^a$ and Fy$^b$. | | |
| | Fy$^x$ reacts weakly with anti-Fy$^b$ serum but not with anti-Fy$^a$ | | |
| | Anti-Fy$^3$ reacts similarly to mixture of anti-Fy$^a$ and anti-Fy$^b$, but absorption tests fail to isolate either antibody | | |
| | Anti-Fy$^3$ not denatured by enzymes but gene Fy$^3$ postulated as but absorption tests fail to isolate either antibody | | |
| | Anti-Fy$^3$ not denatured by enzymes but gene Fy$^3$ postulated as | | |
| | Anti-Fy$^5$ also described | | |

3. The tubes are shaken to mix, incubated at 37°C for 30 minutes, and washed 3 times in 0.85% saline.

4. The saline is thoroughly removed from the last washing by decantation and blotting, and 2 drops of antiglobulin serum added.

5. The tubes are shaken to mix and centrifuged.

## KIDD BLOOD GROUP SYSTEM

This system is characterized by two alleles $JK^a$ and $JK^b$. The antibodies formed in this system are characterized by often being complement-dependent and rarely found in a pure form. They also deteriorate quickly and are frequently implicated in delayed hemolytic transfusion reactions even though the pretransfusion tests did not detect any abnormality.

Sera suspected of containing Kidd antibodies should be tested fresh while complement activity remains. Anti-$JK^a$ $JK^b$ formed by individuals of type $JK^{(a-b-)}$ cross-reacts with $JK^{(a+b-)}$ $JK^{(a-b+)}$ and $JK^{(a+b+)}$ cells.

The common properties of the Kidd blood group system are shown in Table 10-26.

## LUTHERAN BLOOD GROUP SYSTEM

Recent studies have disclosed new high frequency red cell antigens related to the Lutheran blood group. The common properties of the system are shown in Table 10-27.

### Genetic Pathway[6]

Marsh[6] has suggested that a precursor substance (I) forms a second precursor substance (II). Some of the precursor II material could then be used by $Au^a$ (Auberger) genes to make $Au^a$ antigen, and some could be converted into a third precursor (III), which could be used as substrate by $Lu^b$, $Lu^b$, Lu4, Lu5, Lu6, Lu7 and (Lu8 and Lu9—?) genes for the manufacture of their respective antigens. Precursor substance III is, in this hypothesis, believed to be Lu3.

If the presence of a dominant gene could block the precursor I conversion to precursor II, the cells would all type as $Lu^{(a-b-)}$, Lu $-3$, $-4$, $-5$, $-6$, $-7$ ($-8$, $-9$) and $Au^{(a-)}$. If a recessive gene in the homozygous state blocks the development of precursor II to precursor III, the cells would cell type as $Lu^{(a-b-)}$, Lu $-3$, $-4$, $-5$, $-6$, $-7$, ($-8$, $-9$) and $Au^{(a+)}$.

TABLE 10-26. Common Properties of the Kidd Blood Group System.

| Genes | JKª, JKᵇ | | |
|---|---|---|---|
| Frequency and genotype | | CAUCASIAN (%) | NEGROID (%) |
| | JK$^{(a+b-)}$ | 25 | 57 |
| | JK$^{(a+b+)}$ | 50 | 34 |
| | JK$^{(a-b+)}$ | 25 | 9 |
| | JK$^{(a-b-)}$ | — | — |

| | |
|---|---|
| Optimal temperature | 37°C. |
| Natural or immune form | Immune |
| Serological behavior | Most antibodies react best by antiglobulin technique |
| | Some JKª antibodies and a few JKᵇ antibodies hemolyse in saline at 37°C. A few anti-JKª examples are known to react in saline and albumin at 22°C and 37°C, and anti-JKᵇ has not been reported to react under these conditions |
| | Enzyme activity when followed by antiglobulin test enhances Kidd antibodies (ficin and trypsin) |
| | Anti-JKª JKᵇ reacts soley by the antiglobulin test. |
| Immunoglobulin | Most Kidd antibodies IgG in form, although a few IgM forms are known |
| Clinical importance | Hemolytic transfusion reactions, especially delayed reactions |
| | Hemolytic disease of the new born (by both anti-JKª and JKᵇ) usually mild |
| Miscellaneous | System exhibits dosage effect |
| | Kidd antibodies often found in association with antibodies belonging to other blood group systems. |
| | Titer of Kidd antibodies falls rapidly in vivo and may be difficult to detect by routine crossmatching methods |

## OTHER BLOOD GROUPS

### Diego (Di)

Two antibodies in this system have been described, anti-Diª and anti-Diᵇ. These antibodies react by the antiglobulin test and are not apparently enhanced by complement. The antigens of this system are found primarily in people of Mongolian extraction, although anti-Diª was first found in Venezuela where it had been responsible for a case of hemolytic disease of the newborn. The antigen Diª is developed at birth and the corresponding antibody has been responsible for hemolytic disease of the newborn.

### Cartwright (Yt)

This is a common system, the antigen being present in about 98% of the population. The antibody may be naturally occurring reacting in saline at room temperature as well as by the antiglobulin test. Comple-

TABLE 10-27. Common Properties of the Lutheran Blood Group System.

| Antigens | Lu$^a$ Lu$^b$, Lu4*, Lu5*, Lu6, Lu7*, Lu8*, Lu9, Lu11*, Lu12* (Au$^a$)* | |
|---|---|---|
| Frequency and genotype | CAUCASIAN (%) | NEGROID (%) |
| Lu$^{(a+b-)}$ | 0.2 | 4 |
| Lu$^{(a+b+)}$ | 7.5 | 4 |
| Lu$^{(a-b+)}$ | 92.3 | 96 |
| Lu$^{(a-b-)}$ | — | — |

| | |
|---|---|
| Optimal temperature | 14-37°C |
| Natural or immune form | Occasional immune forms present but most antibodies exist in natural form |
| Serological behavior | Anti-Lu$^b$ reacts best by antiglobulin technique |
| | Some forms of antibody also react in saline at room temperature and 37°C |
| | Antibody does not react in albumin at 20°C and only weakly in albumin at 37°C |
| | Anti-Lu$^a$ reacts over wide thermal range in saline, albumin and by antiglobulin method |
| Immunoglobulin | IgM, IgG and IgA |
| Clinical importance | Mild hemolytic disease of newborn (anti-Lu$^b$) |
| | Hemolytic transfusion reactions (anti-Lu$^a$ and Lu$^b$) |
| Miscellaneous | *Common antigens Lu4, Lu5, Lu7, Lu8, Lu11 and Lu12 related to Lutheran, in lacking on Lu$^{(a-b-)}$ cells but have not been proved to be controlled by Lutheran locus. |
| | Antigen Au$^a$ also related to Lutheran, but controlling gene believed not part of Lutheran complex |

ment may be bound by the antibody, and it can be partly IgG or wholly IgG. Anti-Yt$^b$ has not been implicated in clinical problems and Anti-Yt$^a$ is believed to be only weakly effective in causing red cell destruction. The antigen Yt$^b$ is believed to have an incidence of approximately 8%.

### Dombrock (Do)

This system is an independent blood group characterized by the antigen Do$^a$. The corresponding allele Do$^b$ has been postulated but not reported to date. Anti-Do$^a$ has been found in previously transfused individuals. The antibody has been found to react to the antiglobulin test and by enzymes methods.

### Xg$^a$

Only one antigen, determined by the gene Xg$^a$ has been described, but an allele Xg is postulated. The striking feature of this system is that the genes are carried on the X chromosome, so that males have only one gene for the blood group system instead of the pair of genes they naturally possess for other systems. Anti-Xg$^a$ is usually detected by the antiglobulin test, and one example has been reported to be saline-reactive. It appears that anti-Xg$^a$ is a weak antibody and is not a cause of serious in vivo reactions when transfused into Xg$^{a+}$ individuals.

### Colton (Co)

The system is characterized by antigens Co$^a$ and Co$^b$  The corresponding antibodies reacting by the antiglobulin method and by enzymes have been described.

### I Blood Group System

The system differs from most other high incidence blood groups in several ways. The antigen is poorly developed at birth and no one has yet been found lacking in traces of the antigen.

Cord cells appear to react most weakly when tested against powerful anti-I. It appears that its antigenic strength becomes fully developed by the age of 18 months  The antigen can be classified according to its strength of reaction as follows:

$$i_1 \; i_2 \; i(cord) \; I \; (int) \; I$$

Weak ——————————▶ Strong

Antibodies having specificity to the i and I antigen are well documented. Anti-I reacts with all adult cells, but only weak reactions or negative reactions are seen when tested against cord cells. Most examples react at 4°C or at room temperature, but some antibodies do exist in the incomplete form and may be detected by the antiglobulin method. In situations in which other high incidence antibodies have to be excluded, the autoagglutinin control is the test of choice, being positive with anti-I, but usually negative with systems such as Yt$^a$ etc. Enzyme reactions usually enhance the antibodies.

Auto anti-I is often present in the serum of individuals with acquired hemolytic anemia. The naturally occurring form of this antibody is seen in the serum of i$_1$ or i$_2$ adults when demonstrated by ficin. It does not cross the placenta and is usually IgM in form. The anti-I found in "cold type" acquired hemolytic anemia is often characterized by weak positive direct antiglobulin tests and by a wide thermal reacting range, although stronger reactions are found at 4°C than at 37°C.

Some so-called "nonspecific" cold antibodies have been characterized by a mixture of anti-I and anti-i. Although anti-PP$_1$p$^k$ is usually associated with the Donath-Landsteiner antibody of paroxysmal cold hemoglobinuria, anti-I is also occasionally present.

Anti-i is rare. Its clinical significance almost entirely is in its presence in the serum of infectious mononucleosis, reticuloses, and alcoholic cirrhosis patients. Anti-i reacts strongly with adult i and i cord cells and weakly with I adult cells.

The influence of the I system with the ABO and the P blood groups has been well established. This association has been manifested by the finding of four antigenic sites, IH, IA, IB and IP. The respective antibodies can be detected on the cells only when the combination of I and the corresponding ABH substance can be shown. Thus anti-IB will react only against group B cells that are I-positive, and anti-IH will react best against Group O cells that are I-positive; Group A and B I-positive cells will react weakly against anti-IH due to small amounts of intracellular H substance.

## Other Rare and Unusual Antigens

### Low Incidence (Private Systems)

*Levay.* This system reacts best by saline techniques at 37°C *Wright* (Wr). The incidence approximates 0.01%. Anti-Wr$^a$ has been reported to be responsible for hemolytic disease of the newborn and can be detected with the antiglobulin test. Occasionally, the antibody occurs naturally, and it then reacts as a saline agglutinin at room temperature.

*Swann* (SW). The antigen Sw$^a$ has a frequency of 0.0016. Anti-Sw$^a$ was first detected in a patient with acquired hemolytic anemia (cold antibody type) and is usually associated with anti-Wr$^a$, and occasionally with anti-Vw and Anti-Mi$^a$.

Other low incidence antigens include Jobbins, Becker, Ven, Romunde, Chr$^a$, Berrens, Batty, Good, Traversu, Webb, Kamhuber, Radin, Jn$^a$, Heibel, Torkildsen, Biles, Bishop, Box, Griffiths, Hunt, Lewis II, and Wulfsberg, It is very likely that many more private low incidence antigens will be reported. In the majority of the systems listed, one or only a few reports have been recorded in the literature, and there are likely to be countless more systems to be discovered to perplex the blood banker.

### High Incidence (Public Antigens)

*Vel.* This system (like all public systems) is characterized by the extremely high frequency found in the general population. Approximately 4 out of 10,000 individuals are Vel-negative. The antigens comprising the system appear to be subdivided into at least 5 types, although only Vel 1 and Vel 2 are clearly defined. The corresponding antibodies appear to be reactive by antiglobulin tests, and some anti-Vel 1 have reacted by saline, albumin and enzyme methods.

*Gerbich* (Ge). The corresponding rare antibody has been reported as being saline-reactive at room temperature, and by the two-stage anti-globulin test. The antibody is believed to be naturally occurring, although one individual was thought to have experienced a mild transfusion reaction due to anti-Ge that reacted more strongly in the antiglobulin test.

Other high incidence antigens include Chido, Sd$^a$, Cad, Augustine, Minnie Peal Davis, York, Stirling, Gregory, Langereis, Sp$_1$ Gn$^a$, So$^a$ and Lan.

## REFERENCES

1. Beatty, K. M., and Zuelzer, W. W.: A serum factor reacting with acriflavin causing an error in ABO cell grouping. Transfusion, *8*: 254, 1968.
2. Marsh, W. L.: Anti Lu5, anti Lu6, anti-Lu7 Three antigens defining high frequency antigens related to the Lutheran blood group system. Transfusion, *12*: 27, 1972.
3. Race, R. R.: Modern concepts of the blood group systems. Ann. N.Y. Acad. Sci. *127*: 884, 1965.
4. Race, R. R., and Sanger, R.: Blood Groups in Man. ed. 5, p. 158. Philadelphia, F. A. Davis, 1970.
5. Race, R. R., and Sanger, R.: Blood Groups in Man. ed. 5, p. 280. Philadelphia, F. A, Davis, 1970.
6. Rosenfield, R. E., Allen, F. H., Jr., Swisher, S. N., and Kochwa, S. A.: A review of Rh serology and presentation of a new terminology. Transfusion, *2*: 287, 1962.

# 11

# *Other Blood Banking Procedures*

### ELUTION OF ANTIBODIES

*Principle.* The antibody is removed from the coated red cell surface by the action of heat or by organic methods, and its specificity is determined. The red cell can then be typed correctly.

Elution techniques may be used to

1. Verify the diagnosis of hemolytic disease of the newborn due to ABO blood group incompatibility;

2. Identify the antibody causing hemolytic disease of the newborn from the infant's cells if the maternal serum is unavailable;

3. Aid in the identification of the antibody coating transfused red cells which is responsible for a transfusion reaction;

4. Identify specific isoantibodies at nonspecific autoantibodies from the red cells of patient's with autoimmune hemolytic disease;

5. Identify mixtures of antibodies by absorption techniques.

**Method 1**

*Reagents and Apparatus*
1. Saline
2. Centrifuge
3. 37°C and 56°C Waterbath
4. Pasteur pipets
5. Anti-human globulin serum
6. Test cells

*Method*
1. The test cells are washed 5 times in at least 10 volumes of saline.

2. An equal volume of saline is added to the packed washed cells to make a 50% suspension.

3. This suspension is incubated at 56°C for 20 minutes, agitating at least every 5 minutes.

4. The cells are centrifuged at 3,000 rpm for 3 minutes; the super-

natant saline is removed and tested for the presence of the antibody by the indirect anti-human globulin technique described on page 395.

## Method 2

### Reagents and Apparatus
1. Saline
2. Deep freeze
3. 50% Ethyl alcohol
4. Centrifuge
5. 37°C Waterbath
6. Test cells

### Method
1. The test cells are washed 5 times in saline, packed and the supernatant discarded.

2. The cells are lysed by alternate freezing and thawing (placing in the deep freeze and immersing in a 37°C waterbath)

3. 10 Volumes of 50% ethyl alcohol, which has been precooled to −6°C, is added to 1 volume of the lysed test cells, mixed and left in the deep freeze at −20°C for 2 hours.

4. The mixture is centrifuged at 3,000 rpm for 5 minutes and the supernatant removed.

5. The sediment is broken up and washed in excess of distilled water.

6. An equal volume of saline is added to the sediment and the mixture left at 37°C for 30 minutes.

7. The mixture is centrifuged and the supernatant removed and tested for the presence of antibodies.

## Method 3

### Reagents and Apparatus
1. Saline
2. Diethyl ether
3. Centrifuge
4. Pasteur pipets
5. 37°C Waterbath
6. Test cells

### Method
1. 1 Volume of saline is added to 1 volume of washed packed test cells.

2. 2 Volumes of diethyl ether is added to the mixture, the tube stoppered and mixed for 1 minute.

3. The cell-ether mixture is centrifuged at 3,000 rpm for 10 minutes,

the top two layers discarded and the hemoglobin-stained bottom layer kept and tested for the antibody.

*Notes*

1. Elutions can be used to identify antibodies that are coating cord red cells in hemolytic disease of the newborn.

2. The method can also be used to demonstrate antibodies in cases of hemolytic anemias having a positive anti-human globulin test.

3. Additional uses of the technique are to assist in typing coated cells in the confirmation of D$^u$ typing, and in cases of transfusion reaction.


# ABSORPTION OF ANTIBODIES

*Principle.* Nonspecific agglutinins that produce problems in crossmatching blood can be removed by means of absorbing them from the serum by allowing the blood to clot at the optimum temperature of the antibody. More complete absorption can be carried out by the addition of excess cells to the serum.

Absorption techniques are helpful in:

1. Removing nonspecific antibodies;

2. Separating mixtures of antibodies to aid in their identification;

3. Determining the presence of a specific isoantibody as well as a nonspecific autoantibody in the serum of a patient with acquired hemolytic anemia.

*Reagents and Apparatus*

1. Saline
2. Centrifuge
3. 37°C Waterbath or refrigerator
4. Test serum or cells

## Method 1 (When More Than One Antibody Is Suspected)

1. The test cells are washed 4 times in saline. The residual saline is decanted and an equal volume of the test serum is added to the washed cell button. If absorption is to be carried out at refrigerator temperature, the cells and serum should be first chilled before mixing together.

2. The cell-serum mixture is incubated at the optimal temperature of the antibody for 30 minutes (cold nonspecific antibodies are incubated at 4°C and Rhesus antibodies at 37°C) and the mixture is continually shaken to mix.

3. The cells are centrifuged at 2,000 rpm for 2 minutes to remove the absorbed sera. The serum is tested for complete absorption by adding the appropriate cells and carrying out an anti-human globulin test.

*Note*

1. Frequently, absorption techniques are required to be repeated on several occasions to completely rid the serum of unwanted antibodies.

2. Variation in the length of time that each absorption is carried out depends on the strength of the antibody present.

## Method 2 (Nonspecific Cold Antibodies)

1. EDTA anticoagulated and clotted specimens of patient's blood are collected.

2. The clotted sample is immediately placed at 4°C and the anticoagulated sample at 37°C for 30 minutes respectively. This is carried out so that the cold agglutinin will remain in the plasma of the warm specimen but will be absorbed by the cells of the cold specimens.

3. Centrifuge the anticoagulated blood at 2,000 rpm for 2 minutes keeping it at 37°C (warm the centrifuge cups in order to maintain the 37°C temperature.)

4. Separate the serum from the clotted sample and remove the plasma from the EDTA anticoagulated blood.

5. Wash the anticoagulated cells at least 3 times in large volumes of warm saline, decant after the last wash, so that the cell button is dry.

6. Prepare a 2% saline suspension of these washed cells in saline.

7. Add 2 volumes of absorbed serum to 1 volume of the 2%-cell suspension.

8. Centrifuge (Serofuge) at 3,600 rpm for 15 seconds, gently dislodge the cells and examine for macroscopic agglutination. If agglutination is present, remove residual antibody by adding 1 volume of serum to 1 volume of washed packed cells, mix and incubate at 4°C for 30 minutes.

9. Centrifuge as in step 8 above and retest.

10. Continue to retest and reabsorb serum until all the antibody is removed.

*Note* It is necessary to use fresh warm cells in order to absorb efficiently. Do not reuse cells by washing them with warm saline.

## THE USE OF ENZYMES IN ABSORPTION PROCEDURES

Anti-M, anti-N, anti-S, anti-Fy$^a$ and anti-Fy$^b$ typing reagents can be prepared from raw serum by absorption with any ficin-treated cells of appropriate ABO group. This is possible because the enzyme destroys M, N, S, Fy$^a$ and Fy$^b$ antigenic sites. For example, a Group O anti-Fy$^a$ serum can be absorbed with Group AB Fy$^{(a+b-)}$ ficin-treated cells. The enzyme destroys the Fy$^a$ site absorbing the anti-A and anti-B antibodies but leaving anti-Fyᵃ in the serum. The practical advantage of the procedure is that the number of absorptions can be reduced. This procedure cannot be used to prepare anti-s or anti-U reagents, since ficin does not destroy the s or U receptor sites.


# CROSSMATCHING TECHNIQUES

*Principle.* The term "crossmatch" refers to the procedure in which cells and serum are observed for possible agglutination. In transfusion therapy, the crossmatch tests the donor's cells against the patient's serum (the major side) and the donor's serum against the patient's cells (the minor side). There are many crossmatch procedures listed in blood bank manuals. All differ in the establishing of condition, temperature, media of suspending cells, serum-cell volume ratios and time. The following procedures are given as a guide and can be modified in the light of competence and experience.

### Reagents and Apparatus
1. Donor's cells and serum
2. Patient's cells and serum
3. Saline
4. 30% Bovine albumin
5. Anti-human globulin serum
6. Tubes—10 × 75 mm
7. 37°C Waterbath
8. Pasteur pipets

### Method (Major Side)
1. Two drops of patient's serum is placed in a tube and 1 drop of a 5% saline suspension of donor's cells is added.

2. The tube is centrifuged at 1,000 rpm for 1 minute, observed for agglutination, and the red cell button gently resuspended.

3. Step 1 is repeated and 3 drops of 30% albumin is added to the tube. Incubate for 30 or 60 minutes at 37°C and examine microscopically for agglutination, using the technique described in handling the Pasteur pipet on page 375. *Do not* centrifuge the tube before examining the tube for agglutination.

4. If no agglutination is present in 2, this tube is also incubated for 30 or 60 minutes at room temperature and examined in the same way as described in 3.

5. On the residue of the cells in the tube from step 3, carry out an anti-human globulin test as described on page 395.

***Notes***

1. Agglutination in any one of the three testing media indicates that the blood is incompatible with the patient.

2. *Evidence of hemolysis in place of or with agglutination also denotes that the blood is incompatible.*

3. Both positive and negative controls of the anti-human globulin test should *always* be set up along with the test. Because it is common to encounter cold or warm autoantibodies in the patient's serum, a control should be set up, using the patient's own cells and serum. The same method should be used for this control as for the crossmatch.

4. The use of 30% albumin in place of 22% albumin is merely a personal preference. Either can be used with equal success, but if the technologist uses 22% albumin, the volume used will increase from 3 drops to approximately 5 drops. To achieve the desired albumin concentration in the test, sufficient albumin should be added to produce a protein concentration of 13 to 17%.

5. The minor crossmatch has been purposely omitted, because it is felt that routine screening of the blood donors is at least as satisfactory and practical. The minor side of the crossmatch will detect incompatibilities if the donor's serum contains atypical antibodies. However, routine screening would in most cases save time by detecting these antibodies prior to crossmatching. Another use of the minor crossmatch is in checking the ABO type of the patient.

6. The immediate centrifuge technique (step 2) often detects anti-M, anti-N, anti-P and cold autoantibodies and serves as a final confirmation of ABO grouping.

7. The incubation of a saline suspension of cells and patient's serum at room temperature is included, so that anti-Lewis, anti-M, anti-N and anti-P, if present, will have enhanced reactivity.

8. The high protein or albumin phase at 37°C enhances agglutination within the Rhesus blood group system, and the albumin-fortified indirect anti-human globulin test detects most of the remainder of the clinically significant antibodies.

9. The time allowed for compatibility testing is governed by the urgency of the need for blood. Many opinions exist as to the optimal incubation time, and periods from 15 minutes up to 2 hours have been suggested by various workers.

In general, incubation periods of either 30 or 60 minutes have been found to be most sensitive to antibody uptake by the clinically important blood group systems. Incubation periods of 15 minutes should be avoided since it has been shown that, while antibody binding is present, it is more difficult to detect and frequently presents as a weaker reaction that could be easily missed. This is particularly true of systems other than ABO and Rhesus.

Incubation periods of 45 minutes should likewise be avoided, since Kell antibodies, and possibly other antiglobulin-reacting systems, become self-eluting at this time, and are most easily detected at 30 minutes or after 1-hour incubation.

## In Vivo Crossmatch

*Principle.* If the compatibility of a unit of blood is in doubt (as is occasionally seen in hemolytic anemias), the estimation of the red cell survival of a small aliquot of the cells can be quickly assessed by examination of the patient's plasma for hemoglobin. Although isotope studies remain a more definitive test, there is often insufficient time for $Cr^{51}$ tagging to be carried out. In situations in which transfusions are lifesaving to the patient but incompatibility exists, the attending physician must decide on the course of action. The following procedure can be used to remove some of the threat to the patient in such circumstances and should always be carried out. The procedure is limited in that it cannot be carried out if the patient has a preexisting hemoglobinemia.

### Method

1. The patient's hematocrit is determined from a venous sample of blood. Save the centrifuged blood.

2. Set up the unit of blood with a saline infusion using a standard Y-transfusion set.

3. Infuse approximately 20 ml of whole blood into the patient.

4. Infuse saline at approximately 20 drops per minute for about 15 minutes.

5. Determine the patient's hematocrit from a venous sample obtained from the arm opposite the infusion.

6. Examine the postinfusion plasma from the hematocrit and compare with the preinfusion plasma. If the postinfusion sample shows an increase in free hemoglobin, continue to transfuse the blood slowly while monitoring the patients' vital signs.

The presence of visible free plasma hemoglobin indicates that the in vivo crossmatch is incompatible and should be immediately discontinued.

### Note

1. Approximately 5 ml of whole blood when hemolysed in vivo will produce a plasma hemoglobin of 20 mg/100 ml plasma. Such plasma will macroscopically be a faint pink color.

2. 25 ml of whole blood when transfused will normally liberate 100 mg hemoglobin/100 ml of plasma and will macroscopically be red in color.

3. An alternative procedure is to determine the plasma hemoglobin quantitatively (p. 16). This, however, may be impractical and will depend upon the availability of the test.

# 12

# *Obstetrical Studies*

## PRENATAL STUDIES

*History.* A transfusion and obstetrical history on all patients should be obtained.

*Sample Required.* Clotted blood

*Tests Performed*

a. **Initial visit**
   1. ABO grouping
   2. Rh typing
   3. Antibody screening test
   4. Antibody identification
   5. Antibody titer (if antibody demonstrated is known to cause hemolytic disease of the newborn)

b. **Following visits.** Carry out tests 3 to 5 above if indicated

*Serological Tests on Newborn Infants*

The following should be carried out on well-washed cord blood at the time of delivery (cord cells are washed to remove Wharton's jelly).

   1. ABO forward grouping only; reverse or backtyping is not done.
   2. Rh typing (D) with controls.
   3. Direct antiglobulin test.

*Notes*

1. If the direct antiglobulin test is positive, determine the Rhesus typing using saline agglutinating anti-$Rh_0$ (D) sera.

2. Occasionally the cells of an $Rh_0$ (D)-positive infant will be so completely coated with specific maternal antibody that the antigenic sites on the cells are blocked and cannot react with the antisera. This results in a false-negative typing. This can be suspected when the direct antiglobulin test is strongly positive and the maternal serum contains anti-$Rh_0$ (D). In most instances the correct Rh type of the infant can be resolved by using a washed saline suspension of cells and saline agglutinating antisera.

In addition, an eluate may be prepared from the infant's red cells in order to correctly ascertain the Rh type of the infant. If the eluate contains anti-Rh$_0$ (D), the infant's red cells are Rh$_0$ (D)-positive.

## SEROLOGICAL TESTS IN SUSPECTED HEMOLYTIC DISEASE OF THE NEWBORN

### Antibody Titer

*Principle.* The titer of an antibody is the measure of the amount of the antibody present. A titer is expressed as the reciprocal of the greatest dilution of the patient's serum which has sufficient antibody present to react with the corresponding antigen. Only antibodies that are clinically significant should be serologically quantitated; all antibodies do not carry the same implication for predicting the possibility of hemolytic disease of the newborn.

The relationship between the degree of which Rhesus-positive red cells are coated with antibody and the rate of their destruction is not uniform. There frequently is little relationship between the antibody titer in the maternal serum and the severity of the disease.

### Method 1 (Saline Titration)

#### Reagents and Apparatus
1. Tubes—12 × 75 mm
2. 0.85% Saline
3. Pipets—0.1 ml and 0.2 ml
4. Patient's serum
5. Fresh washed 2% saline suspension of red cells of appropriate type
6. Centrifuge (Serofuge)

#### Method
1. Set up 11 tubes as shown in Table 12-1.

The patient's saline-serum dilution should be well-mixed prior to adding the saline suspension of cells.

2. Shake all the tubes to mix and incubate at room temperature for 60 minutes.

3. Centrifuge at 3,600 rpm for 15 seconds, gently dislodge the cells, and examine for microscopic agglutination.

4. Read the titer by first examining tube 11 working down to tube 1. This will prevent a prozone titer being misread.

5. Grade the degree of agglutination (p. 378). The end point is taken as the tube containing the greatest dilution of serum causing microscopic agglutination.

TABLE 12-1.

| TUBE | SALINE (ML) | PATIENT'S SERUM (ML) | WASHED 2% SALINE SUSPENSION OF CELLS (ML) | TITER |
|---|---|---|---|---|
| 1 | — | 0.1 | 0.1 | 1 |
| 2 | 0.1 | 0.1 | 0.1 | 2 |
| 3 | 0.1 | 0.1 ml from total of tube 2 | 0.1 | 4 |
| 4 | 0.1 | 0.1 ml from total of tube 3 | 0.1 | 8 |
| 5 | 0.1 | 0.1 ml from total of tube 4 | 0.1 | 16 |
| 6 | 0.1 | 0.1 ml from total of tube 5 | 0.1 | 32 |
| 7 | 0.1 | 0.1 ml from total of tube 6 | 0.1 | 64 |
| 8 | 0.1 | 0.1 ml from total of tube 7 | 0.1 | 128 |
| 9 | 0.1 | 0.1 ml from total of tube 8 | 0.1 | 256 |
| 10 | 0.1 | 0.1 ml from total of tube 9 | 0.1 | 512 |
| 11 | 0.1 | 0.1 ml from *total of tube 10 | 0.1 | 1024 |

* Discard 0.1 ml from tube 11

## Method 2 (Albumin-Antiglobulin Titer)

### Reagents and Apparatus

1. Carry out steps 1 through 5 as in the saline method but use 30% albumin in place of saline in tubes 2 through 11.

2. After grading the degree of agglutination (step 5 above), the cells are washed 3 times in large volumes of saline.

3. Decant the residual saline completely after the last wash and add 2 drops of antiglobulin serum to the cell button in each tube.

4. Centrifuge (Serofuge) at 3,600 rpm for 15 seconds and gently dislodge the cells.

5. Examine macroscopically or using a low power hand lens, reading the first results in tube 11 and working down to tube 1.

## Control of Errors in Titrations

1. Carry out a saline and albumin-antiglobulin titration on the first sample during each pregnancy, when antibodies are identified.

2. This serum sample should be stored frozen, and retested together

* Available from Dade Serums, Miami, Florida

with the new serum sample. If possible, the same individuals cells should be used to ensure that identical conditions are maintained.

### Titration of Natural Antibodies of the ABO System

1. Set up the following tubes as in Table 12-2, making sure to mix the contents of the tubes before subsampling 0.1 ml to the next tube. Add a saline suspension of appropriate cells ($A_1$ or B) to each tube after all the dilutions have been made.

2. Shake the tubes. Incubate at room temperature for 10 to 15 minutes, centrifuge (Serofuge) at 3,600 rpm for 15 seconds.

3. Gently resuspend the cells and examine for agglutination.

### Titration of Immune Antibodies of the ABO System

1. 0.1 ml of Neutrab to 0.5 ml of patient's serum, and allow to stand for 5 to 10 minutes at room temperature.

2. Carry out step 1 as in the saline titration using the Neutrab-serum mixture in place of the straight serum.

3. Shake the tubes and incubate at 37°C for 30 minutes.

TABLE 12-2.

| TUBE | SALINE (ML) | SALINE (ML) | WASHED 2% SALINE CELL SUSPENSION (ML) | TITER |
|---|---|---|---|---|
| 1 | — | 0.1 | 0.1 | 1 |
| 2 | 0.1 | 0.1 mix | 0.1 | 2 |
| 3 | 0.1 | 0.1 ml from tube 2 | 0.1 | 4 |
| 4 | 0.1 | 0.1 ml from tube 3 | 0.1 | 8 |
| 5 | 0.1 | 0.1 ml from tube 4 | 0.1 | 16 |
| 6 | 0.1 | 0.1 ml from tube 5 | 0.1 | 32 |
| 7 | 0.1 | 0.1 ml from tube 6 | 0.1 | 64 |
| 8 | 0.1 | 0.1 ml from tube 7 | 0.1 | 128 |
| 9 | 0.1 | 0.1 ml from tube 8 | 0.1 | 256 |
| 10 | 0.1 | 0.1 ml from tube 9 | 0.1 | 512 |
| 11 | 0.1 | 0.1 ml from tube 10 | 0.1* | 1024 |

*Discard 0.1 ml from tube 11

4. Wash the cells 3 times in large volumes of saline, making sure to completely decant the residual saline between washings.

5. Add 2 drops of antiglobulin serum to each tube and centrifuge (Serofuge) at 3,600 rpm for 15 seconds.

6. Gently resuspend the cells and observe for agglutination macroscopically or using a low power hand lens.

7. Anti-human control cells may be used to confirm the reactivity of the system in those tubes in which no agglutination is observed (see p. 392).

### Amniocentesis

Spectrophotometric examination of amniotic fluid has allowed a more accurate prognosis of the degree of disease in the fetus, differentiating patients whose infants will be severely affected with hemolytic disease from those who are either Rhesus-negative or midly affected.

The optical density of filtered centrifuged amniotic fluid is plotted from 750 to 365 $\mu$ on semilogarithmic paper. A rise in optical density at 450 $\mu$ occurs in a mother carrying an infant with severe hemolytic disease. The increase in optical density ("bilirubin bulge") can be estimated by joining up the smooth curve on each side of the bulge. The rise in optical density for the "bulge" at 450 $\mu$ is recorded.

Amniocentesis is repeated at regular intervals throughout the gestation and the rise in optical density plotted against the gestation time. Since there is a tendency for the amount of bile pigment to decrease in mild cases of hemolytic disease as the pregnancy advances, interpretation of the significance of the optical density at 450 $\mu$ varies according to the period of gestation.

## SEROLOGICAL TESTS NECESSARY FOR EXCHANGE TRANSFUSION

### Tests on Maternal Serum

1. ABO group
2. Rhesus typing
3. Antibody screening test
4. Antibody identification

### Tests on Cord Blood

1. ABO group (front type only)
2. Rhesus typing
3. Direct Coombs' (if strongly positive elution and antibody identification)
4. Antibody screening (indirect antiglobulin test)

**Tests on Donor Blood**

1. ABO group
2. Rhesus typing ($Rh_o$-D)
3. If hemolytic disease of the newborn is due to a factor other than $Rh_o$ (D) type for the antigen concerned (e.g., $Fy^a$, K, etc.), The typing must be negative with respect to the irregular antibody in the maternal serum.
4. Antibody screening test
5. Screen for anti-A and anti-B if low titered blood is to be used

*Crossmatch*

1. The maternal serum should be used for crossmatching for the first exchange.
2. Use postexchange sample for each additional exchange.
3. *Do not crossmatch donor cells against infant serum* unless maternal serum is unavailable (e.g., baby transferred to hospital from another hospital).

*Selection of Blood for Exchange Transfusion.* Select the blood which does not possess the antigen to which the mother has developed an antibody (Table 12-3 and Table 12-4).

*Rh Immune Globulin Crossmatch*

Rh immune globulin is a purified preparation of $Rh_o$ (D) used as a prophylactic treatment for Rh hemolytic disease of the newborn. It is injected intramuscularly to a mother not previously sensitized to anti-$Rh_o$ (D) by pregnancy or transfusion, within 72 hours of delivery of an $Rh_o$ (D)-positive infant. This injection destroys any $Rh_o$ (D) cells that may have reached the maternal circulation and thus prevents isoimmunization. This crossmatch is essentially a minor side compatibility test.

*Method*

1. The following tubes are set up as shown in Table 12-5.
2. Incubate all tubes at 37°C for 1 hour.

TABLE 12.3 Selection of Blood for Exchange Transfusion (ABO Disease).

| TYPE DISEASE | MATERNAL GROUP ABO | RHESUS | INFANT GROUP ABO | RHESUS | EXCHANGE WITH: |
|---|---|---|---|---|---|
| ABO hemolytic | O | Positive | A,B,AB | Positive | low titer O Rh-positive |
| disease of | O | Positive | A,B,AB | Negative | low titer O Rh-negative |
| the newborn | O | Negative | A,B,AB | Negative | low titer O Rh-negative |
| | *O | Negative | A,B,AB | Positive | low titer O Rh-negative |
| | | * ABO and Rh Disease can coexist | | | |

TABLE 12-4. Selection of Blood for Exchange Transfusion (Rh Disease).

| TYPE DISEASE | MATERNAL GROUP ABO | RHESUS | INFANT GROUP ABO | RHESUS | EXCHANGE WITH: |
|---|---|---|---|---|---|
| Rh° (D) | O | Negative | O | Positive | O Rh-negative |
| hemolytic | A or AB | Negative | A | Positive | A Rh-negative |
| disease of | B or AB | Negative | B | Positive | B Rh-negative |
| the newborn | AB | Negative | AB | Positive | AB Rh-negative |
| | O | Negative | A | Positive | low titered O Rh-negative |
| | O | Negative | B | Positive | low titered O Rh-negative |
| | O | Negative | AB | Positive | low titered O Rh-negative |
| | A | Negative | AB | Positive | A Rh-negative |
| | B | Negative | AB | Positive | B Rh-negative |
| | A | Negative | B | Positive | low titered O Rh-negative |
| | B | Negative | A | Positive | low titered O Rh-negative |
| | A | Negative | O | Positive | O Rh-negative |
| | B | Negative | O | Positive | O Rh-negative |

3. Centrifuge (Serofuge) at 3,600 rpm for 15 seconds and examine macroscopically.

4. Resuspend cell buttons and wash thoroughly 3 times with large volumes of saline.

5. Decant the last saline wash so that a dry cell button remains, and add 2 drops of antiglobulin serum to each tube.

6. Centrifuge (Serofuge) at 3,600 rpm for 15 seconds and examine for agglutination under a low power hand lens.

TABLE 12-5.

| TUBE | 1 | 2 | 3 | 4 | 5 |
|---|---|---|---|---|---|
| 2% Patient's cells (vols) | 1 | — | 1 | — | — |
| Rh-immune globulin (vols) | 2 | 2 | — | — | — |
| 30% Albumin (vols) | 3 | 3 | 2 | 3 | 3 |
| 2% O Rh-positive cells (vols) | — | 1 | — | 1 | 1 |
| 1:100 Saline dilution of commercial anti-D (vols) | — | — | — | 2 | — |
| Saline (vols) | — | — | — | — | 2 |

Key:
Tube 1. Rh-Immune globulin crossmatch
Tube 2. Rh-Immune globulin positive control
Tube 3. Albumin control
Tube 4. Positive-antiglobulin control
Tube 5. Negative-antiglobulin control

## CLINICAL CONSIDERATIONS

### Erythroblastosis Fetalis (Hemolytic Disease of the Newborn)

This disease is due to the destruction of fetal cells by maternal antibodies. Small numbers of fetal cells are thought to cross the placenta and enter the maternal circulation during pregnancy. If the fetus possesses a cell antigen which the mother lacks, the maternal blood produces an antibody, which, in turn, can cross the placenta, enter the fetal circulation and destroy the fetal red cells.

At birth, the infant's cells may be blocked by adsorbed maternal antibodies. This occurs when the antigen receptors on the cells are saturated with incomplete antibodies. In such cases, the addition of albumin to the cells may cause agglutination. Occasionally, the blocking action may be so complete that the infant's cells do not react with high protein anti-D, and the cells type as Rhesus-negative. If this occurs, the cells should be typed with a complete anti-D, or the blocking antibody should be eluted from the cells as described on page 442. *A technologist should be acutely aware and distrustful of results showing jaundiced infants who are typed as Rhesus-negative and have Rhesus-negative mothers.*

ABO disease frequently affects the first-born infant. The direct anti-human globulin test on the infant's cells is weakly positive or even negative. The presence of an immune anti-A or anti-B in the maternal circulation and also the elution of an incompatible antibody from the fetal cells (anti-A eluted from a group A cell) aids in the diagnosis.

TABLE 12-6. Diseases Associated with Blood Groups.

| DISEASE | BLOOD GROUP | COMMENT |
|---|---|---|
| Duodenal ulcer | O | 40% More common in secretors |
| Gastric ulcer | O | |
| Carcinoma of the stomach | A | 20% More common in secretors |
| Pernicious anemia | A | 25% More common in secretors |
| Diabetes | A | |
| Carcinoma of the salivary glands | A | |
| Rheumatic fever | Nonsecretors of ABH substance | |
| Broncho-pneumonia | A | |
| Adenoma of the pituitary | O | |

Frequently, the offending antibody can be detected in the infant's serum by using the indirect anti-human globulin test.

Hemolytic disease due to the Rhesus blood group does not affect the first-born child. The direct anti-human globulin test on the infant's cells is always positive. The presence of an immune Rhesus antibody in the maternal serum suggests that possible sensitization has occurred, although maternal antibody carry-over from a previous pregnancy cannot be excluded. If the maternal genotype has a C or E gene, it may be a protective influence for the infant. The potency of the D antigen varies in the red cells of different genotypes. $R_2$ (cDE) genes react more strongly than do $R_1$ genes (CDe) to anti-D. Infants who are $R_2$ are more likely to be severely affected because of their genetic makeup. Hemolytic disease of the newborn has also been caused by other blood group systems; the next most common systems are the Kell and Duffy groups. Other diseases that have been correlated with blood groups are found in Table 12-6.

It is not implied that individuals of these blood groups will ultimately be stricken with these diseases. They are listed to show that a statistically greater number of individuals with each of these diseases possess the listed blood groups.

# Appendix

## NORMAL VALUES

| | |
|---|---|
| Hemoglobin—Adult male | 12.5-18.0 g% |
| —Adult female | 11.5-16.0 g% |
| —Infant | 14.0-22.0 g% |
| Hemoglobin Iron Content | 0.340 g% hemoglobin |
| Hemoglobin Oxygen Capacity | 1.34 ml/g hemoglobin |
| Plasma Hemoglobin | 1.0-5.0 mg% |
| Alkali Denaturation (hemoglobin F) | 100 seconds |
| Red Cell Count—Adult male | 4,500,000-6,500,000/cu mm |
| —Adult female | 4,000,000-6,000,000/cu mm |
| —Infants | 6,500,000-7,250,000/cu mm |
| Reticulocytes—Adults | 0.2-2.0% |
| —Infants | 2.0-6.0% |
| Hematocrit—Adult male | 40-54% |
| —Adult female | 37-47% |
| —Infants | 44-64% |
| Mean Cell Volume (MCV) | 76-96 cu $\mu$ |
| Mean Cell Hemoglobin (MCH) | 27-32 $\mu\mu$g |
| Mean Cell Hemoglobin Concentration (MCHC) | 32-36% |
| White Cell Count—Adults | 5,000-10,000/cu mm |
| —Infants | 9,000-38,000/cu mm |
| Differential White Cell Count— | |
| Adults—Neutrophils | 50-75% (2,500-7,500/cu mm) |
| —Bands | 0-3% (0-300/cu mm) |
| —Eosinophils | 1-6% (40-440/cu mm) |
| —Basophils | 0-1% (0-100/cu mm) |
| —Monocytes | 2-10% (200-800/cu mm) |
| —Lymphocytes | 20-40% (1,500-3,500/cu mm) |
| Children—Neutrophils | 20-50% |
| Lymphocytes | 30-60% |
| Infants—Neutrophils | 30-60% |
| —Lymphocytes | 40-70% |
| Arneth-Cooke Count—Group I | 10-12% |
| —Group II | 25-30% |
| —Group III | 47-53% |
| —Group IV | 16-19% |
| —Group V | 2-3% |

Differential Bone Marrow Count—

| | |
|---|---|
| Reticulum Cells | 0-2% |
| Hemocytoblasts | 0-1% |
| Myeloblasts | 0-3.5% |
| Promyelocytes | 0-5% |
| Myelocytes—Neutrophil | 5-20% |
| —Eosinophil | 0-3% |
| —Basophil | 0-1% |
| Metamyelocytes | 10-30% |
| Polymorphonuclear—Neutrophil | 7-25% |
| —Eosinophil | 0-3% |
| —Basophils | 0-1% |
| Lymphocytes | 5-20% |
| Monocytes | 0-1% |
| Megakaryocytes | 0-1% |
| Plasma cells | 0-4% |
| Rubriblasts | 0-5% |
| Prorubricytes | 0-5% |
| Rubricytes | 2-20% |
| Metarubricytes | 2-10% |
| Myeloid/Erythroid | 2/1-5/1 |

Osmotic Fragility (Immediate)

| % Saline | % Hemolysis |
|---|---|
| 0.3 | 97-100 |
| 0.35 | 90-97 |
| 0.4 | 50-95 |
| 0.45 | 5-45 |
| 0.5 | 0-6 |
| 0.55 | 0- |

Osmotic Fragility (incubated 24 hours)

| % Saline | % Hemolysis |
|---|---|
| 0.2 | 95-100 |
| 0.3 | 85-100 |
| 0.35 | 75-100 |
| 0.4 | 65-100 |
| 0.45 | 55-100 |
| 0.5 | 40-85 |
| 0.55 | 15-70 |
| 0.6 | 0-40 |
| 0.65 | 0-10 |
| 0.7 | 0-5 |

Mechanical Fragility    2-5% blood hemoglobin
0-5 mg plasma hemoglobin

Autohemolysis (at 24 hours)

| | |
|---|---|
| Without glucose | 0.05-0.5% |
| With glucose | 0-0.4% |
| (at 48 hours) | |
| Without glucose | 0.4-4.5% |
| With glucose | 0.03-0.4% |
| Red Cell Glutathione | 45-100 mg% |

Glucose-6-Phosphate Dehydrogenase
Decolorization    100 minutes

| | |
|---|---|
| Serum Bilirubin (total) | |
| Adult | 0.3-0.8 mg% |
| Infant | 0.5-2.5 mg% |
| Red Cell Acetylcholinesterase | 0.5-1.0 units |
| Red Cell Survival (Cr$^{51}$) Half-life | 28-38 days |
| (Ashby) Half-life | 40-60 days |
| Stercobilinogen | 30-220 mg% |
| Bleeding Time (Ivy) | 2-7 minutes |
| Bleeding Time (Duke) | 0-5 minutes |
| Bleeding Time (Borchgrevink and Waaler) | |
| Primary time | 3-11 minutes |
| Secondary time | 0-9 minutes |
| Coagulation Time (Lee and White) | 6-10 minutes |
| (Siliconized) | 18-25 minutes |
| (Dale and Laidlaw) | 1-3 minutes |
| Tourniquet Test (Positive pressure) | 0-10 petechiae |
| (Negative pressure) | 200-350 mm |
| Platelet Adhesiveness (In vitro) | 28-68% |
| (In vivo) | 24-58% |
| Clot Retraction | 38-97% |
| Platelet Counts—Indirect method | 150,000-500,000/cu mm |
| —Direct method | 150,000-400,000/cu mm |
| One-stage Prothrombin | 11-15 seconds |
| Prothrombin and Proconvertin (P and P) | 30-40 seconds |
| Thrombotest | 20-45 seconds |
| Stypven Time | 11-15 seconds |
| Prothrombin (Owren) | 18-22 seconds |
| Prothrombin Consumption Index | 0-30% |
| Serum Prothrombin | >30 seconds |
| Partial Thromboplastin Time (PTT) | 60-100 seconds |
| Activated Partial Thromboplastin Time | 30-45 seconds |
| Thromboplastin Generation Test (Hicks and Pitney) | <14 seconds |
| Thromboplastin Generation Test (Biggs) | <14 seconds |
| Factor VIII Assay | 70-145% |
| Platelet Factor 3 Assay | 9-16 seconds after 4 minutes incubation |
| Siderocytes | 0.4-0.6% |
| Leukocyte Alkaline Phosphatase | 8-100 |
| Sedimentation Rate (Wintrobe) | |
| Male | 4-7 mm in 1 hour |
| Female | 5-10 mm in 1 hour |
| Sedimentation Rate (Westergren) | |
| Male | 0-9 mm in 1 hour |
| Female | 0-20 mm in 1 hour |
| Sedimentation Rate (Landau) | |
| Male | 0-5 mm in 1 hour |
| Female | 0-8 mm in 1 hour |
| Heterophil Test (Presumptive) | 1:7-1:56 |
| Blood Viscosity | 4.8-5.2 times as viscous as distilled water |

# REGISTRY QUESTIONS

1. Hemoglobin occurs normally in the circulating blood as:
   - (a) Oxyhemoglobin
   - (b) Sulfhemoglobin
   - (c) Methemoglobin
2. In the Spencer bright-line hemocytometer, the chamber depth is 0.1 mm. What is the volume over 16 of the smallest squares in the ruled area?
   - (a) 0.004 cu mm
   - (b) 0.910 cu mm
   - (c) 0.025 cu mm
   - (d) 0.020 cu mm
3. When blood is drawn to the 1.0 mark in the white pipet and diluting fluid to the 11.0 mark, the blood is diluted:
   - (a) 1 to 20
   - (b) 1 to 10
   - (c) 1 to 40
   - (d) 1 to 200
4. In the red cell fragility test, the cells of a normal person begin to hemolyze at a salt concentration of:
   - (a) 0.50%
   - (b) 0.44%
   - (c) 0.34%
   - (d) 0.30%
5. The clot retraction time is related to:
   - (a) White cell count
   - (b) Platelet count
   - (c) Coagulation time
   - (d) Prothrombin time
6. Which of the following is not a method for determining the sedimentation rate?
   - (a) Cutler
   - (b) Westergren
   - (c) Tallquist
   - (d) Wintrobe-Landsberg
7. The weight of hemoglobin in the average red cell is:
   - (a) 30 $\mu\mu$ g
   - (b) 22 $\mu\mu$ g
   - (c) 36 $\mu\mu$ g
8. The immediate precursor of the blood platelet is the:
   - (a) Metamyelocyte
   - (b) Osteoblast
   - (c) Myeloblast
   - (d) Megakaryoblast
   - (e) Megakaryocyte
9. The most accepted theory of blood maturation is:
   - (a) Dualist theory
   - (b) Trialist theory
   - (c) Monophyletic theory
   - (d) Howell's theory

10. A Tart cell differs from an LE cell in that the ingesting cell is:
    (a) A lymphocyte
    (b) A neutrophil
    (c) A thrombocyte
    (d) A monocyte
11. Two main groups of hemolytic anemia are recognized. They are:
    (a) Acholuric jaundice and sickle cell anemia
    (b) Congenital and acquired
    (c) Transfusion reactions and hemolysis due to specific drugs
    (d) Antigen sensitization and thalassemia
12. Sickle cell anemia is due to an abnormality in the patient's:
    (a) Red cell stroma
    (b) Plasma
    (c) Serum
    (d) Hemoglobin
    (e) None of the above
13. The osmotic fragility in sickle cell anemia is:
    (a) Increased
    (b) Decreased
    (c) Not altered
    (d) Variable
    (e) Depends on the method used
14. Megalobastic anemias are nearly always:
    (a) Microcytic
    (b) Polychromatic
    (c) Neurocytic
    (d) Macrocytic
15. Basophilic stippling in red cells is found in cases of:
    (a) Malaria
    (b) Hemophilia
    (c) Lead poisoning
    (d) Infectious mononucleosis
16. Positive peroxidase reactions are found in:
    (a) Early red cells
    (b) Lymphocytes
    (c) Granulocytes
17. In acute myeloid leukemia, the predominant and diagnostic cell in the bone marrow is:
    (a) Lymphocyte
    (b) Metamyelocyte
    (c) Myelocyte
    (d) Megakaryoblast
    (e) Myeloblast
18. One of the functions of a lymphocyte is:
    (a) Transportation of oxygen
    (b) Antibody formation
    (c) Phagocytosis
    (d) Connected with blood coagulation
    (e) Connected with the pH of the blood

19. Feulgen is specific for:
    (a) Iron
    (b) Peroxidase
    (c) DNA
    (d) RNA
    (e) LE cells
20. A hematocytoblast is:
    (a) A normal mature white cell
    (b) An immature white cell
    (c) A normal mature red cell
    (d) An immature red cell
    (e) A stem cell capable of forming either a red or a white cell
21. Smudge cells are characteristically found in:
    (a) Acute granulocyte leukemia
    (b) Iron deficiency anemia
    (c) Sprue
    (d) Naegli monocytic leukemia
    (e) Chronic lymphatic leukemia
22. The anticoagulant used in Wintrobe's sedimentation rate test is:
    (a) Calcium phosphate
    (b) 3.8% Sodium citrate
    (c) 1.34% Sodium oxalate
    (d) Sodium fluoride
    (e) Heller's and Paul's mixture
23. The diagnostic laboratory test for paroxysmal nocturnal hemoglobinurea is:
    (a) Donath-Landsteiner test
    (b) Indirect Coombs' test
    (c) Direct Coombs' test
    (d) Ham's test
    (e) Gamma globulin neutralization test
24. When separating hemoglobins by electrophoresis, the type of hemoglobin listed below moves faster than HbF:
    (a) HbG
    (b) HbD
    (c) HbA
    (d) HbC
    (e) HbE
25. Polycythemia is a disease in which there is:
    (a) An increase in the number of platelets and white cells
    (b) An increase in the number of red cells and platelets and a decrease in the number of white cells.
    (c) A decrease in the red cells and an increase in white cell precursors
    (d) An increase in granulocytes and a decrease in both platelets and red cells
26. Poikilocytosis refers to a variation in the:
    (a) Structure of the red cell
    (b) Size of the platelets
    (c) Shape of the red cells
    (d) Size of the red cells
    (e) None of the above

27. The dominating feature of the peripheral blood smear from a person having thalassemia is:
    (a) Target cells
    (b) Elliptocytes
    (c) Poikilocytes
    (d) Macrocytes
    (e) Microcytes
28. The normal activated partial thromboplastin time is:
    (a) 60-100 seconds
    (b) 12-15 seconds
    (c) 35-45 seconds
    (d) None of these
29. These cells have a decreased resistance to hypotonic saline:
    (a) Poikilocytes
    (b) Spherocytes
    (c) Microcytes
    (d) Macrocytes
    (e) Schistocytes
30. When fresh plasma is adsorbed with barium sulfate, the following factors are left in the plasma:
    (a) IX & VII
    (b) VIII & V
    (c) XII & IV
    (d) IV & VI
    (e) III & I
31. The normal Ivy bleeding time is:
    (a) 0-10 minutes
    (b) 1-7 minutes
    (c) 5-10 minutes
    (d) 12-15 minutes
    (e) 0-1 minute
32. The prothrombin consumption test is affected by the following factors:
    (a) I
    (b) Platelet numbers and function
    (c) VIII and III and IV
    (d) IV
    (e) VI
33. The clot retraction is affected by the following factors:
    (a) VIII
    (b) IX
    (c) X
    (d) I
    (e) XII
34. The normal recalcification time is:
    (a) 3-5 minutes
    (b) 90-120 seconds
    (c) 10-15 seconds
    (d) 1-3 minutes
35. The optimal pH of the test solution in coagulation work is:
    (a) 6.8
    (b) 7.8

(c) 6.35

(d) 7.35

(e) None of the above

36. A myelocyte usually has:

(a) 3-4 nuceoli in the nucleus

(b) No nucleoli in the nucleus

(c) Many coarse blue-black granules overlaying a deeply basophilic cytoplasm

(d) A multilobed nucleus

(e) A vacuolated cytoplasm devoid of granules

37. When investigating a case of suspected erythroblastosis, an indirect Coombs' test should be done on the:

(a) Mother's serum

(b) Mother's cells

(c) Infant's cells

(d) None of the above

38. The Anti-D agglutinin is the same as:

(a) Anti-RH°

(b) Anti-Hr°

(c) Anti-rh

(d) Anti-rh″

(e) None of the above

39. Group O blood with Anti-A hemolysins should not be used for a recipient of group:

(a) A or B

(b) A or AB

(c) B or AB

(d) O

40. An infant with erythroblastosis fetalis due to ABO incompatibility should receive:

(a) Group O blood Rh-negative

(b) Group O blood Rh-positive

(c) Group O blood of the same Rh type as his own

(d) Type-specific blood

41. The purpose of group-specific substances, when added to O Rh-negative blood, is to:

(a) Decrease the titer of Rh antibodies

(b) Prevent allergic reactions

(c) Reduce naturally occurring Anti-A and Anti-B

(d) Reduce immune antibodies

42. The siblings of a mating in which the parents are Group A and Group B could be either:

(a) AB

(b) A

(c) B

(d) O

(e) Any of the above

43. The direct Coombs' test in ABO hemolytic disease is often:

(a) Negative

(b) Positive

(c) Found to exhibit prozone

(d) Found to be of no value

44. A true Rhesus-negative will have the genotype:
    (a) cde/Cde
    (b) Cde/Cde
    (c) CDe/cde
    (d) cde/cde
45. An agglutinoid is an example of:
    (a) A complete antibody
    (b) An incomplete antibody
    (c) A bivalent antibody
    (d) A precipitin
    (e) A lysin
46. Anti-human antibodies will agglutinate only:
    (a) Group O human red cells
    (b) Group A human red cells
    (c) All human red cells
47. A person who has only naturally occurring anti-A in the plasma is:
    (a) Type B
    (b) Type A
    (c) Type AB
    (d) Type A₁
    (e) Type O
48. A person who is type AB has the following agglutinogen in the red cells:
    (a) A
    (b) None
    (c) A and B
    (d) B
49. R₁r red cells have the genotype of:
    (a) cde/cde
    (b) Cde/Cde
    (c) CDe/CDe
    (d) CDe/cde
    (e) cdE/CDe
50. If a person is a secretor, he will always be:
    (a) Group O
    (b) Le⁽ᵃ⁺⁾
    (c) Le⁽ᵃ⁻⁾
    (d) Group A
    (e) None of the above

## ANSWERS TO REGISTRY QUESTIONS

| | | | | |
|---|---|---|---|---|
| 1. a | 11. b | 21. e | 31. b | 41. d |
| 2. a | 12. d | 22. e | 32. b | 42. e |
| 3. b | 13. b | 23. d | 33. d | 43. a |
| 4. b | 14. d | 24. c | 34. b | 44. d |
| 5. b | 15. c | 25. b | 35. d | 45. b |
| 6. c | 16. c | 26. c | 36. a | 46. c |
| 7. a | 17. e | 27. a | 37. a | 47. a |
| 8. e | 18. b | 28. c | 38. a | 48. c |
| 9. c | 19. c | 29. b | 39. b | 49. d |
| 10. c | 20. e | 30. b | 40. c | 50. b |

# Index